Changing the Stigma of Mental Health Among African Americans:

Moving From Denial to Acceptance

LaVelle Hendricks
Texas A&M University, Commerce, USA

Dimitra Smith
Texas A&M University, Commerce, USA

IGI Global
PUBLISHER of TIMELY KNOWLEDGE

A volume in the Advances in Psychology, Mental Health, and Behavioral Studies (APMHBS) Book Series

Published in the United States of America by
IGI Global
Information Science Reference (an imprint of IGI Global)
701 E. Chocolate Avenue
Hershey PA, USA 17033
Tel: 717-533-8845
Fax: 717-533-8661
E-mail: cust@igi-global.com
Web site: http://www.igi-global.com

Library of Congress Cataloging-in-Publication Data

Names: Hendricks, LaVelle, 1964- editor. | Smith, Dimitra Jackson, 1981- editor.
Title: Changing the stigma of mental health among African Americans : moving from denial to acceptance / edited by LaVelle Hendricks, Dimitra Smith.
Description: Hershey, PA : Information Science Reference, 2024. | Includes bibliographical references and index. | Summary: "Mental health among African Americans historically has been kept in the closet and covered in the quilt of denial. Thus, African Americans remain shielded from treatment that is readily available to allow them to become healthy and whole. Bringing awareness of mental health issues among African Americans to light. The focus is recognizing treatment as a strength and not a weakness. Issues of mental health in the African American community is essential in preparing African Americans to be productive citizens"-- Provided by publisher.
Identifiers: LCCN 2023012722 (print) | LCCN 2023012723 (ebook) | ISBN 9781668489185 (hardcover) | ISBN 9781668489192 (paperback) | ISBN 9781668489208 (ebook)
Subjects: LCSH: African Americans--Mental health. | African Americans--Mental health services.
Classification: LCC RC451.5.B53 C43 2024 (print) | LCC RC451.5.B53 (ebook) | DDC 362.2089/96073--dc23/eng/20230503
LC record available at https://lccn.loc.gov/2023012722
LC ebook record available at https://lccn.loc.gov/2023012723

This book is published in the IGI Global book series Advances in Psychology, Mental Health, and Behavioral Studies (APMHBS) (ISSN: 2475-6660; eISSN: 2475-6679)

British Cataloguing in Publication Data
A Cataloguing in Publication record for this book is available from the British Library.
All work contributed to this book is new, previously-unpublished material.
The views expressed in this book are those of the authors, but not necessarily of the publisher.
For electronic access to this publication, please contact: eresources@igi-global.com.

Advances in Psychology, Mental Health, and Behavioral Studies (APMHBS) Book Series

ISSN:2475-6660
EISSN:2475-6679

Editor-in-Chief: Harish C. Chandan, Argosy University, USA, Bryan Christiansen, Southern New Hampshire University, USA

MISSION

The complexity of the human mind has puzzled researchers and physicians for centuries. While widely studied, the brain still remains largely misunderstood.

The **Advances in Psychology, Mental Health, and Behavioral Studies (APMHBS)** book series presents comprehensive research publications focusing on topics relating to the human psyche, cognition, psychiatric care, mental and developmental disorders, as well as human behavior and interaction. Featuring diverse and innovative research, publications within APMHBS are ideally designed for use by mental health professionals, academicians, researchers, and upper-level students..

COVERAGE

- Personality Disorders
- Human Interaction
- Addiction
- Socialization
- Treatment & Care
- Emotional Health
- Substance Abuse
- Developmental Disorders
- Trauma & Stress
- Counseling & Therapy

IGI Global is currently accepting manuscripts for publication within this series. To submit a proposal for a volume in this series, please contact our Acquisition Editors at Acquisitions@igi-global.com or visit: http://www.igi-global.com/publish/.

The Advances in Psychology, Mental Health, and Behavioral Studies (APMHBS) Book Series (ISSN 2475-6660) is published by IGI Global, 701 E. Chocolate Avenue, Hershey, PA 17033-1240, USA, www.igi-global.com. This series is composed of titles available for purchase individually; each title is edited to be contextually exclusive from any other title within the series. For pricing and ordering information please visit http://www.igi-global.com/book-series/advances-psychology-mental-health-behavioral/110200. Postmaster: Send all address changes to above address.

Titles in this Series

For a list of additional titles in this series, please visit:
http://www.igi-global.com/book-series/advances-psychology-mental-health-behavioral/110200

Facilitating Social Justice, Service Delivery, and Advocacy Through Multicultural Counseling Copetencies
Keith B. Wilson (University of Kentucky, USA) and Si-Yi Chao (University of Kentucky, USA)
Information Science Reference • © 2023 • 369pp • H/C (ISBN: 9781668461556) • US $215.00

Handbook of Research on Current Trends in Asian Education, Psychology, and Sociology
Kittisak Jermsittiparsert (Dhurakij Pundit University, Thailand) and Pannee Suanpang (Suan Dusit University, Thailand)
Information Science Reference • © 2023 • 400pp • H/C (ISBN: 9781668473757) • US $270.00

Combining Exercise and Psychotherapy to Treat Mental Health
Lara Carneiro (United Arab Emirates University, AI) and Felipe Schuch (Universidade Federal de Santa Maria, Brazil)
Medical Information Science Reference • © 2023 • 300pp • H/C (ISBN: 9781668460405) • US $325.00

Stabilization Approaches That Empower Clients Through Mental Health Crises
Isabel Logan (Eastern Connecticut State University, USA) and Cheryl A. Green (Southern Connecticut State University, USA)
Medical Information Science Reference • © 2023 • 320pp • H/C (ISBN: 9781799882282) • US $360.00

Exploring the Benefit of Creative Arts Therapies for Children, Adolescents, and Adults
Nava R. Silton (Marymount Manhattan College, USA)
Information Science Reference • © 2023 • 293pp • H/C (ISBN: 9781668478561) • US $215.00

For an entire list of titles in this series, please visit:
http://www.igi-global.com/book-series/advances-psychology-mental-health-behavioral/110200

IGI Global
PUBLISHER of TIMELY KNOWLEDGE

701 East Chocolate Avenue, Hershey, PA 17033, USA
Tel: 717-533-8845 x100 • Fax: 717-533-8661
E-Mail: cust@igi-global.com • www.igi-global.com

Table of Contents

Preface xv

Section 1
Foundations of Mental Health Disorders

Chapter 1
Borderline Personality Disorder 1
Anissa Guerin, Texas A&M University, Commerce, USA

Chapter 2
Post-Traumatic Stress Disorder in African-Americans 23
LaShondra P. Manning, Tarleton State University, USA

Chapter 3
Insomnia Disorder Among African-Americans 43
Kayla Denise Solomon, Texas A&M University, Commerce, USA

Chapter 4
Eating Disorders Among African-Americans 64
Marcella Smith, Texas A&M University, Commerce, USA

Chapter 5
Factitious Disorder Among the African-American Population 91
LaVelle Hendricks, Texas A&M University, Commerce, USA
Dimitra Smith, Texas A&M University, Commerce, USA
Karl Mitchell, Texas A&M University, Commerce, USA
Elizabeth Hudson, Texas A&M University, Commerce, USA
Jovaria Baig, Texas A&M University, Commerce, USA

Chapter 6
Obsessive-Compulsive Disorder and the African-American Experience 112
Marian Edwards Ellis, Clarksville Independent School District, USA

Chapter 7
Paranoia Disorder and the African-American Community 135
Dimitra Smith, Texas A&M University, Commerce, USA
LaVelle Hendricks, Texas A&M University, Commerce, USA
John Kuykendall, University of Indianapolis, USA
David Tolliver, Texas A&M University, Commerce, USA

Chapter 8
Narcissistic Personality Disorder and the African-American Culture 146
James M. Devlin, Texas A&M University, Commerce, USA
Marvin Dale Bellows, Texas A&M University, Commerce, USA
Samone Donald, Texas A&M University, Commerce, USA

Chapter 9
Major Depressive Disorder Among African-Americans 163
Elizabeth Wachira, Texas A&M University, Commerce, USA
Priscilla W. Wachira, Texas Woman's University, USA
Rahmatu Kassimu, Dr. K.'s Health Minute, USA

Section 2
Addressing Mental Health in the African-American Community

Chapter 10
Promoting Black or African-American Men's Mental Health Through Empowering Masculinity 183
Daniel Bates, Truman State University, USA

Chapter 11
Schizophrenia: Impact and Disparities in the Black Community 216
Avril W. Knox, Texas A&M University, Commerce, USA

Chapter 12
The Neurodevelopment of the Brain 242
Marcus Karltonian Bills, Best Alcohol & Drug Services, USA

Chapter 13
Drug and Alcohol Use Among Blacks: Mental Health Implications 252
Gracie Brownell, Texas A&M University, Commerce, USA

Chapter 14
The Impact of the Psychoeducational Approach: Changing the Stigma of Mental Health 283
Sindu Padmanabhan, Bharathiar University, India

Compilation of References 295

About the Contributors 360

Index 365

Detailed Table of Contents

Preface xv

Section 1
Foundations of Mental Health Disorders

Chapter 1
Borderline Personality Disorder..1
Anissa Guerin, Texas A&M University, Commerce, USA

Borderline personality disorder (BPD) is characterized as a psychological disorder with a characteristic pervasive pattern of instability in affect regulation, impulse control, interpersonal relationships, self-image, and occupational attainment. Patients with BDP are often depicted as difficult because of aggressive outbursts, health-sabotaging behaviors, and high healthcare utilization. Despite that several evidence-based psychotherapies are recommended for BPD, neither psychotropic drugs nor medications for this condition have been approved by the FDA and none are known to be efficient treatments. Moreover, it is unclear how satisfactorily clinical—or research—diagnoses actually capture the experiences of African Americans who identify with BPD. Further research and development of care pathways for African Americans with BPD would help to ensure available resources are used effectively and services are suited to their specific needs.

Chapter 2
Post-Traumatic Stress Disorder in African-Americans..23
LaShondra P. Manning, Tarleton State University, USA

Post-traumatic stress disorder (PTSD) is a psychiatric disorder that occurs when people have experienced or been exposed to a traumatic event. PTSD is important to assess in African American clients due to systemic and constant traumas that dates back to slavery. This multigenerational trauma is demonstrated as many African Americans experience socioeconomic disadvantages with increased exposure to poverty and crime. Additionally, mental health stigma microaggressions, and lack of knowledge often serves as common barriers that prevents African Americans from seeking mental health treatment. To supplement traditional theories, mental health professionals should rely upon movement therapy, Ubuntu practices, emancipation circles, and the church to augment mental health treatment.

Chapter 3
Insomnia Disorder Among African-Americans..43
Kayla Denise Solomon, Texas A&M University, Commerce, USA

In this chapter, the author addresses the sleep disturbance of insomnia, which is defined within the chapter. The signs and symptoms related to insomnia were addressed to provide individuals with knowledge to be more aware of any potential cues. The chapter also address African American views on mental health, as well as the risk factors for being more susceptible to experiencing insomnia and its impact. The chapter closes out by acknowledging effective treatment options for Insomnia that can be utilized by the African American community and discusses the need for additional future research.

Chapter 4
Eating Disorders Among African-Americans...64
Marcella Smith, Texas A&M University, Commerce, USA

Eating disorders affects 20 million women and 10 million men in the United States at some point in their lives. The purpose of this chapter was to explore eating disorders among African Americans. Historically, eating disorders were perceived to be prevalent in European American females from upper socio-economic status. However, there is mounting evidence that eating disorders are no longer limited to the European American population; in recent years, several community surveys have revealed the prevalence of eating disorders among ethnic minorities in Western nations. It is critical that clinicians take a holistic approach and seek to comprehend the entire experiences of African American clients, which involves not only their physical health but also their emotional lives and the numerous ways in which racism, discrimination, poverty, trauma, and adverse childhood experiences can lead to eating disorders. It is critical to understand the probable causes and symptoms of eating disorders in African American clients, so they do not suffer in silence.

Chapter 5
Factitious Disorder Among the African-American Population 91
LaVelle Hendricks, Texas A&M University, Commerce, USA
Dimitra Smith, Texas A&M University, Commerce, USA
Karl Mitchell, Texas A&M University, Commerce, USA
Elizabeth Hudson, Texas A&M University, Commerce, USA
Jovaria Baig, Texas A&M University, Commerce, USA

Factitious disorder, also known as Munchausen syndrome, is a mental health condition in which a person intentionally exaggerates physical or psychological symptoms in themselves or in someone else. The rationale behind this behavior is to assume the role of a sick person and receive attention, sympathy, or emotional support from others. People with factitious disorder may go to great lengths to produce or falsify symptoms, such as taking medication, inducing vomiting, tampering with medical devices, or lying about their medical history. They may also seek out medical procedures, hospitalizations, or surgeries that are not necessary or that pose a significant risk to their health.

Chapter 6
Obsessive-Compulsive Disorder and the African-American Experience..........112
Marian Edwards Ellis, Clarksville Independent School District, USA

The purpose of this chapter is to examine obsessive-compulsive disorder (OCD) and its debilitating effects on millions of people world-wide, specifically, African Americans. OCD is often times comorbid and affects various ages, genders, races, ethnicities, in the areas of one's mental health, physical health, social life, family relationships, and employment. Findings include causation and contributory factors such as but not limited to discrimination, racism, environment, lack of knowledge, mistrust in healthcare, mistrust in research studies, bias curriculum, and/or neurological impairments. Another purpose of this study is to awaken the need for mental health services in the African American culture and reduce the stigma attached.

Chapter 7
Paranoia Disorder and the African-American Community 135
Dimitra Smith, Texas A&M University, Commerce, USA
LaVelle Hendricks, Texas A&M University, Commerce, USA
John Kuykendall, University of Indianapolis, USA
David Tolliver, Texas A&M University, Commerce, USA

African Americans have experienced grave inequities in healthcare. These inequities have extended to mental health and continue to be a concern for African Americans. Paranoia is a mental health challenge that exists among African Americans, for varying reasons, including impacts from slavery, trauma, and current systematic discrimination. Due to low representation of healthcare providers among the African American community and African American distrust in the medical community, African Americans often turn to their church and the spiritual community for healing and support.

Chapter 8
Narcissistic Personality Disorder and the African-American Culture............... 146
James M. Devlin, Texas A&M University, Commerce, USA
Marvin Dale Bellows, Texas A&M University, Commerce, USA
Samone Donald, Texas A&M University, Commerce, USA

The present chapter covers the diagnostic criteria related the Narcissistic Personality Disorder (NPD) and takes into consideration the African American culture. The chapter presents specific information related to NPD and its elements as presented in the Diagnostic Statistical Manual V-Text Revisions (DSM-V-TR, American Psychology Association [APA]). Furthermore, the authors of this chapter present historically and contemporary issues of the African American Culture into the scope of diagnostic measures and specifically NPD. The authors also present alternative to diagnostic classifications as it relates to the African American culture and community.

Chapter 9
Major Depressive Disorder Among African-Americans 163
Elizabeth Wachira, Texas A&M University, Commerce, USA
Priscilla W. Wachira, Texas Woman's University, USA
Rahmatu Kassimu, Dr. K.'s Health Minute, USA

Major depressive depression is a common but serious mood disorder, and the leading cause of disability globally. It is associated with poorer physical health and higher rates of disability, as traumatic experiences can trigger a depressive episode. This chapter presents an overview of major depressive disorder, and highlights the pathways that lead to African Americans being disproportionately affected. It discusses the social determinants of health among African Americans that lead to depression being underreported and undertreated in this demographic group. This discussion extends to reinforce once again how systemic racism "a pandemic in a pandemic" shape the availability, quality, and use of mental healthcare access. The chapter concludes with a discussion on lessons learned and recommendations on how to aid in equitable and targeted interventions that are culturally relevant and attentive to the unique needs of this population.

Section 2
Addressing Mental Health in the African-American Community

Chapter 10
Promoting Black or African-American Men's Mental Health Through Empowering Masculinity 183
Daniel Bates, Truman State University, USA

There is a critical need for community advocates to understand the mental health needs of Black or African American (BA) men and the hesitancy in regard to accessing mental health services. Traditional, western masculinity powerfully influences how BA men perceive mental health struggles and vice versa, how reaching out for help and support affects an individual is perceived as being a man. Racial discrimination, marginalization and institutional oppression need to be taken into account when exploring mental health among BA men, especially in how these experiences interact with the enactment of masculinity. There is a great need for those who work with BA men to be aware of the mental health trends of this population, and the sociopolitical dynamics in the United States that contribute to them, equipped to effectively employ gender-adapted strategies with BA men, and familiar with evidenced-based approaches for promoting BA men's health and wellbeing in a way that is culturally responsive.

Chapter 11
Schizophrenia: Impact and Disparities in the Black Community 216
Avril W. Knox, Texas A&M University, Commerce, USA

Schizophrenia is a chronic psychotic illness that compromises a patient's ability to think clearly and maintain emotional stability. A patient's disease frequently makes interacting with others and forming enduring relationships challenging. It impacts a person's thoughts, feelings, and behavior as a severe mental disease. The diagnosis of schizophrenia among African Americans seeking mental health treatment is thus one of the most prominent and prevalent inequities. Environmental risk factors may be a part of the incidence rise. Black people's schizophrenia diagnoses may be biased, which can significantly impact the treatment provided. Determining and reducing diagnostic bias has been a critical strategy for reducing disparities in Black People's mental health outcomes.

Chapter 12
The Neurodevelopment of the Brain..242
Marcus Karltonian Bills, Best Alcohol & Drug Services, USA

The pleasure pathway is a form of the limbic part of the brain that is responsible for behaviors. The brain is a very interesting phenomenon. It is comprised of various parts that consist of neurotransmitters (serotonin, dopamine, and norepinephrine, just to name a few). Serotonin's chemical function is to carry messages between nerve cells in the brain and throughout your body. Serotonin plays a key role in such body functions as mood, sleep, digestion, nausea, wound healing, bone health, blood clotting, and sexual desire; in essence, sending signals of the state of well-being. The dopamine neurotransmitter sends signals of pleasure or euphoria to the nerves cells that your body makes. Norepinephrine sends chemicals of adrenaline; it is also known as the fight or flight neurotransmitter. It increases the breathing rate, relaxes the intestinal muscles, increases the heart rate, and increases the blood sugar levels. As a neurotransmitter in your brain and spinal cord, it increases alertness, arousal, and attention for the individual to protect themselves from harm.

Chapter 13
Drug and Alcohol Use Among Blacks: Mental Health Implications 252
Gracie Brownell, Texas A&M University, Commerce, USA

Drugs and alcohol abuse is a global social problem with negative consequences on personal, community, and societal levels. Earlier research has shown that Blacks use drugs and alcohol less than their white and Hispanic counterparts. However, evidence also shows that there are more negative and severe drugs and alcohol-induced consequences among Blacks in the United States. This disconnect between the low prevalence and higher negative outcomes is worsened by lack of culturally appropriate and timely interventions. This chapter has four main sections. The first part begins with a case study and covers the causes of drugs and alcohol use among Black and the factors that contribute to drug use and abuse, the second part is devoted to the consequences or outcomes that result from drug and alcohol abuse, while the third and fourth sections address treatment options available to this population and mental health perceptions.

Chapter 14
The Impact of the Psychoeducational Approach: Changing the Stigma of Mental Health 283
Sindu Padmanabhan, Bharathiar University, India

People who suffer from mental diseases may encounter stigma; they could be treated differently, judged negatively, or made to feel undeserving or lower than others. Stigma can lead to discrimination, which can make mental illness worse. It arises as a result of misunderstandings and false information about mental illness, as well as some people's unfavorable opinions or beliefs (prejudice). This could lead to discrimination against people who have mental illnesses. The lives of many people can be changed by helping to understand what emotions are, how to detect them, what they mean, and how to cope with them healthily with the help of psychoeducation. The initial step is to educate oneself on the basics of mental illness. Make sure there is a safe space where individuals feel appreciated, where they can be honest about their struggles, and where they can express their emotions. Ask them if they feel that receiving treatment for a mental disorder will harm them. If necessary, add counseling and other forms of support services to the medical care.

Compilation of References 295

About the Contributors 360

Index 365

Preface

It is clear that the prevalence of mental health and substance use has continued to expand over the past several years, with more individuals than ever requiring professional interventions. Unfortunately, deteriorating mental health and increased substance use have disproportionately impacted communities of color, often coinciding with a hesitancy to acknowledge the need for mental health care, as well as a lack of options for culturally informed professional assistance.

Dr. Maya Angelou once said, "When people show you who they are, believe them the first time." A powerful quote reminding us of the nature of our actions, and what they share about who we are and without denial, how we are doing. Unfortunately, in today's volatile world, many are still searching for who they are, or perhaps even more concerning, because of denial, fear, or stigmatization, are not willing to share who they are or the struggles they face. This is amplified throughout our communities of color as we witness deep political divides, hostilities toward different cultures, and increased targeted violence. For members of racial and ethnic minority groups who are increasingly suffering and experiencing a lack of mental health resources, stigma can add to the difficulty for people of color to not only acknowledge mental health issues but to overcome the denial to seek help.

Stigma continues to prevent many in the African American population from reaching out for professional assistance. Yet for some, a return to being well balanced and mentally healthy may only come through recognizing the need to seek professional assistance. The reality may be that addressing issues directly head on is necessary for African Americans who suffer chronic mental health challenges to find relief, and even thrive. For those who are hesitant to acknowledge their pain, falling to fear or underestimating the power of stigma, there must be culturally informed action that emphasizes the understanding that seeking mental health is a strength and not a weakness, with ongoing advocacy from those in the community to seek help. In this book, Dr. LaVelle Hendricks and Dr. Dimitra Smith bring together experts from across the nation to help not only those suffering, but better prepare those who are committed to intervening for the good of all. Written from a culturally informed perspective, this book takes a comprehensive, tailored approach to targeting educators, researchers, practitioners, the African American spiritual community, and others concerned about psychological well-being in the African American population. The individual chapters collectively address the importance of recognition of needs and the true strength and value of seeking help, while providing direct guidance for impactful intervention.

As our schools, colleges, and universities continue to see higher rates of anxiety, depression, substance abuse, and overall poor mental health, there must be an acknowledgment that this problem exists across students from early elementary through completion of the highest degrees. University administrators and other leaders in the African American community must take the opportunity to lead, by recognizing the needs on their own campuses and speaking out. Dr. LaVelle Hendricks and Dr. Dimitra Smith adeptly signal a call to action, offering clarity, insight, and hope within an empathetic context, to identify and provide treatment for those in need. Throughout the chapters we see there must be validation of our students' suffering, and work to decrease stigmatization—normalizing the additional struggles experienced by people of color, and the unique challenges faced by our African American students. Bringing experts in the field together, these editors have provided resources for our students of color, as well as for faculty and staff, along with well-trained professionals, skillfully outlining approaches to help our society to better meet the needs of students in the classroom as it relates to mental health.

One wonders if that was a part of Maya Angelo's message when she stated, "There are people who go through life burdened by ignorance because they refuse to see. When they do not recognize the truth that they belong to their community and their community belongs to them … it is because they refuse to see." This book, under the careful guidance of the co-editors, helps us all to be better able to see, identify, destigmatize, and treat mental health and substance abuse issues in the African American community.

Tammi Vacha-Haase
Texas A&M University, Commerce, USA

Section 1

Foundations of Mental Health Disorders

Chapter 1
Borderline Personality Disorder

Anissa Guerin
Texas A&M University, Commerce, USA

ABSTRACT

Borderline personality disorder (BPD) is characterized as a psychological disorder with a characteristic pervasive pattern of instability in affect regulation, impulse control, interpersonal relationships, self-image, and occupational attainment. Patients with BDP are often depicted as difficult because of aggressive outbursts, health-sabotaging behaviors, and high healthcare utilization. Despite that several evidence-based psychotherapies are recommended for BPD, neither psychotropic drugs nor medications for this condition have been approved by the FDA and none are known to be efficient treatments. Moreover, it is unclear how satisfactorily clinical—or research—diagnoses actually capture the experiences of African Americans who identify with BPD. Further research and development of care pathways for African Americans with BPD would help to ensure available resources are used effectively and services are suited to their specific needs.

INTRODUCTION

The term 'borderline personality' was proposed in the United States by Adolph Stern in 1938 (National Collaborating Centre for Mental Health, 2019). Stern described it as a group of patients who 'fit frankly neither into the psychotic nor into the psychoneurotic group' and introduced the term 'borderline' to describe what he observed because it 'bordered' on other conditions (National Collaborating Centre for Mental Health, 2019). The term 'borderline personality organization' was introduced by Otto Kernberg (1975) to refer to a consistent pattern of functioning behavior characterized by instability and reflecting disturbed psychological self-

DOI: 10.4018/978-1-6684-8918-5.ch001

organization (National Collaborating Centre for Mental Health, 2019). Whatever the purported underlying psychological structures, the cluster of symptoms and behavior associated with borderline personality were becoming more widely recognized and included striking fluctuations from periods of confidence to times of absolute despair, markedly unstable self-image, rapid changes in mood, with fears of abandonment and rejection, and a strong tendency towards suicidal thinking and self-harm (National Collaborating Centre for Mental Health, 2019). Gunderson and Kolb (1978) first outlined the traits that constitute borderline personality disorder, and these traits have now been integrated into the modern psychiatric categories used by mental health specialists.

BORDERLINE PERSONALITY DISORDER

Borderline personality disorder (BPD) is a psychological disorder with a characteristic pervasive pattern of instability in affect regulation, impulse control, interpersonal relationships, and self-image (Mendez-Miller, 2022). Patients with borderline personality disorder are often characterized as difficult because of aggressive outbursts, health-sabotaging behaviors (i.e., exercising on an injury), and high healthcare utilization (Mendez-Miller, 2022). Borderline personality disorder is associated with significant impairment, especially in relation to the capacity to sustain stable relationships because of personal and emotional instability (Chapman et. al., 2023). Interpersonally, they have abandonment and trust issues. "Borderlines" are emotionally unstable, often overreacting to the smallest of things. They have an inconsistent self-image, inappropriate rage, chaotic relationships that mostly end badly, and some self-injure or are suicidal (McCloud, 2013). Furthermore, the severity of symptoms and behaviors that characterize borderline personality disorder correlates with the severity of personal, social, and occupational impairments (National Collaborating Centre for Mental Health, 2019).

Borderline personality disorder (BPD) affects approximately 1-6% of the population, which equates to 14 million Americans (Mendez-Miller, 2022). Specifically, according to the National Education Alliance of Borderline Personality Disorder (2019), borderline personality disorder is more common than many well-known disorders such as schizophrenia. In addition, 20% of inpatients admitted to psychiatric hospitals have BPD, and 10% of outpatients have been diagnosed with BPD. Furthermore, 10% of adults with BPD commit suicide, 55-85% of adults with BPD self-injure their bodies, and the heritability of this illness is estimated to be up to 68% (McCloud, 2013). According to National Collaborating Centre for Mental Health (2009), it is important to note there is a substantial amount of literature that proves borderline personality disorder overlaps considerably with other categories of personality disorders, with 'pure' borderline personality disorder only occurring in 3% to 10% of cases. The level of research studies overlap with other personality disorders including histrionic, narcissistic, and antisocial is very high. In addition, there is considerable overlap between borderline personality disorder and mood and anxiety disorders (National Collaborating Centre for Mental Health, 2009).

Figure 1. Signs of Borderline Personality Disorder
(Gen Psych, 2018)

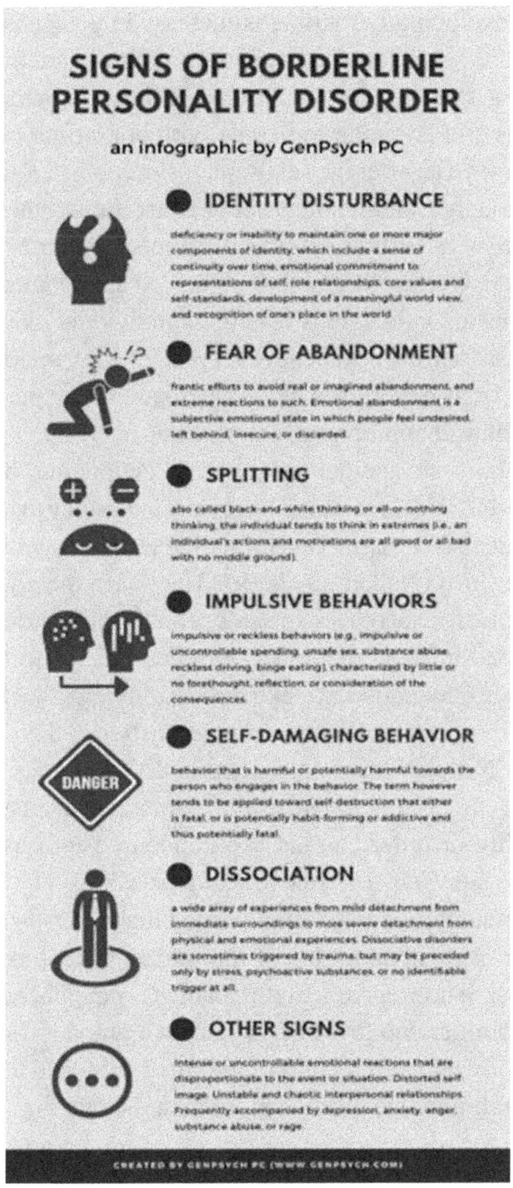
SIGNS OF BORDERLINE PERSONALITY DISORDER
an infographic by GenPsych PC
IDENTITY DISTURBANCE
FEAR OF ABANDONMENT
SPLITTING
IMPULSIVE BEHAVIORS
SELF-DAMAGING BEHAVIOR
DANGER
DISSOCIATION
OTHER SIGNS

General Symptoms

Individuals who have a biologically grounded emotional sensitivity and are reared in an invalidating environment are thought to be borderline, which is thought to be created by a confluence of hereditary and environmental elements (McCloud, 2013). Many, but not all, people with borderline personality disorder recurrently harm themselves, usually to provide relief from intolerable distress, which for many can lead to significant physical impairment and disability (National Collaborating Centre for Mental Health, 2009).

The chance of developing borderline is increased by negative experiences like sexual abuse, and the hereditary component that predicts borderline risk is less strong in those who have experienced certain traumas (Chapman et. al., 2023). Moreover, suicide is still common in people with borderline personality disorder and may occur several years after the first sign of symptoms. (Paris & Zweig-Frank, 2001). Behavior, thoughts, and feelings about oneself and others are all impacted by BPD. Individuals with BPD frequently experience a fear of abandonment and will do whatever it takes to avoid actual or perceived abandonment. This can result in tumultuous and heated interactions where the individual may one moment hold someone in high regard and the next believe they have no regard for them. In addition, those who have BPD may experience mood fluctuations that persist for a few hours to a few days, as well as inappropriate, extreme anger.

Emptiness sensations are another trait of BPD. People may become disoriented and engage in dangerous and threatening behaviors when they lose touch with reality. Uncertainty and indecisiveness in general can lead to frequent changes in work, friends, and relationships (Neil et al., 2019). They have the ability to abruptly go from intense-to-intense hate of others. Instable relationships and emotional suffering can result from these shifting emotions (Zenscott, 2022). Borderline personality disorder patients also frequently have extreme worldviews, such as all good or all negative. They may behave impulsively or dangerously, and their ideals and interests might shift quickly (National Institute of Health, 2022).

Although these general symptoms are all relevant and can be generally applied, borderline personality disorder can also be condensed into four different types: impulsive, discouraged, self-destructive, and petulant. These four borderline personality disorder subtypes are so well defined that a person only exhibits traits that match into one of them and none of the others. Even though it's a lot more complicated than that, it does act as a useful manual for mental health professionals, patients, and their families and loved ones. It's uncommon to find someone whose symptoms split equally between all four of the categories, and the majority of BPD patients will likely fall into one of them more than the others.

Impulsive Borderline Personality Disorders

Despite the fact that borderline personality disorder is in general characterized by a pervasive pattern of impulsivity and instability of interpersonal relationships, impulsive BPD is a subtype of BPD characterized by acting on impulses and engaging in high-risk behaviors while having difficulty controlling such urges. The broad definition of impulsivity is the desire for instant satisfaction without respect to prior knowledge or contemplation of potential repercussions, as well as without having made any prior plans to engage in the conduct. Impulsive activities can be trivial and safe (like taking a spontaneous drive) or extremely risky and perhaps lethal habits and routines. The boundary between being impulsive and discouraged is they are much more vibrant; this personality can be bubbly, flirtatious, and charismatic (Thriveworks, 2023). They have an act now think later approach to most things in life and tend to make rash, foolish life decisions that they will later regret (Thriveworks, 2023). The impulsive borderline personality disorder patient appears constantly conflicted. They start to experience issues with the entire world. They develop sadistic impulses and seek solace in other people's suffering. Impulsive BPD patients develop anti-social behavior. They are far more likely to find themselves in legal or financial troubles than other BPD sufferers, and do most of the things they do simply to take an edge off that boredom or emptiness they feel inside for much of the time (Lavendar, 2013). People with impulsive BPD may engage in these activities to connect with others, to feel immediate satisfaction, to obtain other people's attention, even if other people's attention is often superficial rather than deep or meaningful (Medsafe, 2023).

Discouraged "Quiet" Borderline Personality Disorder

The discouraged borderline type, also known as quiet BPD or high-functioning BPD, combines avoidance with dependency on others. The devoted and modest nature of those with BPD is often so great that they may even cling to others. Their connections, especially romantic ones, have a significant impact on how they define themselves. (Guarnotta, 2013). Those with discouraged BPD frequently struggle to manage when a close relationship ends, which destabilizes their entire universe. They may experience insecurity, helplessness, and uncertainty due to their fear of abandonment. Discouraged borderlines also frequently experience feelings of hopelessness and depression. They lack initiative and ambition, and they struggle to complete even simple tasks. They thus depend on others to the point of unhealthy reliance. They feel unwelcome and think as such; avoiding social connections is the result of all of this. They erroneously believe nobody wants to be around them. In relationships, they frequently seek self-worth and become very dependent on others.

Those with a depressed borderline personality disorder will do all in their power to maintain a relationship. They do not want the relationship to end since it is a form of isolation protection. They act in a specific way to win people over. Individuals that suffer from this BPD type, find it difficult to express their anger since it goes against how they see themselves, and they could consequently channel their rage internally and commit suicide and/or participate in self-harm (Guarnotta, 2013).

Self-Destructive Borderline Personality Disorders

Those who display self-destructive borderline symptoms are, as the term implies, their own worst enemies. When they seem to be moving forward in life, they often undermine themselves since they are prone to all kinds of risky conduct (Pugle, 2022). People with self-destructive borderline systems lack a strong sense of self, and because they are so reliant on other people, their fear of abandonment frequently spirals out of control. Borderline self-destructive men and women are typically irritable, resentful, and filled with wrath that they may or may not express. They believe no one cares about them, and they have little regard for their own needs. They feel a hole in their relationships. Due to their unstable emotions, those with Self-Destructive Borderline Personality Disorder are at a significant risk of taking their own lives. Unconscious and unacknowledged desires are mostly to blame for their difficulties, which can make it challenging for them to get the most out of treatment (Pugle, 2022). The desire to destroy oneself is a trait of BPD that serves as a roadblock to accomplishment. There is continuous discussion over whether this is something that is internalized as a maladaptive defense mechanism or something that is taught from an external source (Fox, 2023).

Petulant Borderline Personality Disorders

Individuals with petulant borderline tendencies frequently exhibit defensiveness, stubbornness, and a refusal to accept when they are mistaken as a result of their propensity to be obstinate and rebellious. Even though they can have wonderful relationships, they are usually complicated, and they frequently use passive-aggressive tactics to strike out at those who offend them (Bridges to Recovery, n.d.). Petulant borderline people are unpredictable and hard to get along with. They are frequently irritable, prone to anger and frustration outbursts, impatient with others, and easily demoralized when they don't get their way (Bridges to Recovery, n.d.). Unpredictable, angry, impatient, grumbling, rebellious, dissatisfied, obstinate, gloomy, and resentful are also some adjectives that describe them (Thriveworks, 2023).

Figure 2. Signs and symptoms
(Pugle, 2021)

Signs and Symptoms of

Four Subtypes of BPD

Impulsive

Superficial	Unreliable
Irritable	Easily distracted
Chaotic	Seductive
Easily annoyed	Charismatic
Fearful	Engaging
Suicidal	

Discouraged "Quiet"

Avoidant	Humble
Depressed	Helpless
Hopeless	Vulnerable
Submissive	Clingy
Loyal	Codepende

Self-Destructive

Moody	Self-focused
Bitter	Directing anger inward
Self-loathing	Submissive
	Suicidal

Petulant

Pessimistic	Stubborn
Unpredictable	Rebellious
Defiant	Cynical
Impatient	Resentful
Irritable	Easily offended

CAUSES OF BORDERLINE PERSONALITY DISORDER

Although studies indicate that social, environmental, and genetic variables may raise the chance of having borderline personality disorder, researchers are unsure of what causes it. In fact, some professionals contend that BPD is a neurodevelopmental disorder that results from maladaptive (responses that make it more difficult to adapt) reactions to stress and trauma. Additionally, compared to other personality disorders, mood disorders, or psychosis, BPD is more likely to be associated with childhood trauma as previously stated. Over 5,000 individuals were studied, and 71.1% of those with BPD had at least one traumatic event as a kid (Sandoiu, 2019). Some additional factors include:

- **Family history:** Individuals may be more likely to acquire borderline personality disorder if they have a close relative (such as a parent or sibling) who has the condition (NIH, 2022).
- **Brain structure and function:** may alter in patients with borderline personality disorder, particularly in the regions of the brain responsible for impulse control and emotion regulation, according to research (NIH, 2022). The investigations, however, do not show whether these alterations were factors in the sickness or if they were brought on by the ailment (NIH, 2022).
- **Environmental, cultural, and social factors**: A large number of patients with borderline personality disorder describe going through terrible life events, such as being abused, abandoned, or going through adversity as a youngster (NIH, 2022). Others could have been exposed to unsteady, invalidated connections or disputes. (NIH, 2022).

UNPACKING MENTAL HEALTH STIGMA AMONG AFRICAN AMERICANS

Although Black Americans have a diverse variety of attitudes on mental health care, some people are discouraged from seeking help because of the stigma associated with mental illness (Morin, 2022). It is crucial to consider how stigma and the factors that contribute to it might make it challenging for people to seek out a mental health expert. Several studies have shown that there is a significant stigma around mental illness in the Black community. An opinion survey conducted in the 1990s revealed that 63% of African Americans thought depression was a sign of personal weakness and only 31% thought it was a medical condition (Thompson-Sanders et al., 2004). In 2018, 50% of Black and African Americans with serious mental illness did not receive mental health treatment (Lee, 2022). The cultural stigma surrounding mental illness is partially responsible, according to a 2013 study published in Nursing Research (Lee, 2022). In 2013, a cross-sectional survey of African Americans aged 25 to 72 found that both men and women were not open to discussing their psychological issues and were concerned about the stigma surrounding mental illness. (Ward EC et. al., 2013).

According to research, the Black community is likely to believe mental illness brings shame and disgrace (Morin, 2020). African Americans and their families are also more inclined to conceal their disease (Ward & Heidrich, 2009). People in the Black community could be more inclined to think that since they have overcome so much difficulty, they are strong and that no one has the right to tell them they are flawed, since they may view a mental health issue as a weakness (Morin, 2020). According to a 2009 study, the majority of African Americans do not stigmatize mental illness. In addition, a considerable number of individuals decide against getting a diagnosis and instead turn to their religious group for assistance (Morin, 2020). The church or other religious organizations may serve as an important gathering place and a source of support for many African American communities in the United States. Spirituality and faith can facilitate healing and play a significant role in a therapy strategy. For instance, religious groups and spiritual authorities can offer assistance and lessen loneliness. Yet, those whose everyday functioning is hampered by mental health problems should not use this method as its sole choice (NAMI, 2023).

Treatment Determent

Many Black Americans who suffer from mental illnesses are not even aware that they may be diagnosed, much less that they can be effectively treated with psychology. African Americans frequently lack understanding about mental health issues and their remedies since it is taboo to talk openly about mental illness (Williams, 2011). Many African Americans are also worried about how well treatments work, which may be brought on by both a lack of information and cultural prejudices. Ambivalence about getting help might result from concerns about conflicting with the ideals or worldview of the doctor, and this may be especially true for those who hold the common belief that mental health therapy was created by white people for white people (Williams, 2011). In 2015, about 86% of psychologists in the United States were white, and by 2018, only 7% of psychiatrists were Black (Green & Hawkins, 2020). The lack of diversity in the mental health field presents a challenge for clients who prefer a provider they feel is culturally competent (Lee, 2020). It also presents a problem for those hoping to avoid the pitfalls of psychiatry's alleged racist history, racially biased treatment, and potential malpractice due to negligence (Raz, 2020). African Americans view the typical psychologist as an older, white male who would be insensitive to the social and economic realities of their lives (Williams, 2011). However, despite the fact that African Americans are underrepresented in the field of psychology, they are disproportionately represented among clinicians with a master's degree, such as clinical social workers and professional counselors. These therapists are quite beneficial for a variety of issues, such as family issues and various mental health requirements (Williams, 2011). As a result, African Americans should seek treatment through these channels, as they can be of tremendous help.

Access and Insurance

Black individuals have a disproportionate number of risk factors for mental illness, such as poverty, homelessness, and violence, as well as major barriers to receiving quality mental health treatment (Lee, 2020). Black people encounter major mental health disorders 20% more frequently than white Americans do, according to the National Institute on Minority Health and Health Disparities (2020). Approximately 23% of Black Americans and 10% of White Americans are estimated to be living in poverty (Lee, 2020). Some Black individuals lack insurance and are unable to afford therapy because of economic imbalances brought on by systematic racism, according to Calixte (2013). According to the U.S. Census, 6% of white Americans and almost 11% of Black Americans did not have health insurance (Berchick et. al., 2018). According to a 2013 study published in *Health Affairs*, it looked back over a ten-year period and determined people without health insurance who sought specialist care for mental illness encountered obstacles such as rising treatment costs (Mcalpine & Blewett, 2010). Since coverage restrictions limit the types of treatments available, having health insurance does not guarantee access to sufficient care (Mcalpine & Blewett, 2010). In 2017, 44% of Black Americans compared to 34% of White Americans, respectively, were covered by Medicaid or other public health care (U.S. Department of Health and Human Services, 2021). As Miles (2021) suggested, individuals with Medicaid coverage may not have access to well-trained and experienced clinicians. Furthermore, those that are Black and impoverished have less access to different treatment methods and providers that use a variety of theoretical approaches to serve a diverse client base (Lee, 2020).

Racial Inequities

Due to racial disparities in employment, education, and housing, many Black Americans now live in environments that are hazardous to their health. According to Miles (2021), if you're Black and poor, your priorities are far more likely to be your daily requirements for survival than your mental health. Most Medicaid customers sought mental health therapy to comply with legal obligations and were compelled into treatment by the judicial system. It is more common for African Americans with mental health issues to end up in jail than to be directed to community-based treatment programs (Johnson, 2014).

Impoverished African Americans may also be more susceptible to malpractice since many communities' mental health institutions employ doctors based on their ability to pay rather than those with more education and expertise (Lee, 2020). Conflicts with the law can serve as an entry point for mental health care because white people sometimes misinterpret the violent or criminal conduct of African Americans who are suffering from mental illness (Lee, 2022). The Black community needs greater mental health education, according to many experts, but addressing past trauma with policy is the only way to make lasting change. All Americans will need to examine implicit prejudice and white supremacy in order to address structural racism and the racial disparities in healthcare. Until more resources are allocated to enhancing living conditions within their communities, Black Americans' mental health won't get any better. Greater diversity within the mental health field will grant Black clients access to culturally competent providers and incentivize the completion of treatment. (Lee, 2022).

BORDERLINE PERSONALITY DISORDER AMONGST AFRICAN AMERICANS

The issue of racial differences in borderline personality disorder has not been examined and research on racial differences in the experience and expression of emotion has been mixed (Newhill et. al., 2009). Thus, there is mounting evidence that borderline personality characteristics and borderline personality disorder are not exclusive to white females, as was previously believed. This may be due to the fact that people of color were consistently ignored in psychological research, which is consistent with the disparities in attention to minority health matters in general (Sue, 1999). Further, there is evidence that the presentation and experience of borderline personality varies by ethnicity, necessitating further investigation of the disorder in the minority population (Walton, 2014). If important racial differences exist in how BPD is manifested and experienced by the people who suffer from this illness, such information could be vital to developing specialized, culturally sensitive treatments for this population (Newhill et. al., 2009).

Despite the lack of research and evidence, the affective and behavioral symptoms of borderline personality were studied in seventeen African Americans and twenty-seven White Americans within a 2009 study (Newhill et. al., 2009). Results indicated that African Americans experience greater affective intensity and emotional dysregulation, fewer self-harming behaviors, and more thoughts of interpersonal aggression than Whites (Newhill et. al., 2009). Interestingly, African Americans also reported experiencing much more positive effects, and were significantly less likely to report engaging in self-harming behaviors (Newhill et. al., 2009). Although differences in affective symptoms were attenuated to non-significant levels when accounting for substance use problems and treatment context, which may in themselves reflect a difference in the presentation of the illness, differences in behavioral symptomatology remained robust after adjusting for these potential confounder (Newhill et. al., 2009). These findings suggest that the experience of BPD may differ in important and significant ways depending on the cultural background of the individual. Research regarding borderline personality disorder should look to extend generality, particularly across socioeconomic, racial and ethnic groups. Implications for future research and directions for developing culturally relevant treatments are desperately needed (Newhill et. al., 2009).

TREATMENT

Despite the fact that several evidence-based psychotherapies are recommended for BPD, neither psychotropic drugs nor medications for the condition that have been approved by the FDA and are known to be efficient treatments for BPD. With the proper therapy, the majority of patients have symptom alleviation, and after a year and two years, remission rates are 85% and 99%, respectively. For that reason, evidence-based borderline treatment receives insufficient public funding and support (Ellilot, Ragsdale, 2022).

Psychotherapy

The initial course of treatment for borderline personality disorder is psychotherapy. Another word for psychotherapy is talk therapy. It serves as a pillar of care for borderline personality disorder. Therapists could adjust the therapy's format to better meet your needs. The goal of psychotherapy is to help patients concentrate on their current level of functioning, learn how to manage difficult emotions, and minimize impulsivity by encouraging experiencing observation rather than acting on it. In addition, work on relationships by being conscious of their own, while also considering other people's feelings. (Mayo Clinic, 2023).

Types of Psychotherapy

Dialectical behavior therapy (DBT). DBT is a type of treatment that combines group and individual sessions to address borderline personality disorder. DBT teaches you how to control your emotions, endure discomfort, and strengthen relationships through a skills-based approach. (Mayo Clinic, 2023)._It has effectively reduced suicide attempts and psychiatric hospitalizations in those with borderline personality disorder. In a randomized controlled trial comparing fluoxetine (Prozac) therapy with dialectical behavior therapy, the medication-only group was observed to have significantly higher rates of suicide attempts (Mendez-Miller, 2022).

Schema-focused therapy (SFT). SFT is individual or group sessions of therapy. It can assist individuals in identifying unmet needs that have given rise to unhealthy life habits that, while once beneficial for survival, are now detrimental to many aspects of adult life (Mayo Clinic, 2023). In order to encourage healthy living patterns, this therapy focuses on assisting individuals in meeting daily life demands (Mayo Clinic, 2023).

Mentalization-based therapy (MBT). MBT is a form of talk therapy that helps clients to identify their own thoughts and feelings at any given moment and form a different perspective. It tries to lessen impulsivity and emotional lability by improving a person's comprehension of how mental states affect behavior. Studies have shown that towards the end of mentalization-based therapy, self-harm and suicidality have decreased. Thinking before action is emphasized in MBT (Mayo Clinic, 2023).

Systems training for emotional predictability and problem-solving (STEPPS). Patients with borderline personality disorder (BPD) can benefit from the group therapy program called STEPPS (Mayo Clinic, 2023). Both patients and therapists were meant to find the application very easy to use. Patients learn emotion control and behavior management techniques during STEPPS. The 20-week therapy program involves working in groups that include family, caretakers, friends, or significant others. And other forms of psychotherapy are utilized in conjunction with STEPPS (Mayo Clinic, 2023).

Transference-focused psychotherapy (TFP). TFP, which is also known as psychodynamic psychotherapy, attempts to improve understanding of a person's emotions and interpersonal issues by fostering a close bond between them and the therapist (Mayo Clinic, 2023). Transference-focused psychotherapy (TFP) uses the person/therapist relationship as a vehicle for healing issues relating to others and the self (McIntyre, 2022). TFP can be applied in a group or individual setting and to a range of personality disorders (McIntyre, 2022). One then uses these realizations in ongoing circumstances (Mayo Clinic, 2023).

Medications

No medications have been FDA-approved to treat borderline personality disorder. Medications such as SSRIs, mood stabilizers, and antipsychotics have shown limited effectiveness in trials aiming at the control of symptoms such as anxiety, sleep disturbance, depression, or psychotic symptoms (Chapman et. al., 2022). Symptoms such as anxiety can be challenging to treat because patients may label their internal experiences with the word anxiety, even if that is not the best way to identify what they are experiencing (Chapman et. al., 2022). Thus, "anxiety" may need to be accurately re-labeled, with treatment recommendations stemming from the patient's specific internal experience (Chapman et. al., 2022). The exception to the misleading use of the word anxiety is that patients with borderline personality disorder often have a fear of being alone; in other words, they have attachment-related anxiety (Chapman et. al., 2022). However, attachment-related anxiety is not necessarily similar in etiology or treatment to recognized anxiety disorders (Chapman et. al., 2022).

Hospitalization

Most inpatient hospitalizations occur due to concern that the patient may be at risk of harming themselves or someone else, and the patient is discharged once that risk has passed (Salters-Pedneault, 2020). Patients with borderline personality disorder do not typically require hospitalization; however, inpatient care may be required in certain situations, such as imminent risk of high lethality behaviors due to overt suicidal ideation or impulsivity, severe social stressors causing intense negative thoughts or transient psychosis, rapid escalation in the severity of self-injurious behavior, and decompensation of comorbid psychiatric diagnoses or severe substance abuse. The traditional belief that prolonged (longer than one week) inpatient hospitalization is counterproductive or even deleterious for patients with borderline personality disorder was not supported in a most recent study (Chapman, 2022).

A psychiatric inpatient hospitalization may occur voluntarily or involuntarily. A voluntary hospitalization occurs when the patient recognizes that patients need more help than can be provided through outpatient treatment (Salters-Pedneault, 2020). For example, an individual may recognize that he is having a period of very strong symptoms that he cannot handle on his own and that he needs more than once or twice-a-week therapy to keep himself safe (Chapman et. al., 2022). In the past, inpatient treatment for BPD may could last months or even years, but now inpatient treatment is generally much shorter, depending on the needs of the individual involved (Salters-Pedneault, 2020). In this case, the patient and the therapist may decide together that inpatient treatment is best (Salters-Pedneault, 2020).

An involuntary hospitalization occurs when the patient is not willing to be admitted to the hospital, but the treatment providers have deemed this level of care necessary (Chapman et. al., 2022). For example, if someone is expressing intent to commit suicide, but refuses to be hospitalized for safety, her treatment providers are required to pursue involuntary hospitalization (also called "commitment") (Salters-Pedneault, 2020).

RECOVERY, COPING, AND SUPPORT

It takes time for individuals to learn how to control their feelings, ideas, and actions. The majority of patients make significant improvements, however certain BPD symptoms may never fully go away. Some people could go through phases when their symptoms get better or worse. However, treatment can increase a person's capacity for function and boost their self-esteem. People who seek the advice of a mental health professional with experience treating borderline personality disorder have the best chance of success. For those who are impacted as well as those around them, borderline personality disorder symptoms can be unpleasant and difficult. Even if they are aware that their feelings, ideas, and actions are hurtful to themselves or others, they may nevertheless feel powerless to control them. According to MayoClinic (2023), in addition to getting professional treatment, individuals can help manage and cope with their condition by:

- Learning about the disorder so that they understand its causes and treatments.
- Learning to recognize what may trigger angry outbursts or impulsive behavior.
- Seeking professional help and sticking to the treatment plan by attending all therapy sessions and taking medications as directed.
- Working with the mental health provider to develop a plan for what to do the next time a crisis occurs.
- Receiving treatment for related problems, such as substance abuse.
- Consider involving family and friends in the treatment plan to help them understand and support you.
- Managing intense emotions by practicing coping skills, such as the use of breathing techniques and mindfulness meditation.
- Setting limits and boundaries for yourself and others by learning how to appropriately express emotions in a manner that doesn't push others away or trigger abandonment or instability.
- Do not make assumptions about what people are feeling or thinking about you.
- Reaching out to others with the disorder to share insights and experiences.
- Build a support system of people who can understand and respect you.
- Keeping up a healthy lifestyle, such as eating a healthy diet, being physically active and engaging in social activities.

- Don't blame yourself for the disorder but recognize your responsibility to get it treated.

PREPARING FOR DOCTOR APPOINTMENTS

A primary care physician is a good place for people to start. The doctor may recommend patients see a psychologist or psychiatrist after an initial session if they need mental health services. To assist patients in getting ready for their visit, according to MayoClinic (2023), before any appointments patients should make a list of:

- Any symptoms you or people close to you have noticed, and for how long.
- Key personal information, including traumatic events in your past and any current major stressors.
- Your medical information, including other physical or mental health conditions.
- All medications you take, including prescription and over-the-counter medications, vitamins and other supplements, and the doses.
- Questions you want to ask your doctor so that you can make the most of your appointment. Take a family member or friend along, if possible. Someone who has known you for a long time may be able to share important information with the doctor or mental health provider, with your permission.

Table 1. Questions to ask your medical provider (Verywellmind, 2023)

QUESTIONS to ask medical health provider
About Symptoms
□ How long have I likely had BPD? □ How does BPD affect my relationships? □ Should I bring someone to my appointment with me who can describe the symptoms they observe? □ Will my symptoms likely come back from time to time?
About Causes & Risk Factors
□ What are the main risk factors for developing BPD? □ Does it put me at risk for having other mental health or physical health issues? □ Does my childhood likely have anything to do with BPD? □ Could my other health issues or mental health conditions contribute to BPD?
About Diagnosis
□ How is BPD diagnosed? □ Is there a test for me to take and what can I expect during it? □ How do you rule out other possible conditions that have similar symptoms to BPD? □ Do I have any other mental illnesses?
About Treatment
□ Are there any medications that can help reduce my symptoms? □ Which might be right for me? □ Should I see a therapist? If so, what kind of therapy? □ How much improvement can I expect to see from treatment? □ Will it ever be OK to stop treatment? □ Does BPD ever go away altogether?
About Coping and Living With
□ How will having a diagnosis of BPD affect my life? □ What should I do if I have thoughts of self-harm or suicide? □ Should I tell my employer I have BPD, and if so, how? □ Are there lifestyle changes I should make to manage my symptoms? □ Should my friends and family be told about my diagnosis? □ Is there something my loved ones can do to support me? □ Are there any things I should avoid doing? □ Should I structure my life in any particular way to help manage my symptoms?

CONCLUSION

Among all the subtypes of personality disorder, borderline personality disorder is one of the most controversial. There is very little information relating to this personality disorder and responses to treatment and management (Lindsay, 2007). Moreover, it is unclear how satisfactorily clinical, and/or research diagnoses actually capture the experiences of African Americans who identify with borderline personality disorder (Ramon et al., 2001). There is evidence that the presentation and experience of borderline personality varies by ethnicity, necessitating further investigation of the disorder in the minority population (Walton, 2014). More research into the causes of borderline personality disorder is needed, the results of which may help to develop evidence-based approaches to treatment that are practical and specifically designed for this challenging disorder (Paris, 2005). In addition, concerns have repeatedly been expressed about the quality of services and appropriate access in primary and secondary services for people of color with borderline personality disorder (Paris, 2005). Therefore, it is crucial to establish standards to guarantee that those with this disorder have access to both general and specialized mental health services. Further research and the development of care pathways for African Americans with borderline personality disorder would help to ensure that available resources are used effectively and that services are suited to their specific needs (National Collaborating Centre for Mental Health, 2009). As previously stated, service provision for African Americans with borderline personality disorder varies greatly and acknowledging these factors when deciding the type and intensity of care they should receive is critical for help and healing (National Collaborating Centre for Mental Health, 2009).

Need Help?

If you or someone you know is struggling or in crisis, help is available. Call or text 988 or chat 988lifeline.org, or call the NAMI Helpline at 800-950-6264 or text "HelpLine" to 62640.

To learn how to get support for mental health, drug, and alcohol issues, visit FindSupport.gov.

To locate treatment facilities or providers, visit FindTreatment.gov or call SAMHSA's National Helpline at 800-662-HELP (4357).

(SAMSHA, 2023)

REFERENCES

Berchick, E., Hood, E., & Barnett, J. (2018, September 12). *Health Insurance Coverage in the United States: 2017*. United Stated Cenus Bureau. Retrieved February 28, 2023, from https://www.census.gov/library/publications/2018/demo/p60-264.html

Bridges to Recovery. *Types of Borderline Personality Disorder*. Bridges to Recovery. (n.d.). Retrieved February 28, 2023, from https://www.bridgestorecovery.com/

Chapman, J., Fleisher, C., & Jamil, R. (2022, October 25). *Borderline personality disorder*. National Center for Biotechnology Information. Retrieved February 28, 2023, from https://pubmed.ncbi.nlm.nih.gov/28613633/

Cullors, P., & Johnson, M. (2014, August 1). *Impact of disproportionate incarceration of and violence against black ...* Retrieved February 28, 2023, from http://www.antoniocasella.eu/archipsy/Dignity_2014.pdf

Cuncic, A. (2022, November 8). *What is quiet borderline personality disorder?* Verywell Mind. Retrieved February 28, 2023, from https://www.verywellmind.com/what-is-quiet-borderline-personality-disorder-5115074

De Genna, N. M., & Feske, U. (2013, December 1). Phenomenology of borderline personality disorder: The role of race and socioeconomic status. *The Journal of Nervous and Mental Disease*, *201*(12), 1027–1034. doi:10.1097/NMD.0000000000000053 PMID:24284636

Elliott, M., & Ragsdale, J. M. (2021, September 15). Stress exposure and well-being: Correlates of meeting criteria for bipolar disorder, borderline personality disorder, or both. *Social Psychiatry and Psychiatric Epidemiology*, *57*(9), 1885–1896. doi:10.100700127-021-02172-z PMID:34524518

Facty, N. (2019, April 2). *What is borderline personality disorder - facty health.* Facty Health. Retrieved February 28, 2023, from https://facty.com/conditions/mental-health/what-is-borderline-personality-disorder/

Fox, D. (2022, August 3). *Borderline personality disorder and the danger of self-destruction.* Psychology Today. Retrieved February 28, 2023, from https://www.psychologytoday.com/us/blog/the-complex-diagnosis/202208/borderline-personality-disorder-and-the-danger-self-destruction

GenPsych PC. (2018). *Signs of Borderline Personality Disorder.* Retrieved February 23, 2023, from https://genpsych.com/

Green, C., & Gaston-Hawkins, L. (2020, July 14). *Racism, policing, and covid-19: How do we justify racial disparities in 2020?* Psychiatric Times. Retrieved February 28, 2023, from https://www.psychiatrictimes.com/view/policing-and-covid-19-disparities-how-do-we-justify-racial-disparities-in-2020

Gullestad, F. S., Wilberg, T., Klungsøyr, O., Johansen, M. S., Urnes, O., & Karterud, S. (2011, August 9). Is treatment in a day hospital step-down program superior to outpatient individual psychotherapy for patients with personality disorders? 36 months follow-up of a randomized clinical trial comparing different treatment modalities. *Psychotherapy Research*, *22*(4), 426–441. doi:10.1080/10503307.2012.662608 PMID:22417131

Johnson, T. (2022, January 1). *5 meaningful ways to embrace black mental health this February*. Anxiety and Depression Association of America, ADAA. Retrieved February 28, 2023, from https://adaa.org/living-with-anxiety/personal-stories/5-meaningful-ways-embrace-black-mental-health-february

Kashyap, N. (2022, September 21). *Transference-focused psychotherapy: Using the therapist-individual relationship to heal*. Verywell Health. https://www.verywellhealth.com/transference-focused-psychotherapy-5323806

Klaus, L., Zararini, M., Schmahl, C., Linehan, M., & Bohus, M. (2004, July 31). *Borderline personality disorder - the lancet*. The Lancet. https://www.thelancet.com/journals/lancet/article/PIIS0140-6736(04)16770-6/fulltext

Lancaster, V. (2022, August 3). Borderline personality disorder and the danger of self-destruction. *Psychology Today*. https://www.psychologytoday.com/us/blog/the-complex-diagnosis/202208/borderline-personality-disorder-and-the-danger-self-destruction

Lee, S. (2020, August 6). Racial disparities lead to poor mental health care for Black Americans. *Verywell Mind*. https://www.verywellmind.com/racial-disparities-mental-health-5072490

Lenzenweger, M. F., Lane, M. C., Loranger, A. W., & Kessler, R. C. (2007, January 11). DSM-IV personality disorders in the National Comorbidity Survey Replication. *Biological Psychiatry*, *62*(6), 553–564. doi:10.1016/j.biopsych.2006.09.019 PMID:17217923

Linehan, M. M. (1993, May 14). *Cognitive-behavioral treatment of borderline personality disorder* (2nd ed.). Guildford Press.

McCloud, M. (2013, February 26). Borderline personality afflicts all races and both genders. *Psychology Today*. https://www.psychologytoday.com/us/blog/black-womens-health-and-happiness/201302/borderline-personality-afflicts-all-races-and-both

Meds Safety. (2023, March 14). *Borderline personality disorder*. Meds Safety. https://medssafety.com/borderline-personality-disorder/

Mendez-Miller, M., Naccarato, J., & Radico, J. A. (2022, February 1). Borderline Personality Disorder. *American Family Physician*, *105*(2), 156–161. PMID:35166488

Morin, A. (2020, October 26). Exploring the mental health stigma in black communities. *Verywell Mind*. https://www.verywellmind.com/exploring-the-mental-health-stigma-in-black-communities-5078964

National Alliance of Mental Health. (2022, March 23). *Black/African Americans-Mental Health.* National Alliance of Mental Health. https://nami.org/Your-Journey/Identity-and-Cultural-Dimensions/Black-African-American

National Collaborating Centre for Mental Health. U. K. (2009). Borderline personality disorder: Treatment and management. British Psychological Society.

Newhill, C. E., Eack, S. M., & Conner, K. O. (2009, April 21). *Racial differences between African and White Americans in the presentation of borderline personality disorder - race and Social Problems.* Springer. https://link.springer.com/article/10.1007/s12552-009-9006-2

Paris, J. (2005, June 7). *Borderline personality disorder.* CMAJ. https://www.cmaj.ca/content/172/12/1579

Pugle, M. (2022, September 2). What are the types of borderline personality disorders? *Verywell Health.* https://www.verywellhealth.com/types-of-bpd-5193843

Raz, M. (2020, April 21). Psychiatry under the shadow of White Supremacy. *Nature News.* https://www.nature.com/articles/d41586-020-01126-w

Rowan, K., Alphine, D., & Blewett, L. (2013, October 1). Access and cost barriers to mental health care, by ... - health affairs. *Health Affairs.* https://www.healthaffairs.org/doi/10.1377/hlthaff.2013.0133

Sandoiu, A. (2019, November 21). Borderline personality disorder: Trauma raises risk by 13-fold. *Medical News Today.* https://www.medicalnewstoday.com/articles/327084

Schwartz, B., & Fuller, K. (2022, June 9). *Impulsive borderline personality disorder (BPD).* Choosing Therapy. https://www.choosingtherapy.com/impulsive-borderline-personality-disorder/

Senol, S. (2023, March 28). *Borderline personality disorder.* Encyclopedia Britannica. https://www.britannica.com/science/borderline-personality-disorder

Substance Abuse and Mental Health Service Administration. (2023, April 24). *Borderline personality disorder.* SAMHSA. https://www.samhsa.gov/mental-health/borderline-personality-disorder

Team, O. P. I. (2018, July 16). *What is impulsive borderline personality disorder?* OPI Residential Treatment Center for Young Adults - Private Pay Mental Health Program. https://www.optimumperformanceinstitute.com/bpd-treatment/impulsive-borderline-personality-disorder/

Thompson, V., & Bazile, A. (2004, February 1). *African Americans' perceptions of psychotherapy and psychotherapists*. ResearchGate. https://www.researchgate.net/publication/232423919_African_Americans%27_Perceptions_of_Psychotherapy_and_Psychotherapists

Thriveworks. (2021, August 30). *Borderline personality disorder*. Thriveworks. https://thriveworks.com/borderline-personality-disorder-symptoms-facts/

U.S. Department of Health and Human Services. (n.d.). *Publications about borderline personality disorder*. National Institute of Mental Health. https://www.nimh.nih.gov/health/publications/borderline-personality-disorder-listing

Vance, T. (2019, February 8). *Addressing mental health in the Black Community*. Columbia University Department of Psychiatry. https://www.columbiapsychiatry.org/news/addressing-mental-health-black-community

Verywell Mind. (2023). Doctor discussion guides. *Verywell Mind*. https://www.verywellmind.com/doctor-discussion-guides-4797486

Walton, M. F. (2014). *Betrayal trauma, experiences of racism, resilience, and borderline personality characteristics in African-Americans* (Order No. 3623046). Available from ProQuest Dissertations & Theses Global. (1548306775). https://go.openathens.net/redirector/ace.edu/login?url=https://www.proquest.com/dissertations-theses/betrayal-trauma-experiences-racism-resilience/docview/1548306775/se-2

Ward, E. (2013, June 1). African American men and women's attitude toward mental. *Nursing research*. https://journals.lww.com/nursingresearchonline/Abstract/2013/05000/African_American_Men_and_Women_s_Attitude_Toward.6.aspx

Ward, E. C., & Heidrich, S. M. (2009, July 31). African American women's beliefs about mental illness, stigma, and preferred coping behaviors. *Research in Nursing & Health*, *32*(5), 480–492. doi:10.1002/nur.20344 PMID:19650070

Williams, M. (2022, November 2). Why African Americans avoid psychotherapy. *Psychology Today*. https://www.psychologytoday.com/us/blog/culturally-speaking/201111/why-african-americans-avoid-psychotherapy

Zeinscott, T. (2022, June 30). How to motivate someone with borderline personality disorder? *Heart Eyes Magazine*. https://www.hearteyesmag.com/how-to-motivate-someone-with-borderline-personality-disorder/

Chapter 2
Post-Traumatic Stress Disorder in African-Americans

LaShondra P. Manning
https://orcid.org/0000-0003-0945-1783
Tarleton State University, USA

ABSTRACT

Post-traumatic stress disorder (PTSD) is a psychiatric disorder that occurs when people have experienced or been exposed to a traumatic event. PTSD is important to assess in African American clients due to systemic and constant traumas that dates back to slavery. This multigenerational trauma is demonstrated as many African Americans experience socioeconomic disadvantages with increased exposure to poverty and crime. Additionally, mental health stigma microaggressions, and lack of knowledge often serves as common barriers that prevents African Americans from seeking mental health treatment. To supplement traditional theories, mental health professionals should rely upon movement therapy, Ubuntu practices, emancipation circles, and the church to augment mental health treatment.

INTRODUCTION

'Nobody knows the trouble I've seen, nobody knows my sorrow…' This gospel spiritual song (sung by many African American musicians) exemplifies post-traumatic stress disorder (PTSD) that many African Americans commonly experience. According to the American Psychiatric Association (2022), PTSD is a psychiatric disorder that may occur in people who have experienced or witnessed a traumatic event, series of events, or circumstances. Many studies note that PTSD is prevalent in African Americans at a rate higher than their Caucasian counterparts (Abdullah,

DOI: 10.4018/978-1-6684-8918-5.ch002

Graham-Lo Presti, Tahirkheli, Hughley, and Watson, 2021; Brooks Holliday, Dubowitz, Haas, Ghosh-Dastidar, DeSantis, and Troxel, 2020; Sibrava, Bjornsson, Perez Benitez, Moitra, Weisberg, & Keller, 2019). For example, the prevalence of PTSD in African Americans ranges from 8.7% (Abdullah et al., 2021; Lu et al., 2022) to 9.1% (Gran-Ruaz, Taylor, Jacob, & Williams, 2022), and African American women are most likely to present with a PTSD diagnosis than African American men (Gran-Ruaz et al., 2022). Additionally, PTSD is substantially higher in African American transgender, queer, nonbinary, or agender populations than African American women (Abdullah et al., 2021). Since the onset of COVID-19 and the disproportional impact COVID-19 has had on African Americans, the number of African Americans who have PTSD is probably higher (Gran-Ruaz et al., 2022). While African Americans also present with a higher prevalence of severe mental illnesses (SMIs) such as major depressive disorder, bipolar, and psychotic disorders [*which are often accompanied by PTSD*], the PTSD diagnosis is often overlooked within this population (Lu, Silverstein, Mueser, Minskey, Bullock, Buchbinder, Chen, Eubanks, & Guillaume-Salvant, 2022). Lu and colleagues (2022) also found that most African American clients who presented with SMIs have experienced domestic violence, childhood sexual assault, robbery, physical assault, threat, witnessing community violence, adulthood sexual assault, and sexual abuse, which is highly linked to trauma. PTSD can be generalizable across many populations and applies to African Americans. However, PTSD has to be conceptualized in a way that recognizes the trauma and struggles that historically and currently plague African Americans.

HETEROGENEITY OF AFRICAN AMERICANS

Whereas this chapter will focus on the impact of PTSD on the typical African American experiences in the United States, it would be a disservice not to differentiate the heterogeneity among African Americans living in the nation. The African American population living in the nation. Demographically, African Americans comprise roughly 14% of the United States population, with 87% identifying solely as African American or Black (Gran-Ruaz et al., 2022). However, 8% of people who identify as African American also identify as multiple heritage, with 5% explicitly identifying as Black-Hispanic (Gran-Ruaz et al., 2022). Additionally, 10% of African Americans immigrated from another country, including 46% from the Caribbean or 42% from Africa (Gran-Ruaz et al., 2022). Regardless of African Americans' native land and/or social locations, Crenshaw's intersectionality must be examined to include the oppression [*which leads to trauma*] that "includes the simultaneous experience of racism, sexism, heterosexism, able-bodyism, ageism, classism, religious intolerance, transphobia, and/or xenophobia" while identifying as African American (Bryant-Davis, 2019, p. 400). Besides demographic intersectionality, there also exists an intersectionality of historical events, customs, languages, beliefs, values, and other lived experiences that contribute to those who live outside of the United States or have multiple identities beyond just identifying as African American (Gran-Ruaz et al., 2022).

Specifically, gender identity must be considered within the African-American community because the community is not solely comprised of cisgender males and females. Transgender, nonbinary, gender queer, and agender; TGNC (Abdullah et al., 2021) or lesbian, gay, bisexual, transgender; LGBT people (Bryant-Davis, 2019) people must be included because they are an example of people facing multiple traumas of identifying as African American and gender non-conforming. Likewise, trauma survivors living with a disability within the African-American community cannot be neglected either. African Americans living with disabilities also face multiple traumas of identifying as 'dual-minorities' because their disability status often subjects them to ableism, health care disparities, lack of access to counseling, increased risk factors, decreased resiliency factors as they navigate intersectional social identity and roles (Bryant-Davis, 2019).

RACIAL OR RACE-BASED TRAUMA

Specifically, racial or race-based trauma is often the root of PTSD in African Americans due to the constant racial and systemic injustice of oppression that African Americans face or witness regularly. Racial or race (Sule, Sutton, Jones, Moore, Igbo, Jones, 2017). Racial or race-based trauma is "a traumatic response to an accumulation of negative race-related experiences" (Williams, Printz, & DeLapp, 2018, p. 736). Historically, African Americans [amongst other minorities] have lived with oppression through "enslavement, attempted genocide, mass incarceration and deportation, poverty, raids, systemic discrimination, colonialism, and neo-colonialism" (Bryant-Davis, 2019, p. 404). Additionally, African Americans fought oppression not long ago through the Jim Crow era (Sule et al., 2017). Embedded in oppressive behaviors are discrimination and racism [amongst others], which create a higher susceptibility to PTSD in African Americans.

Post-Traumatic Slave Syndrome

Multigenerational, intergenerational, or historical trauma or disbursement of trauma from one generation to another in African Americans (Campbell, 2019) can often be traced back to slavery in the form of Post Traumatic Slave Syndrome

(PTSS), which is often the catalyst of PTSD in African Americans (Sule, 2017). Multigenerational trauma manifests in African Americans at individual, family, and community levels through the shared experiences of discrimination, persecution, and oppression (Campbell, 2019). Dr. Joy DeGruy defined PTSS as "a theory that explains the etiology of many of the adaptive survival behaviors in African American communities throughout the United States and the Diaspora" (Campbell, 2019). Likewise, PTSS is "a theory explaining various patterned behavioral responses that many African Americans exhibit and identifies chattel slavery as the root cause for these behaviors, beliefs, and emotions" (Sule, 2017, p. 780) that mimics PTSD symptomatology. PTSS has persisted because of DeGruy's MAP: multigenerational trauma combined with continuous oppression, absence of the opportunity to heal or access to the same benefits as society, and PTSS (Campbell, 2019, p. 217).

PTSS is important while conceptualizing African Americans because there are lingering features rooted in slavery with impact, such as vacant esteem and a marked propensity for anger and violence (Campbell, 2019; Sule, 2017). PTSS often results in "unworthiness, anger and violence, distorted self-concept, and exposure to stress" (Sule, 2017, p. 780), which exemplifies the hallmarks of this condition. African Americans' unworthiness results in depression, negative self-perception, and hopelessness (Sule, 2017), often leading to underachievement and feelings of inferiority (Campbell, 2019). Moreover, the anger that often results in violence is rooted in the minimization of the community's history (Sule, 2017), which often leads to "extreme feelings of suspicion perceived negative motivation of others. Violence against self, property, and others is often perpetrated against one another, such as friends, relatives, or acquaintances (Campbell, 2019). Anxiety that occurs in the presence of police officers, mistrust of health practitioners, and anger with society's negligence in responding to injustices against African Americans often result in heightened PTSS and PTSD responses. DeGruy's racist socialization and internalized racism often occur in African Americans as "learned hopelessness, literacy deprivation, distorted self-concept, antipathy or aversion for cultural/ethnic groups, customs of one's heritage, and physical characteristics of one's identified cultural/ethnic group" (Campbell, 2019, p. 218). Seemingly, African Americans may avoid their cultural identity because they are ashamed of their historical past. African Americans are often blamed for their victimization instead of the system accepting blame and trying to rectify the impact of slavery (Sule, 2017).

In the early 1700s, Africans were enslaved and transported from their native homeland to the United States. The cruelty of slavery disconnected Africans from tradition, language, culture, and heritage (Ormond, Barbour, Lewis, Montgomery, & Ponds, 2021). Slavery forced African Americans to work grueling amounts of hours per day. Slavery forced Africans to work grueling amounts of hours per day. Moreover, most African Americans have been told about the impact that slavery had on their family history and ancestry through stories, photographs, artifacts, etc. Thus, the retelling and learning of slavery can contribute to vicarious traumatization in African Americans. Additional trauma has been perpetuated as African Americans have faced separation and judgment physically based on skin complexion, hair texture, and gender roles (Campbell, 2019).

Microaggressions

Often, African Americans are subjected to microaggressions which negatively impact their mental health, resulting in traumatic symptoms (Zoubaa et al., 2022) such as depression or anxiety (Abdullah et al., 2021; Sibrava et al., 2019; Williams, Printz, & DeLapp, 2018). Microaggressions are defined as the intentional or unintentional words, actions, or environments that communicate hostility, insult, or invalidation based upon membership in a marginalized group (Zoubaa et al., 2022) (Zoubaa et al., 2022) which can exist in the forms of microassaults, microinsults, or microinvalidations (Abdullah, 2021). Microaggressions are perpetrated subtly and covertly or blatantly and overtly. After a microaggression, there is often a dilemma on how the survivor should respond to adequately express his/her/their feelings (Zoubaa et al., 2022). The microaggressions that significantly impact African Americans are: "foreigner/not belonging, criminality, sexualization, low achieving/undesirable culture, environmental, and invisibility." Undergirding, the most common types of microaggressions experienced by African Americans are criminality and inferiority (Williams, Printz, & DeLapp, 2018). Microaggressions condone that African Americans are "less-than-human" (Abdullah et al., 2021), rooted in the original version of the United States Constitution that saw an African American male as 3/5 of a man and not a whole man.

When mental health professionals work with African Americans, the impact of microaggressions needs to be assessed because these occurrences are discriminatory events that often trigger negative memories of past personal or group traumatic experiences (Sibrava et al., 2019). Additionally, mental health professionals need to understand the environments where microaggressions occur. According to Abdullah et al. (2021), most microaggressions in the workplace lack African American representation, with African Americans being treated as low achieving, undesirable, less valuable, low status, or nonexistent despite any achievement or societal status that had been gained. So, if microaggressions occur at work, African Americans are subjected to trauma daily in an environment that cannot be avoided. Microaggressions in the workplace conflict with African Americans fulfilling their purpose and performing their job with passion in a setting that fuels their livelihoods. Moreover, mental health professionals must be sure not to perpetuate racism or microaggressions while providing services because that does not alleviate the problem but only contributes to it (Campbell, 2019).

Discrimination and Racism

Discrimination is born from microaggressions. Discrimination is defined as "unjust, prejudicial treatment based on stigmatized status and may occur as the result of an ascribed identity, such as race/ethnicity, sex, or age; or achieved identities, such as social class or education" (Williams, Printz, & DeLapp, 2018). Consequently, African Americans report higher incidences of discrimination than any other minority group, which often results in traumatization that leads to PTSD (Brooks Holliday et al., 2020; Williams, Printz, & DeLapp, 2018). Racism is embedded in discrimination and must be conceptualized when counseling African Americans because of its traumatic impact.

It must be noted that the DSM 5-TR does not explicitly include racism as a part of the PTSD diagnosis. However, the implications of PTSD are experienced by the survivors of racism, which are mainly African Americans. A possibility for racism not being included as part of the PTSD diagnosis could be because PTSD focuses on past events (Abdullah et al., 2021). However, oppression and racism are constantly and continuously accumulating for African Americans, often with no end in sight. Likewise, survivors of racism tend to experience hypervigilance, avoidance, and re-experiencing of the racism [the traumatic event], which constitutes race-based trauma (Abdullah et al., 2021). Regardless of past or current occurrences, these are symptoms of PTSD. Racism should be mentioned because African Americans are constantly "victimized by those who hold power" (Abdullah et al., 2021, p. 245).

Racial and ethnic discrimination is relative in trauma assessment (Zoubaa et al., 2022) because survivors often continuously experience and re-experience rejection, ridicule, threat, violence, and other types of harm which negatively impacts emotional, psychological, and physical health and is considered abuse after occurring regularly (Sibrava et al., 2019; Zoubaa et al., 2022). Common traumatic symptoms that result from discrimination are anxiety, negative affect, and avoidance (Williams, Printz, & DeLapp, 2018; Zoubaa et al., 2022). This constant re-exposure constantly re-traumatizes African Americans and leaves a cumulative effect regardless of whether it happens once or daily (Williams, Printz, & DeLapp, 2018; Zoubaa et al., 2022). Furthermore, the discrimination and racism that African Americans face are often traumatic, manifested physically, psychologically, emotionally, and socioeconomically.

Systemically Socioeconomically Disadvantaged

Often, African Americans are systemically socioeconomically disadvantaged (Brooks Holliday et al., 2020). Historical adversity, which includes slavery, sharecropping, and race-based exclusion from health, educational, social, and economic resources, translates into socioeconomic disparities experienced by African Americans today (Ormond et al., 2021). Many systemic issues still plague African Americans: police brutality, lack of access to affordable and equitable health care, income inequalities, and mass incarceration (Sule, 2017). African Americans often experience disparities in housing and neighborhood quality, income, and educational achievement (Gran-Ruaz et al., 2022), leading to exposure to crime-filled and violent living conditions (Brooks Holliday et al., 2020). More specifically, Sibrava et al. (2019) state that issues that disproportionately impact African-American living conditions that ultimately contribute to PTSD are:

- Socioeconomic factors that may limit resources to cope with traumatic stressors;
- increased exposure to assaultive violence;
- stressors associated with displacement and immigration;
- cultural differences in emotional expression;
- overrepresentation in poorer, disadvantaged, and higher crime communities;
- pervasive marginalization and "invisibility;"
- higher rates of victim blaming following an assault;
- increased rates of incarceration;
- homelessness;
- intimate partner violence; and
- sex trafficking.

Thus, the disparities that lead to the risk of socioeconomic disadvantages for African Americans provide more exposure to trauma due to living in an environment where traumatic events are more likely to occur. In Gran-Ruaz et al.'s (2022) study, 60+% of African Americans and Black Caribbeans saw someone badly injured or involved in a physical fight near their home. Likewise, this population reported being involved in at least one life-threatening car accident (Gran-Ruaz et al., 2022). Half of the Gran-Ruaz et al. (2022) study participants also experienced the unexpected death of a loved one. *(This is not an exhaustive list of all the traumatic events witnessed in the Gran-Ruaz et al. (2022) study).*

More specifically, Lu and associates (2022) also corroborated that African Americans who experienced sudden deaths of loved ones from violence, suicide, or an accident were more prone to PTSD. Thus, multiple traumas often occur in

African Americans that are exacerbated by the neighborhoods or communities where they live. Lastly, African Americans have a higher unemployment rate than their counterparts (Avent Harris, Wahesh, Barrow, & Fripp, 2021). Unemployment makes African Americans susceptible to PTSD because they do not have the insurance or employee assistance program to supplement the possible high costs of counseling (Avent Harris et al., 2021; Ormond et al., 2021). Thus, unemployment contributes to the poverty and trauma cycles that often prevent mental health progress in African Americans from occurring.

The prevalence of trauma that African Americans experience tends to be racially or race-based, occurring at insurmountable rates compared to other ethnic groups. Much of African Americans' trauma tends to occur in microaggressions, discrimination, racism, and being exposed to socioeconomically disadvantaged living conditions [*just to name a few*]. Additionally, the root of trauma for African Americans stems from Post-Traumatic Slave Syndrome, which has been transmitted throughout generations. Therefore, the astounding trauma that African Americans encounter regularly permits PTSD to be diagnosed at alarming rates compared to their counterparts.

CASE STUDY

Marian is a 42-year-old African-American female. She is an attorney at a prestigious law firm in a metropolitan city. Marian is the only African-American attorney employed at the firm, which she is proud of. She is married to Thomas, an engineer, and has two children: a 10-year-old daughter, Zadiya, and an 8-year-old son, Malik. Marian and Thomas are both Ivy League educated and proud of the suburban home and lifestyle they have created for their family. They aim to give Zadiya and Malik everything they did not have growing up, including private school education, the latest clothes and technology, and involvement in extracurricular activities. Marian and Thomas are from humble beginnings and are the most successful out of their siblings. Although Marian and Thomas have offered their parents to come to live with them, both sets of parents have declined the offer. Marian and Thomas pay for their parents' living expenses to show gratitude.

Marian has been referred to counseling by a senior partner at the law firm. The partner was concerned because Marian 'has lost her spark.' Marian's self-esteem has declined; she appears more anxious and hypervigilant than usual. She has been observed as withdrawing from her social circles and not attending social events like usual. The private schools that Zadiya and Malik attend are under investigation for discrimination, which has garnered media attention. Marian also confided in the senior partner that she and Thomas found a noose in their yard with random notes saying they did not belong in the neighborhood. Many of these current events trigger memories for Marian when she was in college in the northeast. She feels like it is 'déjà vu' that she is experiencing the same racist acts against her as her parents and grandparents did whenever they progressed in society. You are Marian's counselor.

1. What information makes PTSD a suitable diagnosis for Marian?
2. How do you conceptualize the trauma that Marian has experienced to inform treatment?
3. How do you personally relate (or not relate) to Marian's trauma? What steps can you take to become more empathetic so that you can provide the best possible mental health services?

AFRICAN AMERICANS VIEWS AND AVOIDANCE OF MENTAL HEALTH TREATMENT

African Americans' perceptions of mental health treatment have been negative due to instances of historical unethical practices that occurred before research and health practices were regulated. While health practitioners would naturally be perceived as trustworthy, many cases prove them to operate differently. Since these negative health cases occurred, that negative perception has seeped into mental health. Mental health is already stigmatized, but it can further seem off-putting when African Americans have been negatively targeted and not received the same treatment as their counterparts.

The Antithesis of Mental Health Equity

Adewale, Ritchie, and Everhart-Skeels (2016) outline the beginning of African Americans' avoidance of mental health treatment as the discipline began to emerge in the United States:

Mental health was first conceived as 'mental hygiene,' a term coined by William Sweetzer in 1843. Mental hygiene predated the end of the Civil War, which ended slavery by 20 years. At the time, mental hygiene was correlated with cleanliness, hygiene, and sanity. During 1860 and 1895, there were high rates of African Americans being diagnosed as insane and institutionalized. Dr. T. O. Powell of the Georgia Lunatic Asylum stigmatized the freedom that slaves enjoyed and said that African Americans were the most clean, hygienic, and sane as slaves. (This train of thought rose to prevent the passing of the 14th amendment, which granted African Americans citizenship). However, many people in the North 'recognized the trauma of war and slavery, the increased poverty, social instability, and racial tensions that attributed to the mental instability that was becoming so prevalent among African Americans' (p. 84). However, institutionalization was counterproductive because many African-American patients performed labor in asylums instead of receiving the mental health care and treatment they needed.

Thus, this was the beginning of the treachery African Americans were leery of because they did not want to become trapped back into slavery or indentured servitude. Likewise, there was no empathy for slaves wanting to escape slavery. Instead, they were diagnosed with "drapetomania," a mental illness, for wanting to escape and enjoy a better life (Campbell, 2019).

The Betrayal of Traditional Healthcare

African Americans' physical health was also medically exploited during slavery because of their 'availability and lack of rights' (Batelaan, 2022, p. 1100). This exploitation continued after slavery, too, in the form of unwarranted experimentation and sterilization (Batelaan, 2022). Mental health treatment is an extension of traditional healthcare, so the Tuskegee Syphilis Study and the Henrietta Lacks case contribute to how African Americans perceive mental health treatment. Thus, these cases are a part of the collective memories and narratives passed down from generation to generation (Frazier, 2020).

From a medical standpoint, the 1930s Tuskegee Syphilis Study endows mistrust because the research was deceptive and not conducted ethically (Ormond et al., 2021). Participants were told they had 'bad blood' instead of syphilis (Laws, 2018; Frazier, 2020). Although penicillin was developed to treat syphilis, the syphilis diagnosis nor the treatment was diagnosed to the participants (Laws, 2018; Frazier, 2020). Instead, they were monitored for 40 years until the truth was reported in the 70s (Laws, 2018; Frazier, 2020). Furthermore, the Tuskegee Syphilis Study underlies the rationale for the lack of African-American participation in clinical trials and organ donation (Laws, 2018; Frazier, 2020).

Another source of mistrust African Americans have for healthcare stems from the Henrietta Lacks case. Jones, Vyhlidall, Bradley-Ewing, Sherman, & Goggin (2017) summarize:

In the 1950s, Henrietta Lacks had cervical cancer and was treated at John Hopkins Hospital. Instead of just receiving treatment, her cervical cancer tissues were used for other purposes, resulting in financial gain. At that time, informed consent was not mandated. Thus, parts of Henrietta Lacks' body were used unbeknownst to her with no immediate financial gains or credit of contribution. Besides informed consent, the ethical principles (non-existent at that time) of respect for person, beneficence, and justice were omitted.

Many medical advances that were developed from Lacks' cells include "the polio vaccine, chemotherapy, cloning, gene mapping, and in vitro fertilization, and have helped develop drugs for herpes, leukemia, influenza, STIs, and Parkinson's" (Batelaan, 2022, p. 1100).

The Tuskegee Syphilis Study and the Henrietta Lacks cases are the hallmarks of contributors to African Americans' mistrust of healthcare and modern medicine. Despite restitutions, these collective memories and narratives add to the perceived or actual trauma that can occur in health care or mental health treatment. These studies also have implications of mental health stigma that many African Americans seek to avoid.

COMMON BARRIERS TO MENTAL HEALTH

African Americans are more likely to experience poverty and unemployment, be victims of homicide, and suffer physical illnesses resulting in death in disproportionate numbers than their counterparts (Avent Harris et al., 2021). Nevertheless, a disproportionate number of African American women are prone to exhibit trauma from rape, domestic violence, and stalking experiences, which often lead to PTSD (Gran-Ruaz et al., 2022). Given the likelihood of these occurrences, it is essential to understand how African Americans approach seeking mental health treatment (Avent Harris et al., 2021). African American adults are half less likely to seek professional mental health treatment when compared with Caucasian American adults. Although African Americans have a higher prevalence of PTSD, they are less likely to seek or receive counseling (Lu et al., 2022). Hence, Gran-Ruaz and colleagues (2022) say that 35.5% of African Americans diagnosed with PTSD sought mental health treatment compared to 53.3% of their Caucasian counterparts diagnosed with PTSD. The low prevalence of African American men seeking counseling mimics their male counterparts but is often lower (Avent Harris et al., 2021). Likewise, older, less educated African-American women are less likely to seek counseling (Avent Harris et al., 2021).

Gran-Ruaz et al. (2022) studied the prevalence of African Americans and Black Caribbeans' rationale for not seeking mental health treatment. Their results provide insight that can be very applicable to the African-American perspective on the lack of mental health treatment-seeking behaviors:

- 23.5% thought the problem/trauma would get better on its own;

- 11.7% attempted to solve the problem/trauma on their own;
- 9.8% did not think treatment would help;
- 6.1% did not know where to go for assistance;
- 4.7% could not afford treatment;
- 4.7% worried about what others would think or were embarrassed;
- 4.0% reported that the problem/trauma got better on its own;
- 2.5% noted that the problem/trauma did not bother them or was not severe enough to seek help and
- 1.0% noted it was inconvenient for them to seek help (Gran-Ruaz et al., 2022).

Thus, the underlying theme that can be gathered from this study is that the participants preferred to rely upon themselves and tended to minimize their issues. These results also corroborate that African Americans are often limited to seeking mental health treatment due to lack of access to mental health care, unemployment, or low income (Sibrava et al., 2019). Therefore, common barriers that prevent African Americans from receiving mental health care include "transportation, finances, disapproval from family members, and a lack of knowledge of accessing treatment" (Lu et al., 2022, p. 2). However, married African Americans with children are more likely to seek mental health treatment (Avent Harris et al., 2021). Thus, among African Americans, more women seek mental health treatment than men, but it is by a tiny margin Gran-Ruaz et al. (2022). Whereas some barriers to mental health treatment for African Americans can be internal, others are external.

Mental Health Stigmas and Microaggressions

Defreitas, Crone, DeLeon, and Ajayi (2018) define mental health stigma as "a negative evaluation of those with mental illness or of mental health treatment" (p.1). Underlying mental health stigma is the perceived stigma from others and the assumptions that an individual has personally made. "What is said in this house, stays in this house" is an adage familiar to many African-American children and adults and is a part of the common stigmatization of mental health. Seemingly, African Americans do not want to infiltrate shame and blame onto their family. African Americans also do not want to be considered 'crazy,' 'insane,' or 'weak' (Ormond et al., 2021). More specifically, perceived stigma consists of negative attitudes that individuals believe society holds about individuals with mental illness (Defreitas et al., 2018). In contrast, personal stigma focuses on an individual's beliefs about individuals with mental illness (Defreitas et al., 2018). Thus, the beliefs in these stigmas prevent people, especially African Americans, from seeking mental health services. Knowing the negative impact of mental health stigma, a solution is to educate people about mental health in layperson's terms to combat the stigma (Defreitas et al., 2018).

Kin to mental health stigma is mental illness microaggressions (Zoubaa et al., 2022) that are just as powerful in preventing people from seeking mental health treatment. In defining mental illness microaggressions, five themes encompass the perceived and personal mental health stigmas. The five themes of mental illness microaggressions are invalidation, assumption of inferiority, fear of mental illness, shaming of mental illness, and second-class citizen (Zoubaa et al., 2022, p. 868). (*It is also important to note the similarities between the racial or race-based microaggressions discussed earlier with these mental illness microaggressions*). The impact of mental illness microaggressions tends to be 'isolation, negative emotions, and treatment non-adherence" (Zoubaa et al., 2022, p. 868), which leads to internalization or personal mental health stigmas.

Mental health stigma and microaggressions are often internalized across all age groups. Whereas these issues impact everyone, they are more prevalent in African Americans.

Lack of Knowledge About Mental Health

A significant contributor to mental health stigma in the African-American community is a lack of knowledge about mental health. For example, many misnomers about mental health are believed to be accurate or facts interpreted as fables. Often, many African Americans do not believe that some mental health diagnoses can be hereditary. Instead, African Americans often believe they have done something to warrant a diagnosis or are somehow at fault. Many African Americans do not think their problem is 'big enough to warrant intervention.' 'Common negative stories, fables, wives' tales, or simple misinformation' is passed on throughout generations and dramatically influences the perception of mental health.

Lastly, it is a misnomer that mental health professionals prescribe medicine. Often, the general population does not know the difference between a psychiatrist, psychologist, counselor, or social worker. Thus, many clients need counseling, a form of talk therapy, to help solve their problems. [*There are different forms of therapy such as EMDR, expressive arts, etc., but many minority clients do not know those other modalities exist*]. Many African Americans think severe mental illness represents all mental health issues, which is inaccurate. There is neglect to consider that mental health occurs in ranges and that not only one symptom constitutes a diagnosis. The mental health diagnosis is not permanent but often temporary because clients are stuck in coping. Likewise, some African Americans believe mental health can heal independently if it is not severe (Ormond et al., 2021). Regardless of the myths, misnomers, or misinformation, African Americans were reluctant even to acknowledge the existence of a possible mental health diagnosis (Zoubaa et al., 2022).

Stigma is the most significant barrier to accessing mental health (Ormond et al., 2021). However, within African American mental health stigma, there are stigmas of not bringing shame to the family or wanting to avoid mental health microaggressions by society. General knowledge about mental health tends also to be lacking in the African-American community. Some misnomers that can be barriers do not understand that some mental health diagnoses are hereditary; their actions did not warrant mental illness. They fear that a counselor will prescribe medication. Despite common myths and misnomers regarding mental health, steps need to be taken to remedy these misconceptions so African Americans can seek professional mental health to decrease the impact of PTSD.

THE IMPACT OF POST-TRAUMATIC STRESS DISORDER ON AFRICAN AMERICANS

The DSM 5-TR reports twelve symptoms that define PTSD. Gran-Ruaz et al. (2022) report that African Americans tend to exhibit four main symptoms that mental health professionals should primarily assess and treat:

(1) trying not to think about what happened;
(2) having repeated unwanted memories related to the event;
(3) purposely staying away from places, people, or activities that remind them of the event; and
(4) getting very upset when reminded of the past traumatic event (p. 7).

Since African Americans are already marginalized, mental health professionals must recognize that PTSD symptoms can be heightened. For example, African Americans are more likely to experience interpersonal trauma, develop severe PTSD symptoms, and face barriers that often inhibit safety, justice, and mental health services (Bryant-Davis, 2019).

Because Caucasian or Asian doctors heavily dominate the health profession, there is often the belief that there is not a prevalence of Black doctors who can identify with them. This belief system trickles down to mental health as the prevalence of Black mental health professionals is disproportionate to the African-American community. Thus, this generalization still influences and impacts African Americans' decision-making about seeking and engaging in healthcare treatment.

TREATMENT OPTIONS FOR POST-TRAUMATIC STRESS DISORDER ON AFRICAN AMERICANS

To increase African Americans' mental health treatment-seeking behaviors, it is essential to promote that African-American mental health professionals are available to serve. Mental health facilities should attempt to culturally match treatment dyads whenever possible (Bryant-Davis, 2023; Defreitas et al., 2018; Ormond et al., 2021). Research documents that African Americans [*amongst other minorities*] prefer mental health professionals with similar demographics and backgrounds because that person is likely to understand them better. However, suppose mental health professionals from the dominant culture treat African-American clients. In that case, they should have an open conversation regarding racial differences and actively discuss ways to (a) reduce the power differential and (b) empower clients to become more knowledgeable advocates within their treatment, especially when they perceive unfair treatment (Sule, 2017). To better assist African-American clients, mental health professionals should be willing to learn aspects of clients' cultures, such as client beliefs, practices, and rituals (Bryant-Davis, 2019). This knowledge can be gained formally through cultural competence training (Bryant-Davis, 2019), such as the 12-Step Program for Silent Racism training in healthcare (Sule, 2017). Nevertheless, cultural competence can also be gained informally through the lens of their client (Bryant-Davis, 2019). It is also essential for mental health professionals to be mindful and assess the impact of PTSS (Sule, 2017). Specifically, mental health professionals can keep PTSS in mind when completing the DSM 5 TR's Cultural Formulation Interview (Sule, 2017).

Once the impact of PTSS has been determined to currently impact African American clients, mental health professionals should set a goal of increasing self-esteem with personal value and self-worth being sub-goals in the treatment plan (Campbell, 2019). To improve self-esteem, it is beneficial to assess clients' perceptions of being valuable and creating value as a part of self-care to relieve stress (Campbell, 2019). Another impact of PTSS on African Americans is racist socialization (Campbell, 2019). Racist socialization has infiltrated self-hatred that devalues homogeneous African-American physical traits to fit the mold of the dominant culture (Campbell, 2019). To reconcile the impact of racist socialization from PTSS, African-American strengths have to be recognized, embraced, and celebrated.

Possible Theoretical Integrations

In addition to utilizing traditional methods for treating PTSD, mental health professionals should be prepared to counsel African Americans with culturally modified trauma-focused disability, sexual orientation, and religion and/or spirituality. To integrate culturally modified treatment approaches, Bryant-Davis (2021) outlines that mental health professionals should promote resilience (i.e., strengths across various areas and identities) in the forms of spirituality, movement, art, and music (Bryant-Davis, 2021). Specifically, Campbell (2019) suggests that mental health professionals integrate dance movement therapy because dance helps participants (a) process trauma by increasing a reintegrated mind and body, (b) generate creative expression to represent suffering or trauma, and (c) collect personal strengths for recovery. Meanwhile, spirituality must also be integrated because this is one of the ways that people tend to find meaning in life and cope with trauma. Specifically, mental health professionals should assess "the impact of the sacred meaning of relationship, nature, children, ancestors, and spirit" (Bryant-Davis, 2021, p. 402) in their African-American clients. Bryant-Davis (2021) says assessing sacred meaning helps understand the oppression that has impacted the client. Bryant-Davis (2019) also suggests that indigenous trauma therapy be integrated with spirituality to help heal trauma at a community level. The mental health professional must be willing to join the client on their life's journey and assess community influences that "flow from cultural proverbs, values, beliefs, stories, spirits, and resilience" (Bryant-Davis, 2019, p. 404).

For mental health professionals who practice from a psychoanalytic or psychodynamic theoretical approach, conceptualizing the client's trauma from an oppressive lens can be natural because these historical approaches are rooted and emerged from the oppression of Jewish people (Bryant-Davis, 2019). Thus, the perspective of historical Jewish oppression can be likened to and aid the understanding of the historical oppression of African Americans because of the similar trauma that survivors experienced. Moreover, feminism can be integrated into psychodynamic or other traditional approaches to empower clients. Eye Movement Desensitization and Reprocessing (EMDR) therapy is a famous theoretical orientation to treat trauma. EMDR can be augmented by integrating religion and spirituality to assist clients presenting "discrimination, poverty, clinician bias, misunderstandings due to language usage, family responsibility, role conflict, racial identity, and identity confusion" (Bryant-Davis, 2019, p. 403). More specifically, the previously mentioned issues fall under the umbrella of oppression that can help alleviate the impact of "immigration, bilingualism, discrimination, marginalization, microaggressions, racism, and sexism" (Bryant-Davis, 2019, p. 403) on the client.

Mental health professionals need to honor the historical struggles within African American culture and turn that into a motivating factor within individual treatment (Bryant-Davis, 2019). One way to do this is through modern, contemporary, and integrative theories such as solution-focused, narrative, feminist, dialectical behavior, acceptance, and commitment therapies, to name a few (Bryant-Davis, 2019).

Bryant-Davis (2019) also provides non-traditional therapeutic options with African influence, which mental health professionals can research and integrate into their work with African Americans. To begin, Bryant-Davis (2019) promotes the Ubuntu model of therapy that utilizes the concepts of harmony and interconnection in all living things to relieve emotional distress that is rooted in spiritual wounds; the family, and not the individual, is the focus, god(s), and ancestors. Thus, Ubuntu therapy involves clients telling their stories and mental health professionals conceptualizing client issues on three levels: connection to God, connection to themselves, and connection to others (Bryant-Davis, 2019). Although individual counseling is advantageous for African Americans, group therapy is also. Group therapy can also be beneficial because African Americans find strength by fellowshipping with one another.

Emotional emancipation circles are one group intervention with African roots (Bryant-Davis, 2019). Emotional emancipation circles are group interventions that use a narrative approach to diminish the traumatic impact of discrimination and dehumanization to cultivate resistance to the lie of Caucasian supremacy (Bryant-Davis, 2019). These evidence-based groups focus on clients sharing their stories of racism and the impact that historical and contemporary racism have on themselves and their relationships while learning emotional wellness skills to promote growth, dignity, and humanity (Bryant-Davis, 2019).

Influence of the African-American Church

Lastly, the influence of the African-American church should be included when examining the impact of mental health on African Americans. When African Americans are typically ready to disclose any mental health struggles, they seek non-professional help such as counsel and solace from family, friends (who will refer or congregate at the church), and spiritual leaders first (Avent Harris et al., 2021). Specifically, African Americans are more likely to engage in religious coping practices like prayer first (Avent Harris et al., 2021; Ormond et al., 2021). Religious coping is "coping in which individuals use religious-based rituals and practices to make sense of and respond to distressing life events and transitions" (Avent Harris et al., 2021, p. 76). Additionally, religious coping can be helpful in the church, where religious healing, faith, and spiritual connectedness are fostered (Campbell, 2019). It seems natural that African Americans would rely upon their faith because that is how they coped with slavery and other sociopolitical events throughout time (Ormond et al., 2021). Another benefit is that seeing a minister is free, especially when you do not have insurance (Ormond et al., 2021). However, despite the hesitancy or resistance to attend counseling, some mental health stigmatization exists as the rationale.

It is essential to consult with historically African American churches because of the prominence and role that the church plays in the lives of African Americans.

Some steps can be taken to help get African Americans on board with addressing mental health, and the church is a foundation to get started. First, mental health organizations can partner with African-American churches to hold mental health conferences where everyone completes mental health assessments (Ormond et al., 2021). Second, mental health organizations can conduct focus groups with a subset of African Americans to understand the barriers to seeking mental health treatment (Ormond et al., 2021). Third, mental health organizations must reassess their services for culturally competent practices considering the whole gamut of the African American experience (Ormond et al., 2021). Then, after current approaches have been fine-tuned, mental health organizations can intentionally and proactively advertise their services to the church (Ormond et al., 2021). Fourth, mental health organizations need to continue partnering with African-American churches to explore the current offerings of the church and how referrals can be made since many congregants may not have insurance or can pay for mental health services (Ormond et al., 2021; Sule, 2017).

CONCLUSION

In conclusion, African Americans are more prone to PTSD than other demographics. Much of the PTSD that African Americans experience is rooted in racial-based trauma manifested by oppression, discrimination, and microaggressions. PTSD is multigenerational, as most cases of PTSD can be linked to PTSS. To progress in the treatment of PTSD, it is essential to understand the mental health stigma that is often undergirded by the lack of knowledge. Besides utilizing traditional theories to conceptualize and help African American clients, movement [*often in dance*], Ubuntu, and group strategies such as emancipation circles should be integrated into counseling. Lastly, mental health organizations must recognize the influence of the African-American church and partner with them to understand any hesitancy so that more people can be reached to heal from their trauma.

REFERENCES

Abdullah, T., Graham-LoPresti, J. R., Tahirkheli, N. N., Hughley, S. M., & Watson, L. J. (2021). Microaggressions and posttraumatic stress disorder symptom scores among Black Americans: Exploring the link. *Traumatology*, *27*(3), 244–253. doi:10.1037/trm0000259

Adewale, V., Ritchie, D., & Everhart Skeels, S. (2016). African American and African perspectives on mental health: A pilot study of the pre and post colonial and slavery influences and their implications on mental health. *Journal of Communication in Healthcare*, *9*(2), 78–89. doi:10.1080/17538068.2016.1170316

Avent Harris, J. R., Wahesh, E., Barrow, M., & Fripp, J. A. (2021). Demographics, stigma and religious coping and Christian African Americans' help seeking. *Counseling and Values*, *66*(1), 73–91. doi:10.1002/cvj.12145

Batelaan, K. (2022). It's not the science we distrust; it's the scientists: Reframing the anti-vaccination movement within Black communities. *Global Public Health: An International Journal for Research, Policy and Practice*, *17*(6), 1099–1112. doi:10.1080/17441692.2021.1912809 PMID:33843472

Brooks Holiday, S., Dubowitz, T., Haas, A., Ghosh-Dastidar, B., DeSantis, A., & Troxel, W. M. (2020). The association between discrimination and PTSD in African Americans: Exploring the role of gender. *Ethnicity & Health*, *25*(5), 717–731. doi:10.1080/13557858.2018.1444150 PMID:29490467

Bryant-Davis, T. (2019). The cultural context of trauma recovery: Considering the posttraumatic stress disorder practice guideline and intersectionality. *Psychotherapy (Chicago, Ill.)*, *56*(3), 400–408. doi:10.1037/pst0000241 PMID:31282715

Campbell, B. (2019). Past, present, future: A program development project exploring Post Traumatic Stress Syndrome (PTSS) using experiential education and dance/movement therapy informed approaches. *American Journal of Dance Therapy*, *41*(2), 214–233. doi:10.100710465-019-09320-8

DeFreitas, S. C., Crone, T., DeLeon, M., & Ajayi, A. (2018). Perceived and personal mental health stigma in Latino and African American college students. *Frontiers in Public Health*, *6*, 1–10. doi:10.3389/fpubh.2018.00049 PMID:29536000

Frazier, C. (2020). It's more than just news: Print media, the Tuskegee syphilis study and collective memory among African Americans. *Journal of Historical Sociology*, *33*(3), 280–296. doi:10.1111/johs.12281

Gran-Ruaz, S. M., Taylor, R. J., Jacob, G., & Williams, M. T. (2022). Lifetime trauma exposure and posttraumatic stress disorder among African Americans and Black Caribbeans by sex and ethnicity. *Frontiers in Psychiatry*, *13*, 1–15. doi:10.3389/fpsyt.2022.889060 PMID:35800025

Jones, B. L., Vyhlidal, C. A., Bradley-Ewing, A., Sherman, A., & Goggin, K. (2017). If we would only ask: How Henrietta Lacks continues to teach us about perceptions of research and genetic research among African Americans today. *Journal of Racial and Ethnic Health Disparities*, *4*(4), 735–745. doi:10.100740615-016-0277-1 PMID:27664025

Laws, T. (2018). Tuskegee as sacred rhetoric: Focal point for the emergent field of African American religion and health. *Journal of Religion and Health*, *57*(1), 408–419. doi:10.100710943-017-0505-y PMID:29064071

Lu, W., Silverstein, S. M., Mueser, K. T., Minsky, S., Bullock, D., Buchbinder, S., Chen, Q., Eubanks, R., & Guillaume-Salvant, A. (2022). Undocumented PTSD among African American clients with serious mental illness in a statewide mental health system. *Psychological Trauma: Theory, Research, Practice, and Policy*, 1–10. doi:10.1037/tra0001243 PMID:35797171

Ormond, A., Barbour, R., Lewis, R. K., Montgomery, A., & Ponds, A. (2021). Results from a community mental health assessment in a historically Black church: A call for action. *Journal of Prevention & Intervention in the Community*, *49*(3), 235–250. doi:10.1080/10852352.2019.1654257 PMID:31460840

Sibrava, N. J., Bjornsson, A., Perez Benitez, C. I., Moitra, E., Weisberg, R. B., & Keller, M. B. (2019). Posttraumatic stress disorder in African American and Latinx adults: Clinical course and the role of racial and ethnic discrimination. *The American Psychologist*, *74*(1), 101–116. doi:10.1037/amp0000339 PMID:30652903

Sule, E., Sutton, R. M., Jones, D., Moore, R., Igbo, I., & Jones, L. A. (2017). The past does matter: A nursing perspective on Post Traumatic Slave Syndrome (PTSS). *Journal of Racial and Ethnic Health Disparities*, *4*(5), 779–783. doi:10.100740615-016-0328-7 PMID:28078658

Williams, M. T., Printz, D. M. B., & DeLapp, R. C. T. (2018). Assessing racial trauma with the trauma symptoms of discrimination scale. *Psychology of Violence*, *8*(6), 735–747. doi:10.1037/vio0000212

Zoubaa, S., Dial, B., Ryan-Jones, L., Shah, V., & Yanos, P. T. (2022). On the relationship between experienced microaggressions and mental health stigma among members of marginalized groups. *Counselling Psychology Quarterly*, *35*(4), 867–879. doi:10.1080/09515070.2021.1968795

Chapter 3
Insomnia Disorder Among African-Americans

Kayla Denise Solomon
Texas A&M University, Commerce, USA

ABSTRACT

In this chapter, the author addresses the sleep disturbance of insomnia, which is defined within the chapter. The signs and symptoms related to insomnia were addressed to provide individuals with knowledge to be more aware of any potential cues. The chapter also address African American views on mental health, as well as the risk factors for being more susceptible to experiencing insomnia and its impact. The chapter closes out by acknowledging effective treatment options for Insomnia that can be utilized by the African American community and discusses the need for additional future research.

INTRODUCTION

Have you ever experienced the overwhelming desire to sleep but you cannot, regardless of the number of hours that continue to tick by on the clock? Sit in place and imagine being so tired your eyes burn from their inability to shut and get rest. Think about how it feels to finally doze off and begin to sleep, your body receiving the necessary rest it needs, then suddenly you're awake again. This type of sleeping experience can be referred to as insomnia. Insomnia is one of the various mental health issues that many different communities face, with most who are affected by it not viewing this as a serious issue and being unaware of how to effectively treat this mental health issue. The presence of insomnia in the population worldwide is astounding, with if being for that up to third of adults experience this type of sleep

DOI: 10.4018/978-1-6684-8918-5.ch003

disorder. It has been found that this type of sleep disturbance "is characterized by chronic difficulties falling asleep, staying asleep and/or nonrestorative sleep that is associated with impairment of daytime functioning" (Stokes et al., 2022). The amount of energy that is restored to the human body in the midst of sleep while the body is necessary for functioning to occur. When we do not rest, we become fatigued, incapable of focusing, and experience negative mood changes, which all impact the quality of life. If an individual continues to experience insomnia without ever seeking any type of treatment, the sleep disturbance will eventually impair a person's daily functioning.

The next question most want to know in regards to insomnia is, "why is it impossible for me to fall asleep?" There are a plethora of reasons that could contribute to the cause of insomnia or other similar sleep disorders, however research supports that the main underlying issues can be related to medical comorbidities such as diabetes or increased blood pressure, as well as other mental health disorders, such as depression and anxiety. Studies suggest that "insomnia was associated with a variety of mental symptoms, and the psychological symptoms were shown to be severe according to the severity of insomnia" (Lee et al., 2022). Being in a state of emotional distress that is accompanied with negative emotions, generally results in distorted thinking patterns, which occupy the mind and make it feel as if there are one million thoughts running per minute that are all creating a sense of uncertainty and bring discomfort. Depression is being in a state of deep sadness, where an individual can experience a loss of interest and self-isolation. It has been found that "depression is a common illness that severely limits psychosocial functioning and diminishes quality of life" (Malhi & Mann, 2018). Anxiety is described as being in a state of worry or unease about an uncertain outcome. When experiencing anxiety, some might notice "feeling of fear that occurs when faced with threatening or stressful situations" (Dean, 2016). The consistent worry and negative thinking patterns associated with both depression and anxiety can disrupt an individual's sleeping. Though some underlying reasons have been identified by researchers as contributing factors, there is no real reason as to why insomnia is experienced, more data must be found to support that there is a specific cause for insomnia.

There are certain things that can make a person more susceptible to experiencing insomnia, though it is something that impacts the masses. Things such as being in a state of distress, recent change in time zones, or inconsistent sleeping habits. However, there is no rhyme or reason behind the age or gender when it comes to those who experience this sleeping disturbance. There are specific signs and symptoms that relate to insomnia, which includes difficulty falling asleep or staying awake, fatigue, poor quality sleep, difficulty with focusing, and changes in mood; individuals can experience a range of the listed symptoms. There are various ways to help prevent insomnia, as well as multiple effective methods for treatments. Prevention includes following a sleeping schedule or creating a calming rest space for sleeping, and treatment options that have been found to be successful include the use of pharmacology treatment through medication and the practice of psychotherapy, most commonly Cognitive Behavioral Therapy (CBT). Though each person's interaction with treatment is different, treatment should be sought out to identify which individualistic plan of action will be the most effective.

Signs and Symptoms

Insomnia has been defined by researchers as "sleep continuity disturbance associated with daytime complaints related to sleepiness, fatigue, somatic symptoms (eg, head or body aches), mood disturbance, compromised cognitive or occupational function, concerns about sleep, or dissatisfaction with sleep" (Perlis et al., 2022). Those who are plagued with the experience of insomnia will be able to note very clear signs and symptoms that this is what they are experiencing, rather than another sleeping disorder. One of the most common signs or symptoms that will stand out is the inability to fall asleep or stay asleep, even though an individual has the potential to be exhausted. Though this is the most common symptom, this must be a reoccurring issue with the symptom being present for a minimum of three months for the sleep disturbance to be classified as insomnia. Additional symptoms that occur include feelings of fatigue, inability to focus, physical signs such as body aches and headache, as well as a potential change in mood. The risk of a change in mood is due to the possibility of developing a mood disturbance, which can include high levels of irritability and aggressiveness. When this happens, it can lead to outward behavioral responses that could negatively affect an individual.

Another sign that insomnia is occurring that must be present is the impairment of daily functioning due to lack of sleep. An impairment of daily functioning can be described as a disability, being that it places limitations on an individual, especially in relation to mental health. Being that insomnia can affect an individual's focus control, it can impact problem-solving skills, which are necessary in multiple aspects of life, as well as multi-tasking abilities. Depending on the career or daily life experience of an individual dealing with insomnia, it can be much more impactful. Lastly, insomnia can impact social cues, including one's ability to assimilate and difficulty with being able to relate to others around them. All of these factors create limitations and impairs an individual's daily functioning, which creates a sense of disability.

Case Studies

The first case study provides a glimpse into a case-control study completed with university medical students to compare the personality profiles between individuals with paradoxical insomnia, psycho-physiological insomnia and normal sleepers. Within the study, 100 participants were split into three groups, with two groups existing of participants struggling with insomnia and one group having sleepers with normal sleeping patterns. For the study, "20 patients with PARA-I, 20 patients with PSY-I and 60 NS patients were recruited and matched across groups for age, gender, education, and previous history of mental and/or physical illness" (Rezaie et al., 2020). Participants were given the MMPI short form to assess their different personality characteristics. The assessment is a 71-question form with yes or no response questions that examines and categorizes different personality traits associated with participants. Participants who were in the groups that were categorized as different insomnia subtypes were provided with polysomnographic techniques throughout the study.

The study produced results that reflected differences that exist between the three participating groups. Supporting the idea that struggling with insomnia can impair daily functioning, the results showed that participants in the insomnia groups both had "increased levels of guardedness, defensiveness and sensation-avoidance" (Rezaie et al., 2020) when compared to those in the normal sleeping group. It was shown that though there was no significant difference in the results of the two insomnia groups, the difference was statistically significant in comparison to the no sleepers group. "The results of the ANOVA showed a significant difference between the mean scores of hysteria, hypochondriasis, and psychopathic deviate across the three groups" (Rezaie et al., 2020). The participants in this case control study support the idea that those with insomnia have a different daily functioning experience.

The second case-control study examines and compares the prevalence of anxiety and depression amongst those who have paradoxical insomnia, psycho-physiological insomnia, and those who were identified as normal sleepers. It is believed by many that anxiety and depression contribute to the presence of insomnia due to the distorted thinking patterns that occur with both disorders. The study was made up of participants who were placed into three different groups, based on if they were identified as having paradoxical insomnia, psycho-physiology insomnia, or being a normal sleeper. For the case-study, "all subjects underwent a multistep screening evaluation, which consisted of a sleep history interview, an overnight PSG, a psychological assessment, and medical history taken with physical examination" (Liao et al., 2018). Participants for the group were also assessed using the Self-Rating Anxiety Scale (SAS) and the Self-Rating Depression Scale (SDS) to identify the existence of anxiety and depression within a participant. The purpose of the cross-sectional case control study was to compare the presence of anxiety and depression in those who struggle with insomnia to those who do not.

The results from the study suggest that there was significantly increased levels of depression and anxiety within participants who were categorized in the insomnia groups. When reviewing the anxiety and depression self-report scale scores, it was found by researchers that there was a significant difference between those labeled as normal sleepers and those placed in the insomnia groups in reference to anxiety and depression. "This study compared anxiety and depression between patients with Para-I, patients with Psy-I, and NS. As expected, both Psy-I and Para-I groups had higher anxiety and depression levels than NS" (Liao, et al., 2018). With there being an increased likelihood of experiencing both anxiety and depression while suffering from insomnia, it confirms the idea that both disorders could be considered contributing factors to the sleeping disturbance.

An additional case-series study was conducted to test the hypothesis that cognitive behavioral therapy for insomnia (CBTi) can provide effective treatment. The study was a case series chart review design where clients were seen over a one-year period. Within the study, clients were provided with an eight-session trial of cognitive behavioral therapy for insomnia or CBTi in conjunction with appropriate medication. Measures used to assess effectiveness included the Insomnia Severity Index, DBAS-16 which is, "a 16-item measure scored on a 1–10 Likert type scale" (Dolan et al., 2010). The Sleep-Wake Activity Inventory and sleep diaries were also utilized in the study. No session within the study was the same; the sessions included a range of activities surrounding the development of good sleep hygiene, discussion of consequences stemming from insomnia, and challenging dysfunctional or irrational beliefs through role-play. At the end of each session, the participants all met with the "supervising physician to discuss progress and medication issues" (Dolan et al., 2010).

The results from the study provided supporting evidence to show that Cognitive Behavioral Therapy is an effective form of treatment for insomnia. Being that within the study participants were tasked with arguing their dysfunctional thoughts and providing evidence to combat these beliefs, it continues to solidify that negative thinking patterns can contribute to the presence of insomnia and eliminating dysfunctional and irrational beliefs can decrease symptoms of insomnia. One of the biggest takeaways from the study is that "CBTi resulted in 'remission' of insomnia in 37.5–66.8% of patients" (Dolan et al., 2010) based on how the term was defined for the study. The data also reflected a decrease in the use of medication for patients who were originally taking sleeping medication at baseline and then were able to discontinue medication at post-treatment. Overall, the study supports that Cognitive Behavioral Therapy is an effective form of treatment for insomnia.

The last case study was a cross-sectional case-controlled study with the purpose of assessing the effectiveness of Group Cognitive Behavioral Therapy (GCBT). Within the study, it consisted of participants that were classified and placed into three groups. One group being those being treated with the sleeping medication zolpidem for sixteen weeks, the second group received zolpidem for four weeks as well as a combination of GCBT for twelve weeks, and the last group was the healthy control group. Group cognitive therapy is the form of talk therapy in groups to encourage advocacy and support amongst group members. For research and to better assess insomnia and potential contributing factors, "participants were evaluated using the Patient Health Questionnaires (Patient Health Questionnaire-9 [PHQ-9] and Patient Health Questionnaire-15 [PHQ-15]), the Dysfunctional Beliefs and Attitudes about Sleep-16 (DBAS-16), and the Pittsburgh Sleep Quality Index (PSQI)" (Mao et al., 2017). Participants were evaluated using the listed measuring instruments before intervention and sixteen weeks post-treatment.

Results from this study show a decrease in the scores of measuring tools, which screen for symptoms related to depression, distorted thinking patterns, disturbed sleeping patterns, and other mental disorders. It was found that when compared to "the zolpidem and healthy control groups, the scale scores of PHQ-9, PHQ-15, DBAS-16 and PSQI were significantly reduced after intervention in the GCBT group" (Mao et al., 2017). Specifically in reference to the use of Group Cognitive Behavioral Therapy, this type of treatment "played a role in altering the dysfunctional beliefs and attitudes about sleep, improving the subjective sleep quality, as well as lowering the somatic and emotional problems in patients" (Mao et al., 2017). The study also supports the idea that the advocacy that naturally is embedded into group therapy is a contributing factor for decreased symptoms. The concept of adjusting the thought and beliefs of an individual has been emphasized across all case studies as an effective method for decreased symptoms related to insomnia.

African American Views on Mental Health

The treatment of mental health issues is something that has come a long way, being that in the earlier years of the introduction to therapeutic practices and services, people did not realize the importance of addressing these types of problems, or they treated them as if they were nonexistent. This is an issue that exists in various ethnic groups and populations; however it is very common to see these types of issues being dismissed within the African American community. The refusal to acknowledge mental health issues stems from the outdated stereotypes that exist within the African American community, which includes that an individual is "crazy" or "touched", if they suffer from any type of mental disturbance or disorder, though the average person suffers from some type of mental health issue, whether it impacts their daily functioning or not. Due to the plight of African Americans, it is hard for the average person to accept or acknowledge a weakness that exists simply due to the "strong" facade many African Americans must maintain.

African Americans have always been at a disadvantage, dating back to slavery and the terrible mistreatment of black people. All that was endured by slaves during that era was traumatizing to those who experienced it firsthand and many generations after, with the trauma spilling into the present day. In those times, African Americans were taught to suffer in silence, out of fear of the punishments that may be given out due to upsetting the "master". Dealing with emotions by internalizing them and not being able to use self-expression to release their thoughts or emotions taught the African American community not to speak on difficult emotions or situations. Though holding in thoughts stems from fear, it developed into a way of life for this community. This same concept of "keeping it in" is something that was later translated across a multitude of topics when it comes to the African American community, including how mental health issues are addressed within families and individually. The trend of not receiving help is passed down from older generations who "do not receive appropriate mental health treatment or recognize the symptoms of mental disorders" (Stansbury et al., 2013). When members of the African American community refuse to acknowledge or address an issue related to mental health, it prevents an individual from receiving effective treatment to improve their daily functioning.

The lack of acknowledgement of issues related to mental health also relates to the internal pressure that a lot of African Americans place on themselves due to the system racism that exists in the U.S., which requires black people to be "perfect" in comparison to their white counterparts, who are allowed by society to have flaws, and it does not hinder them from advancing in life. Accepting the presence of a mental health disorder for an African American person can create a sense of fear that you will be overlooked in society and viewed as less than, because the starting line for African Americans is already pushed farther back than the average person. The fear that the acceptance of a mental health issue can result in a negative impact on a person's life outweighs some people's desire to seek out treatment for areas where they need additional assistance. If the internal pressure of being "better" didn't exist in the African American community due to obvious systemic disadvantages, it could be argued that the views on acknowledging and seeking treatment for mental health disorders would look differently for the African American community.

Another large contributing factor to the negative views that the black community has on the treatment of mental health disorders is the crippling effect of ignorance. There is so much about mental health that is never explored nor discussed in the households of black families, which leaves people with nothing to do other than create their own ideologies. The creation of inaccurate beliefs to what mental health is, and who is identified as struggling with mental health negatively affects the African American community, because general idea amongst a vast amount of members in the community is that you must suffer from a major psychosis disorder, such as bipolar disorder or schizophrenia to be considered as having issues with your mental health, and in those instances you are considered "crazy"; this also extends to being prescribed and consuming medication to aid in assisting with a mental health issue. It is necessary to adjust African American views on mental health because the "more African Americans believe in the effectiveness of mental health treatment, the more likely they will be engaged and involved in treatment" (Stansbury et al., 2013). Disorders such as depression or anxiety aren't treated as if they are real concerns or issues that impact a person's quality of life, most members of the community are told to just "get over it", which can be overall harmful because they too can negatively affect someone.

The last and most importantly known factor that deters African American people from receiving any type of medical assistance, whether it be physical or mental, is the lack of access to quality resources and the fear of mistreatment by medical and mental health professionals. Though professionals are tasked with providing adequate care to all patients who are seeking assistance, it is the common experience of black people to be treated as well or for their health concerns not to be taken seriously. The ability to afford the cost of mental health treatment, even with insurance, is not a luxury that most black households have, being that most African Americans fall within the middle and lower financial classes. This leaves the community relying on receiving treatment from community centers and government run agencies that may not be able to provide the individualized care that is needed to ensure the effectiveness of treatment for a particular client, that could be provided at private practice that offers services at a much higher rate.

Though the views on treatment to mental health in the African American community has historically been negative, it is something that has begun morphing over time with younger generations. With the numbers of Black Mental Health Professionals increasing over the past ten years, so has the knowledge regarding mental health and the distribution of this wealth of information within the community. The increased number of familiar faces when seeking services also provides a sense of comfort and security in being able to receive help from someone who looks like you. As the number of African American mental health professionals continues to rise, there is a strong possibility that it could eventually lead to a trend where mental health is accepted by the black community in all aspects.

Impacts of Insomnia on African Americans

Insomnia can impact people in various ways, but namely in their ability to fall asleep and receive restorative rest, but also daytime functioning. The type of issues that can develop from insomnia include decreased productivity, inability to focus, issues related to mood, the development of other mental health issues, and the use of potentially harmful sleeping aids, such as alcohol and marijuana. Research suggests that insomnia can specifically impact "fatigue, mood disturbance, daytime sleepiness, and impaired social, family, occupational, or academic performance" (Sandlund et al., 2017). When these problems happen, it can bleed into other aspects of an individual's life and create a domino effect of a plethora of various issues. Any of the previously listed factors can impact the life of those with insomnia, however the impact it leaves on those in the African American community is unmatched. Due to the daily experience that the average African American faces, the presence of any of the problems listed above set them apart from their peers, which puts them behind and births the negative stereotypes that are associated with black people.

In relation to decreased productivity and inability to focus, when insomnia occurs and it produces these additional issues, it contributes to a false stereotype that African Americans are lazy and do not believe in hard work. A lack of sleep can begin to cause the body to slowly begin deteriorating and decrease how productive a person is. When a person's productivity decreases, it normally relates to a job or academics. Studies have shown that "reporting sleep difficulties and problems with productivity due to poor sleep. Raising awareness about the importance of sleep in the workplace and a targeted approach to help those in greatest need for assistance improves not only sleep, but also loss of work productivity" (Espie et al., 2018). In a career field, when a person becomes less productive than what is expected of them, it can result in them being demoted in their positions or even possibly losing their jobs. The quick decision for an infraction in a work setting due to a decrease in productivity can be attributed to the negative stereotype that others have of the African American community. In regard to academics, a decreased amount of productivity can lead to failure in academics, being that some may argue that an individual is simply lazy and unmotivated, though they may be experiencing these factors due to insomnia and the inability to receive restorative sleep. Not only can insomnia affect productivity, but it can also impact a person's ability to maintain focus. When a person struggles with focusing, it can also lead to an issue regarding how a person learns. If a person is incapable of absorbing knowledge, this then potentially leads to disruptive behavioral issues, which is one of the most common stereotypes associated with black people.

Another aspect of life that can be impacted by insomnia is a change in mood. Though a change in mood doesn't necessarily mean it will result in a negative mood, that is more common when it is related to a lack of sleep. Studies suggest that the presence of "insomnia symptoms, stress, and pain were associated with greater mood disturbance" (Walsh et al., 2019). Some could be described as rude, mean, or grumpy while trying to engage in daytime functioning. This is the view that the average person has of those within the African American community, so it is detrimental for black people to develop these negative moods, as they are judged much more harshly for experiencing them. A constant negative mood can also impact an individual's interpersonal skills, and then negatively affect their relationships with others. Additionally, experiencing insomnia can also relate to the development of other mental health issues, such as anxiety and depression. These types of disorders have been found to directly link to insomnia, being that when you struggle with insomnia there is never an opportunity to receive restorative sleep, which doesn't allow your brain time to rest. That necessary rest is when your mind is supposed to be shut down and your thoughts shouldn't be flowing; however, if a person never gets the chance to sleep, their brain never shuts off and their potentially negative thoughts and beliefs never cease.

One extremely harmful impact that is common amongst members in the African American community is the use of harmful substances as sleeping aids, such as alcohol use or marijuana. Though the use of alcohol can help a person fall asleep, it also can cause much more harm, including causing even more disruption to a person's sleeping pattern. Mentally, the use of alcohol as a sleeping aid can make an individual more susceptible to developing an alcohol addiction. Alcohol addiction is already common, as it is the number one abused substance however, it can also affect not only the brain and cognitive functioning, but also other internal organs. When the human body abuses alcohol, it can also create problems within your liver, kidneys, heart, and pancreas. Using marijuana as an aid to sleep is not only illegal in many parts of the United States, but it also cultivates another form of addiction, though most people do not believe that you can abuse marijuana. This is a false ideology that has been adopted by a large portion of the African American population. The use of marijuana can create legal issues, due to certain state laws, but it can also affect mood, self-awareness, and cognitive functioning. Research has also found that "alcohol/marijuana sleep aid use is prevalent among college students and is concurrently associated with increased poor sleep quality and pre-sleep arousal" (Williams et al., 2018). Both forms of addiction not only affect cognitive functioning, but they also can impair motor functioning such as standing and walking. If you scratch the surface, the reason why the use of harmful sleeping aids is detrimental is obvious, however when you dig deeper you see these types of addictions can lead to many other issues.

There are many negative impacts that can occur for an individual experiencing insomnia; however they also have the ability to cause a domino effect and lead to a range of other problems. Insomnia not only affects sleep, but when it comes to the impairment of daytime functioning, it impacts individuals in the categories of living, socially, and learning. Due to the possibilities of inability to focus and decrease in productivity, this can impact a person in a learning environment, as well as living in the case that problem-solving skills are impacted. An impact that can affect a person socially includes how a person's mood may be affected, which impacts their ability to form and maintain relationships. The last category of living can be impacted by each previous factor listed above.

Factors/Risks for Insomnia

There are various factors that can make a person more susceptible to developing a sleeping disturbance such as insomnia. Risk factors can be defined as an increased likelihood of experiencing a possible negative outcome. Some identified risk factors include the presence of other mental health disorders, comorbidities, quality of life and stress. The research surrounding risk factors for insomnia is still limited, being that that still isn't an actual cause of insomnia that has been identified. If these factors are identified early, steps can be taken to mediate their presence and in turn, decrease the chances of insomnia. You can also identify the most appropriate form of treatment for your individual needs based on associated risk factors.

One of the known risk factors associated with insomnia is the presence of other mental health disorders and comorbidities. Medical comorbidities that are associated with pain, such as diabetes, which is a common medical condition for members in the African American community. It has also been found that when other mental health disorders such as anxiety and depression are present, it increases the likelihood that an individual could develop the sleeping order of insomnia. It is common that those who suffer from insomnia have the potential to have "developed insomnia in association with another physical or mental health problem" (Leblanc et al., 2009). Due to the dysfunction of thoughts and beliefs when referring to both anxiety and depression, the lack of sleep never allows for restorative sleep to occur and never presents the opportunity for the brain to rest and continued distorted thinking, can keep the mind awake. The chronic pain that could exist from comorbidities and distorted thinking patterns associated with mental health disorders such as anxiety and depression, can cause a disturbance in sleeping.

One of the most known risk factors to being more susceptible to insomnia is a poor quality of life. For African Americans, it is very common for the quality of life to be poor in comparison to other racial communities. The access to resources and calming environments is not always near those in the African American community. Taking the idea that members in the African American community have a higher risk of living in poverty and close quarters, which can result in louder environments which can cause an inconsistent sleeping pattern to be developed. Additionally, a poor quality of life can come in the form of having a decline in physical health as well. Poor physical health can create other medical issues and it has already been suggested by researchers that the presence of comorbidities makes a person more susceptible to experiencing insomnia. Additionally, a poor quality of life can cause a person to be incapable of recognizing signs and symptoms related to insomnia; however, if noticed early on, treatment can be sought to mediate the presence of insomnia.

The last identified risk factor is the presence of excessive stress in an individual's daily life. Stress is an overwhelming amount of pressure that can derive internally or externally from outside factors. Empirical studies suggest that "Perceived stress is strongly associated with sleep problems" (Cardoso et al., 2021). External factors that can cause stress for African Americans, that they face within society, include the stress of finances, fear of being unsuccessful, need to maintain a certain image as to not be judged, as well as going through each day being identified as African Americans. African Americans are already viewed as less than by society, so the external pressure to be what the world expects them to be can be daunting and form stress. The internal pressure related to stress can also stem from the pressures of society to fit in and meet the criteria for what is considered the "standard" for the average person.

Overall, there are a range of risk factors that relate to prevalence of insomnia in an individual. Though there is no identified "cause" of insomnia, there are various factors that make a person much more susceptible to developing the sleep disturbance. Identified factors include the presence of comorbidities and other mental health problems, as well as a poor quality of life and increased levels of stress. If these factors can be identified, an individual can attempt to take preventative measures to decrease the likelihood of experiencing insomnia. Also, in identifying risk factors, it can help a person create an effective individualized plan for treatment.

Theoretical Orientation

A common theoretical orientation that is embedded in treatment for insomnia is Cognitive behavioral therapy The main ideology of cognitive behavioral therapy is that our internal thoughts and feelings can lead to outwardly negative behaviors. In the process of assisting your client, the use of CBT requires the counselor to help in changing the current thinking pattern by aiding the client in reframing their thoughts. "Cognitive research has shown that distortions in processing information about oneself are integral to many behavioral and psychological problems" (Hazlett-Stevens & Craske, 2002). Some believe that when utilizing CBT it is not only the duty of the counselor to provide assistance in helping the client identify their thoughts and behaviors, but also helping the client to find purpose and build self-efficacy, as that can be beneficial in the counseling process. With the combination of identifying and reshaping the client's negative thoughts and feelings and building their confidence while addressing interpersonal and intrapersonal issues, CBT can be effective.

Cognitive Behavioral Therapy (CBT) is a therapeutic approach that connects the link between thoughts, emotions, and outward behaviors. When practicing using CBT, the belief or assumption is that an activating event or experience influences an individual's thoughts, which then affects their emotions and outward behaviors and reactions. It has been found that though this theory is generally considered problem-focused, it allows the client the opportunity to fully process the negative experience before moving on to a solution. During the process of dissecting the thoughts and emotions, it allows the client the chance to understand the "why" behind their behaviors and then reframe those same thoughts. CBT is also considered a brief form of therapy that most people consider to be affordable and effective. Some feel this theoretical approaches' popularity lies in the fact that it can be used for various problems individuals face and the length allows it to be accessible to many.

While utilizing Cognitive Behavioral Therapy (CBT), there are specific techniques that must be used by the counselor to assist in clients. The techniques that are said to be the most beneficial include self-talk, reframing, thought stopping, and cognitive restructuring. It is said that by using the techniques in a session it allows the client the chance to shift their way of thinking from negative to a more positive perspective, however they must first process their problem prior to doing this. When using a technique such as self-talk, it helps the client to learn how to redirect their inner thoughts from negative to positive. Another technique that also does this is thought stopping, which requires the client to stop the current negative thoughts that are running through their minds and alter them to combat the negative emotions and behaviors that arise from those negative thoughts. Research suggests that self-talk, reframing, and thought stopping all share a common goal of cognitive restructuring.

CBT is an approach that examines the connection between thoughts, emotions, feelings, and how they impact our behaviors. This type of therapy is problem-focused, rather than solution so it gives the client the chance to fully explore their presenting issues. Once you begin acknowledging and unpacking the problem, it allows the client room for progression as they can start to reframe their mindset once they are able to identify what is causing a distortion to the client's behaviors. Many professionals believe that CBT is an effective approach to helping clients determine what causes the domino effect to their behaviors. It could be said that this approach teaches clients how to implement these techniques into their daily lives' and continue to progress even after completing therapy.

Effective Treatment for Insomnia in African Americans

Cognitive behavioral therapy (CBT) has been identified by many professionals as an effective approach to treating insomnia. Cognitive behavioral therapy is a form of psychotherapy, which is talk therapy, that gives the client a chance to explore the connection between their thoughts, emotions, and behaviors. When using CBT, this theoretical approach calls for an individual to work on restructuring and reframing their irrational thoughts and beliefs. Being that distorted thinking can cause a disruption in sleeping patterns, eliminating that type of dysfunctional thinking can help to effectively treat insomnia symptoms. Reframing negative thoughts that constantly consume the human mind, will allow for the necessary restorative sleep to occur, because the thought that "too much is on your mind" to fall asleep would no longer be an element that is blocking restful sleep from happening. Cognitive behavioral therapy can be offered in many forms, including both individual and group psychotherapy. Research also suggests that when combining both medication and CBT, we can see positive results. Specific techniques related to CBT that would be beneficial to a person suffering from insomnia includes the use of cognitive restructuring, reframing, positive-self talk, as well as thought stopping as an effective approach to treating insomnia. When using Cognitive behavioral therapy, it also teaches a person resiliency, and it improves a person's quality of life through providing them with skills that can be implemented in their everyday lives.

Though found to be more effective with a combination of other approaches to treatment, providing information about sleep hygiene has also been identified as an effective approach to treating insomnia. Sleep hygiene is simply information regarding sleeping habits and patterns, as well as preventative measures that can be taken to decrease the likelihood of insomnia from occurring. The approach to treatment using sleep hygiene is very educational for the client because they learn more about "practicing behaviors that facilitate sleep and avoiding behaviors that interfere with sleep" (Riedel, 2000). Practicing behaviors that facilitate sleep could include a consistent bedtime, the use of appropriate sleeping aids, and practicing calming or thought clearing exercise prior to attempting to go to sleep. Also, the quality of the sleep obtained, plays a major role in ensuring adequate sleeping hygiene. Guaranteeing that a person will receive a good quality sleep is something that can not necessarily be controlled due to the various external variables that are out of our control, such as living in a peaceful quiet environment versus a loud city environment. With sleep hygiene education, you also learn about avoiding certain behaviors or actions that will increase your chances of experiencing insomnia. Additionally with sleep hygiene, an individual will learn more about pharmacology, and the impacts of medication usage for insomnia.

Sleep restriction therapy refers to a form of therapy that derives from Cognitive behavioral therapy, however it can be used as a stand-alone intervention for effective treatment of insomnia. The use of sleep restriction therapy involves the process of "restricting a patient's time in bed (TIB, sleep window) to match their average (self-report) total sleep duration. The sleep window is then titrated, weekly, based on sleep efficiency (the proportion of TIB spent asleep), in order to arrive at the patient's core sleep requirement" (Kyle et al., 2014). Essentially the purpose is to build a client's sleeping habits and then adjust it based on the needs and requirements for the sleep to be considered restorative. Some believe that sleep restriction therapy can also be detrimental to sleeping patterns, because it eliminates the client from excessive oversleeping as well as daytime napping. The argument that some people try to make is that eliminating those additional opportunities for sleep limit the amount of restorative sleep that can occur; however research suggests that those types of sleep are not restorative. The proposed idea with the use of sleep restriction therapy is that "decreasing the opportunity to sleep over successive nights, it is argued, builds homeostatic sleep pressure, stabilizes circadian control of sleep and wakefulness, and dampens pre-sleep cognitive and physiological (hyper)arousal, leading to shorter sleep latencies and more consolidated, uninterrupted sleep" (Kyle et al., 2014).

Another effective approach to the treatment of insomnia includes the use of mindfulness, which is rooted in improving an individual's quality of life. This specific approach helps to decrease stress and encourages stress management, as well as emotion regulation in an individual. With the use of mindfulness, it "integrates behavioral treatments for insomnia with the principles and practices of mindfulness meditation" (Ong & Sholtes, 2010). When using mindfulness-based therapy, it teaches clients how to be more self-aware of what they are experiencing in the present moment as well as developing different relaxation techniques and exercises that can be implemented in their lives. Specific techniques and exercises include the use of meditation, yoga, progressive muscle relaxation, and different breathing techniques. The main goal behind the use of mindfulness-based therapy for treating insomnia is "to help individuals increase awareness of the mental and physical states that develop with chronic insomnia and to develop adaptive ways of working with these undesirable states" (Ong & Sholtes, 2010). With the combination of all of these strategies when using mindfulness-based therapy, it can help reduce sleep through the night and improve daytime functioning.

An additionally effective approach to treating insomnia is bright light exposure therapy, due to the fact that "light has an important influence on sleep and wakefulness" (Maanen et al., 2016). The process of adding bright natural light or taking it away has the ability to impact sleeping patterns because it has been found to impact circadian rhythm. Factors that impact the effectiveness of this form of therapy include light intensity, color, as well as temperature. In studies relating to the use of bright light exposure to treat insomnia, it was found that "significant moderating effect of light intensity, indicating that studies using a higher light intensity found larger effects" (Maanen et al., 2016). Though some research has been shown to support the effectiveness of bright light exposure therapy, there are limitations that suggest the effects are not as significant for all people. It is possible that "light therapy might be combined with CBT, to see whether there is an additive treatment effect", as it has been found to have positive effects (Maanen et al., 2016).

Another treatment form that has been found to be beneficial is Brief Behavioral therapy, which is an alternative, but simplified version of Cognitive Behavioral therapy. When using brief behavioral therapy, one of the most important actions is to adhere to the steps that must be followed, otherwise it can impact the effectiveness of this form of therapy. Those suffering from insomnia must who are using brief behavioral therapy as treatment would potentially have toad adhere to "not going to bed at night without sleeping, getting up early in the morning, not going to bed during the day, not staying in bed at night after attempting to sleep for 30 minutes, and not doing anything unrelated to sleep or having sex (especially using cell phone and thinking)" (Zheng et al., 2021).

The most common form of treatment for insomnia that is known to a vast majority of society is the use of sleeping aids such as sleeping pills or melatonin; however, the use of any form of medication for treatment of a mental health disorder can be referred to as psychopharmacology. The range of medical treatments for insomnia include sedative medication, hypnotic drugs, antidepressants, antipsychotics and herbal remedies. The biggest factor in ensuring the effectiveness of psychopharmacology, is to have actual knowledge behind medication usage and be actively monitored by a mental health professional. Though psychopharmacology has been identified as a beneficial form of treatment for insomnia, research suggests that it is more effective when combined with Cognitive behavioral therapy.

Though insomnia has the ability to impair daytime functioning and decrease an individual's quality of life, there are effective approaches to treatment that have helped to alleviate symptoms and improve life quality. Some of the treatment types that have been found to be effective include Cognitive behavioral therapy, sleep hygiene education, Sleep restriction therapy, Mindfulness-based therapy, Bright light exposure therapy, Brief behavioral therapy, and the combination of both psychotherapy and medication, which can be referred to as psychopharmacology. Though there are a plethora of approaches to treating insomnia, each type of treatment has different variables that can cause limitations on its effectiveness. Multiple empirical studies have suggested that Cognitive behavioral therapy is the most effective treatment for combating insomnia.

Limitations and Future Research

One of the first limitations that comes to mind when referencing research into insomnia is that there could be cultural factors that discourage the treatment of mental health disorders. Within the African American community, it is common for an individual not to seek services for mental health disorders due to the stigma that is associated with having an official diagnosis. Additionally, in the African American community, some may not even identify insomnia as being a disorder or an impactful issue, though insomnia has the actual ability to affect daytime functioning, as well as mood, ability to focus, productivity, and many other aspects of a person's quality of life. Not only do cultural views on mental health play a role, but also views on receiving assistance due to the typical mistreatment of African American in the health system. It can be argued that with being provided more knowledge and resources, African Americans' views on seeking assistance for mental health issues, such as insomnia, could potentially be altered.

Another possible limitation that could arise when treating insomnia using medication, is the potential risk of overuse. Being that not all sleeping aids require a prescription and can be purchased over the counter, it leaves room for the possible abuse of sleeping medication. Research has found that though sleeping aids are effective for treating insomnia, "these drugs are widely prescribed at the symptomatic level, resulting in potential overuse" (Lader, 1999). Short-term use of sleeping medication that is being monitored and managed by a health professional can help to decrease the likelihood of developing an addiction. The long-term use of sleeping can be harmful as, "the risk/benefit ratio of these drugs becomes less favorable or even adverse as treatment becomes prolonged: efficacy wanes and risks accumulate" (Lader, 1999).

There is no identifiable "cause" for this type of sleeping disturbance. Researchers have yet to find an actual cause for insomnia and its prevalence, though research is still developing on this topic. Because there is no cause that has been directly linked to insomnia, it is difficult to create appropriate preventative measures, being that there is no specific "thing" that must be prevented. There are certain risk factors that have been labeled as making a person more susceptible to experiencing insomnia; however, there is still limited research on this topic. With learning the causes of insomnia, interventions can be applied early to limit the number of symptoms an individual experiences. In time, it is possible that the true cause for insomnia can be identified and explained.

There are still many unanswered questions when it comes to insomnia, how it functions, as well as effective ways to treat the sleeping disorder. Though the information that we have for insomnia is present and accurate, it is still being developed each day. Future research should focus on the cause of insomnia, being that there is no identifiable cause. Additionally, as more studies are done over insomnia, there should be a deeper look into the effectiveness of Cognitive behavioral therapy in comparison to other forms of treatment, being that it has been found to be the most effective out of a variety of other forms of treatment, including the use of medication. Lastly, researchers should try to identify factors that make a person more susceptible to developing an addiction to sleeping medication, so preventative measures can be taken for those who are more likely to abuse sleeping medications.

CONCLUSION

Insomnia can be described as a sleep disturbance that impairs daytime functioning and quality of life. When experiencing insomnia, a person will have difficulty falling asleep, staying asleep, as well as inability to function at a full capacity due to lack of restorative sleep. Insomnia has the ability to seep into various aspects of our lives through the range of impacts that can occur due to insomnia. Looking through the lens of the African American experience, insomnia can at times not be identified as an actual mental health issue, nor are they acknowledged. Due to the general views that African Americans have about mental health, it contributes to why this is a detrimental issue for those in the community. If the current views that African Americans have on mental health are reframed and more knowledge is provided, as well as access to resources, it could encourage members of the community to seek treatment.

Impacts of insomnia for those in the African American community include a possible change in mood, which affects a person socially, as it could impact their ability to develop and maintain relationships with others. Additionally, other impacts include focus control, as well as a decrease in productivity, which can affect a person's job performance or academic performance. Lasty, due to lack of restorative sleep, insomnia can also produce distorted thinking patterns, which can lead to the development of other mental health disorders. Also, specific factors that make an individual more susceptible to experiencing insomnia were discussed. Factors discussed include the presence of comorbidities and other mental health disorders, a poor quality of life as well as an increased amount of life stressors. When risk factors are discovered, a person can navigate these factors to try to decrease the chances of experiencing insomnia.

Different approaches to treatment for insomnia that have been found to be effective were discussed. The most effective treatment approach identified was the use of Cognitive behavioral therapy (CBT). CBT examines the link between thoughts, emotions, and behaviors, and because of this, it teaches an individual how to restructure cognitive functioning, as well as reframe negative irrational thoughts. Though CBT has been identified as the most effective form of treatment, various other approaches have been adopted as well including the use of sleep hygiene education, sleep restriction therapy, mindfulness-based therapy, bright light exposure therapy, brief behavioral therapy and the use of mediation. All treatments have been deemed effective; however, there are certain variables that dictate the level of effectiveness. Though there is a plethora of research regarding insomnia, there are still current limitations to treatment. With future research these limitations should be addressed and resolved to ensure effectiveness.

REFERENCES

Cardoso, A., Almeida, T. C., Ramos, C., Sousa, S., & Brito, J. (2021). Bidirectional relationship between perceived stress and insomnia symptoms: The role of coping and quality of life. *Sleep and Biological Rhythms*, *19*(1), 23–31. doi:10.100741105-020-00284-8

Dean. (2016). Anxiety. *Nursing Standard*, *30*(46), 15–15. doi:10.7748/ns.30.46.15.s17

Dolan, T., Taylor, D. J., Bramoweth, A. D., & Rosenthal, L. D. (2010). Cognitive–behavioral therapy of insomnia: A clinical case series study of patients with co-morbid disorders and using hypnotic medications. *Behaviour Research and Therapy*, *48*(4), 321–327. doi:10.1016/j.brat.2009.12.004 PMID:20074701

Espie, P., Pawlecki, B., Waterfield, D., Fitton, K., Radocchia, M., & Luik, A. I. (2018). Insomnia symptoms and their association with workplace productivity: Cross-sectional and pre-post intervention analyses from a large multinational manufacturing company. *Sleep Health*, *4*(3), 307–312. doi:10.1016/j.sleh.2018.03.003 PMID:29776626

Hazlett-Stevens, H., & Craske, M. (2002). *Brief Cognitive-Behavioral Therapy: Definition and Scientific Foundations*. John Wiley & Sons Ltd.

Kyle, M., Miller, C. B., Rogers, Z., Siriwardena, A. N., MacMahon, K. M., & Espie, C. A. (2014). Sleep restriction therapy for insomnia is associated with reduced objective total sleep time, increased daytime somnolence, and objectively impaired vigilance: Implications for the clinical management of insomnia disorder. *Sleep*, *37*(2), 229–237. doi:10.5665leep.3386 PMID:24497651

Lader. (1999). Limitations on the use of benzodiazepines in anxiety and insomnia: are they justified? *European Neuropsychopharmacology*, *9*, S399–S405. doi:10.1016/S0924-977X(99)00051-6

LeBlanc, M., Mérette, C., Savard, J., Ivers, H., Baillargeon, L., & Morin, C. M.LEBLANC. (2009). Incidence and Risk Factors of Insomnia in a Population-Based Sample. *Sleep*, *32*(8), 1027–1037. doi:10.1093leep/32.8.1027 PMID:19725254

Lee, K., Kwon, Y.-J., Lee, K., Lim, E., Jang, S.-H., & Sohn, I.-K. (2022). Psychological Characteristics of Community People with Insomnia Focused on : Attention deficit hyperactivity symptoms, Depression, Anxiety and Mood Disorder. *Sleep Medicine*, *100*, S134–S135. doi:10.1016/j.sleep.2022.05.368

Liao, Z., Zhu, S., & Li, X. (2018). Anxiety and depression in paradoxical insomnia: A case-control study. *Neuropsychiatric Disease and Treatment, 14*, 231–238. doi:10.2147/NDT.S156058 PMID:29386896

Malhi, & Mann, J. J. (2018). Depression. *The Lancet (British Edition), 392*(10161), 2299–. https://doi.org/ doi:10.1016/S0140-6736(18)31948

Mao, J., Ji, Y., Xu, Y., Tang, G., Yu, Z., Xu, L., Shen, C., & Wang, W. (2017). Group cognitive-behavioral therapy in insomnia: A cross-sectional case-controlled study. *Neuropsychiatric Disease and Treatment, 13*, 2841–2848. doi:10.2147/NDT.S149610 PMID:29200858

Ong, & Sholtes, D. (2010). A mindfulness-based approach to the treatment of insomnia. *Journal of Clinical Psychology, 66*(11), 1175–1184. doi:10.1002/jclp.20736

Perlis, P. D., Riemann, D., Bastien, C. H., Teel, J., & Thase, M. (2022). Insomnia. The Lancet (British Edition), 400(10357), 1047–1060. doi:10.1016/S0140-6736(22)00879-0

Rezaie, Vakili-Amini, Y. Y., Paschall, E. E., & Khazaie, H. H. (2020). Personality profiles in paradoxical insomnia: a case-control study. *Sleep Science (São Paulo, SP), 13*(4), 242–248. https://doi.org/ doi:10.5935/1984-0063.20190148

Riedel, B. W. (2000). Sleep hygiene. In K. L. Lichstein & C. M. Morin (Eds.), *Treatment of Late-life Insomnia* (pp. 125–146). Sage. doi:10.4135/9781452225555.n5

Sandlund, H., Hetta, J., Nilsson, G., Ekstedt, M., & Westman, J. (2017). Group treatment for insomnia and impact on daytime symptomatology associated with insomnia: Analyses from a randomized controlled trial in primary care. *Sleep Medicine, 40*, e291–e292. doi:10.1016/j.sleep.2017.11.856

Stansbury, P., Peterson, T. L., & Beecher, B. (2013). An exploration of mental health literacy among older African Americans. *Aging & Mental Health, 17*(2), 226–232. doi:10.1080/13607863.2012.724652 PMID:23067011

Stokes, P., Bell, K., & Mellman, T. A. (2022). Strategies for Controlling Unwanted Intrusive Thoughts and Insomnia Severity in Urban-Residing Young Adult African Americans. *Behavioral Sleep Medicine, ahead-of-print*(ahead-of-print), 1–8. doi:10.1080/15402002.2022.2057986

van Maanen, M., Meijer, A. M., van der Heijden, K. B., & Oort, F. J. (2016). The effects of light therapy on sleep problems: A systematic review and meta-analysis. *Sleep Medicine Reviews, 29*, 52–62. doi:10.1016/j.smrv.2015.08.009 PMID:26606319

Williams, Perlis, M., Castor, C., Barnes, A., Chung, A., Kalinowski, J., Roseus, J., Rogers, A., & Jean-Louis, G. (2018). 0193 An Exploratory, Descriptive Study Of African American's Experiences Of Insomnia Symptoms And Treatment. *Sleep (New York, N.Y.), 41*(suppl_1), A75–A76. doi:10.1093/sleep/zsy061.192

Zheng, Q., Qin, Y., Lyu, Y., Li, L., Chen, Y., & Yao, Z. (2021). Community promotion and application of Wuqinxi combined with brief behavioral therapy for insomnia: A study protocol. *Medicine, 100*(49), e28046–e28046. doi:10.1097/MD.0000000000028046 PMID:34889248

Chapter 4
Eating Disorders Among African-Americans

Marcella Smith
Texas A&M University, Commerce, USA

ABSTRACT

Eating disorders affects 20 million women and 10 million men in the United States at some point in their lives. The purpose of this chapter was to explore eating disorders among African Americans. Historically, eating disorders were perceived to be prevalent in European American females from upper socio-economic status. However, there is mounting evidence that eating disorders are no longer limited to the European American population; in recent years, several community surveys have revealed the prevalence of eating disorders among ethnic minorities in Western nations. It is critical that clinicians take a holistic approach and seek to comprehend the entire experiences of African American clients, which involves not only their physical health but also their emotional lives and the numerous ways in which racism, discrimination, poverty, trauma, and adverse childhood experiences can lead to eating disorders. It is critical to understand the probable causes and symptoms of eating disorders in African American clients, so they do not suffer in silence.

INTRODUCTION

Eating disorders are severe mental illnesses that can result in life-threatening consequences (Almenara, 2022; Hambleton et al., 2022; Ralph et al., 2022). "Eating disorders are mental disorders characterized by continuous disturbance in eating behavior" (Almenara, 2022, p.1). The most frequent eating disorders include "binge-eating, other specified feeding or eating disorder (OSFED), anorexia nervosa (AN)

DOI: 10.4018/978-1-6684-8918-5.ch004

and bulimia nervosa (BN) which are common in individuals with different body types (Ralph et al., 2022; Sinha & Warfa, 2013). Anorexia nervosa mortality rates are the highest of all mental disorders (Kazdin et al., 2017). Binge-eating disorder can be recurring and is a sincere concern. Binge-eating disorder is described as frequently eating more food than one would eat followed by a feeling of loss of control (Franko et al. 2012; Goode et al., 2019; Scott et al., 2019). Binge-eating disorder is related to binge-eating, emotional eating, and over-eating (Assari, 2018). The clinical criteria for binge-eating disorder involves recurrent binge-eating weekly for at least three months without purging and there is noticeable discomfort due to the binge-eating behavior (American Psychiatric Association, 2013; Udo et al., 2016). These characteristics must occur along with at least three related symptoms such as eating too fast, eating a lot when not hungry, eating past the point of feeling comfortably full, and eating alone due to shame and discomfort after eating too much (American Psychiatric Association, 2013).

PREVALENCE

Eating disorders affect 20 million women (about the population of New York) and 10 million men (about half the population of New York) in the United States at some point in their lives. Anorexia affects 0.5 to 3.5 percent of all women, bulimia affects 1.1 to 4.2 percent of all women, and other specified feeding or eating disorder affects 2 to 5% of all women (Thompson, 2016). Furthermore, eating disorders are the 12th leading disorder in young females from affluent countries (Kazdin et al., 2017). There is mounting evidence that eating disorders are no longer limited to the European American population; in recent years, several community surveys have revealed the prevalence of eating disorders among ethnic minorities in Western nations (Sinha & Warfa, 2013). Eating disorders affect people of all ages, genders, socioeconomic, and cultures (Hambleton et al., 2022). Binge-eating disorder is one of the most common eating disorders and is prevalent among different racial and ethnic groups (Franko et al., 2012; Goode et al., 2019). Binge-eating disorder affects 0.85 and 2.6% of the U.S. population (Kessler et al., 2013; Udo & Grilo, 2018).

Eating disorders have historically been thought to mostly afflict women. Indeed, women had greater lifetime, 12-month, and point prevalence of eating disorders than males. This finding, however, differs depending on the kind of eating disorder. Male patients are often thought to account for 10% of those with anorexia nervosa or bulimia nervosa (American Psychiatric Association, 2013). However, other studies indicate that approximately 25% of individuals with anorexia nervosa or bulimia nervosa are men and that men account for 36% of individuals with all typical binge-eating disorders (Galmiche et al., 2019). Eating disorders are already quite frequent as early as the teenage years, ranging from 6% to 8% in numerous studies. These findings are consistent with previous research indicating the early start of eating disorders, particularly anorexia nervosa and bulimia nervosa (Javaras et al., 2015; Micali et al., 2013). For instance, in recent research, 75% of individuals with anorexia nervosa developed it before the age of 22. Similarly, 83.3 percent of the participants had bulimia nervosa at an early age (before the age of 24) (Volpe et al., 2016). The onset of binge eating disorder (Kessler et al., 2013) is more spaced out over time and the risk of onset is consistent throughout adolescence compared with bulimia nervosa and anorexia nervosa (Galmiche et al., 2019).

The Effects of Eating Disorders

Eating disorders have some of the highest mortality rates of all mental health disorders and come with serious personal, interpersonal, social, and economic hardships (van Hoeken & Hoek, 2020; Weigel et al., 2019). People with eating disorders can suffer from other psychological, social, and functional challenges. Furthermore, they can also experience mental and medical comorbidities (Hambleton et al., 2022; Jahraus, 2018; Udo & Grilo, 2019). Moreover, binge-eating disorder is linked to various somatic and psychiatric coexisting conditions such as obesity, substance abuse, and mood disorders (American Psychiatric Association, 2013; Franko et al. 2012; Thornton et al., 2017; Welch et al., 2016) and diminished quality of life, and high death rates (Kazdin et al., 2017). Research shows that 55-95% of individuals with eating disorders also have some sort of psychiatric comorbidities at some point. Eating disorder mortality rates are remarkably greater than the general population with the highest rates in anorexia nervosa because of how it affects the cardiovascular system and suicide (Hambleton et al., 2022).

Mortality rates are high in bulimia nervosa and other specified feeding and eating disorders. Suicide rates are heightened over the eating disorder scale with higher rates in people with some form of comorbid psychiatric disorder (Mayes et al. 2014; Smith et al., 2018). Approximately 75% of individuals with eating disorders are not obtaining treatment, as a result of comorbidities, which may affect motivation and the capacity to make appointments (Hambleton et al., 2022). Medical comorbidities occurring with eating disorders can be mild to severe and potentially fatal (Jahraus, 2018). Thus, understanding how co-occurring medical comorbidities and difficulties affect eating disorders is crucial to therapy and rehabilitation. Comorbidities might emerge before or after the beginning of the eating disorder, or they can be caused by symptoms and behaviors associated with the eating disorder (Van Alsten & Duncan, 2020). This is exacerbated further by the fact that eating disorders and comorbidities may have a reciprocal connection in which the existence of one influences the pathophysiology, treatment, and results of the other (Hambleton et al., 2022).

THE IMPACT OF MENTAL HEALTH ON AFRICAN AMERICANS

Historically, eating disorders were perceived to be prevalent in European American females from upper socio-economic status (Kroon Van Diest et al., 2014; Ross, 2019). However, research suggests that African American and ethnic minority females in the United States experience eating disorders as well (Kroon Van Diest et al., 2014; Lydecker & Grilo, 2016; Udo et al., 2016). According to Scott et al. (2019), national studies found equivalent rates of binge-eating disorder in African American and European American participants. Similarly, Crow's (2014) study found that binge-eating disorder was the most common eating disorder among both African American and Caribbean Black participants and bulimia nervosa was the second most common. In North America, an increasingly diversified picture of eating disorders is emerging. In recent years, the demographics of people who appear with eating disorders have changed both globally and within Western, high-income countries, where eating disorders were initially diagnosed. Recent data suggests that ethnic and racial minority groups in the United States are more likely to experience eating disorders than other groups, and that the prevalence of clinical eating disorders among these populations is rising (Pike et al. 2014).

Body Image

The prevalence of eating disorders in African American women is much higher than in African American men. In addition, the importance of values connected to body image is another sociocultural aspect in understanding and treating binge-eating disorders in African American women. African American women with binge-eating disorder may be more accepting of a bigger, full-figured physical frame, which can be associated with binge-eating. As a result, binge-eating disorder may be an acceptable or preferred coping mechanism among African American women, as the related bigger frame is neither unpleasant nor a barrier to binge-eating. According to these findings, therapy should include a discussion of alternate coping techniques. Similarly, AfricanAmerican women may regard a bigger physical frame as a representation of strength and power to counteract weakness and anguish. The media and African American popular culture are dominated by bigger-sized women, which encourages both the tolerance of greater size and the corresponding ideas of strength. Furthermore, some African American women may overeat on purpose to achieve the culturally desirable, bigger, and curvier frame. Additionally, for African American women, hair and skin tone may take precedence over typical body image issues associated with European American women (Awad et al., 2015; Scott et al., 2019). African American females are often presumed to be less affected by body dissatisfaction based on the assumption that African American culture is more accepting of larger or curvier body types compared to the dominant culture (Ross, 2019).

Although some reports indicate that anorexia nervosa is not as common in African American females compared to European American females; African American females engage in more frequent binge-eating compared to European females (Ross, 2019). A 2011 study found similar rates of eating disorders among Latino, African American, and European American groups. Furthermore, this study revealed that rates of bulimia nervosa may be much greater among Latinos and African Americans than among European Americans, particularly among men. What is interesting is that binge-eating did not vary between the groups (Pike et al., 2014). On the contrary, African American women with clinically significant binge-eating disorders reported more binge-eating episodes than their European American counterparts, with African American females having two more episodes per week (Scott et al., 2019). Anorexia nervosa prevalence is steady in North America and Western Europe; however, bulimia nervosa prevalence may be rising among African American and Latina populations in North America while declining among European Americans (Pike et al., 2014). Because women are more likely than males to suffer from eating disorders, feminist researchers have claimed that the human body is a mirror of society and that eating disorders are a symptom of inequality and gendered norms (Flowers et al. 2012).

Additionally, African American females who acquire African American cultural beliefs and conventions related to eating habits and body type could also be at risk for obesity. African American females, on the other hand, maybe more likely to engage in greater dieting habits and feel dissatisfied with their bodies if they have been raised to follow European American cultural standards on thinness (Talleyrand, 2011). African Americans, in general, have fewer issues with body dissatisfaction, dieting, and dietary restraint compared to European Americans but have similar rates of binge-eating and bulimia (Kroon Van Diest et al., 2014). Compared to European American females, African American females may be less likely to engage in extreme dieting behaviors or feel dissatisfied with their bodies, but they may be more likely to adopt poor eating habits that can result in obesity and obesity-related health issues, such as diabetes. A survey of European American and African American adolescents showed that African American females were more likely to be overweight and exhibit behaviors (such as bingeing) that are indicative of weight gain compared to European American females. For African American females, this risk may be associated with the fact that larger body types are accepted in African American culture and that there may not be social demands to be thin (Talleyrand, 2011).

Emotional Responses

Depression, anxiety, and worry are the most common emotional responses among families impacted by eating disorders (Karlstad et al., 2022). Depression is related to more serious symptoms of binge-eating in African American females such as recurrent binge-eating and almost one fourth of African American females with depression may engage in some type of binge- eating. This puts African American females at a higher risk of becoming obese (Scott, et al., 2019). African American females have greater levels of depression compared to European American females. Ross (2019) study of depression and coping behaviors in African American and European American women found that women who experienced greater rates of depression were more likely to experience some form of eating disorder. In addition, females with reoccurring binge-eating had high rates of psychological distress (Ross, 2019). An African American participant, Lisa, reported problematic eating practices to handle stress. She and some of her female peers would binge eat together. She characterized her group of friends as accomplished African American women who utilized eating to relax. She indicated,

I eat to manage emotions and to cope, definitely. It calms me, you know? Have a hard day at work? Grab a bag of chips or ice cream. . . . My friends and I would totally pig out and just eat like crazy foods and then get a dessert or whatever and then we would be like oh well. We referred to our sessions as confessions of fat women.... (Godbolt et al., 2022, p. 624)

Although many women cope with stress by eating, the forms of eating disorders differ by race, with European American women being more likely to suffer from anorexia and bulimia and African American women suffering from binge-eating disorders (Lydecker & Grilo, 2016). Questionable eating behaviors may occur as a way of coping with stress and stress may cause existing eating disorders to get worse (Ross, 2019). Godbolt et al. (2022) found more than 50% of the African American females admitted to using disordered eating behaviors including binge- eating as a coping technique to deal with the stresses of daily living. One participant highlighted a healthy coping strategy like "going to the gym with a friend to relieve stress" (p. 623) but she also highlighted the difficulties in deciding on whether to exercise or eat "a tray of cupcakes" (p. 623). Other participants were aware of their overeating in reaction to daily stress and reported that their self-esteem, stress, and overall mental health suffered as they felt they were losing control. One of the participants, Mia stated,

I overeat because of stress but I don't know if I consider it binge-eating. I don't eat a half a gallon of ice cream. Instead, I eat more than I know that it takes to be full. Instead of eating 2 or 3 slices of pizza, I might eat 4 or 5. Recently I have eaten until I was sick afterwards.... (Godbolt et al., 2022, p. 623)

African American females are more likely than European American females to be at risk of poverty, which is a common cause of stress. Binge-eating disorders (also known as disorganized eating) are characterized by frequent periods of disorderly eating behaviors that result in more food consumed in a brief period (American Psychiatric Association, 2013). Researchers predicted that African American women may use binge-eating as a poor coping technique to deal with stress caused by racism, sexism, stereotyped expectations of Black women, and/or other traumatic events (Talleyrand, Gordon, Daquin & Johnson, 2017). Thus, African American women who use binge-eating as a way of dealing with stress may inadvertently increase their risk of obesity and other unfavorable health effects (Godbolt et al., 2022). There is little research on binge-eating in African American women as a response to stress, racism, and sexism (Sbrocco et al., 2012). African American women who feel obligated to demonstrate strength are also more likely to consume food to cope with stress and to be overweight (Godbolt et al., 2022).

Indeed, stress perceptions are linked to increased binge-eating, hunger, and attempts to limit and regulate eating (Groesz et al., 2012). Specific forms of stress combined with food as a coping method may be causing binge-eating and binge-eating disorders. According to studies, there is a relationship between stress, specific types of coping, increased hunger, the temptation to eat, and binge-eating disorder among African American women (Groesz et al., 2012; Sulkowski et al., 2011; Scott et al., 2019). One participant, Bianca, disclosed that her response to emotional stress often drove her to binge-eating:

It's difficult being a Black woman, especially on this campus. I remember before one episode, I got so upset when one of my White classmates gave me a look of disgust and rolled her eyes at me. I didn't want to say something because then people would think I am just that big Black girl. So, I went to my room, cried, and ate pizza. (Godbolt et al., 2020, p. 625)

In addition, African American women who are better able to understand and express their feelings, a critical coping skill, have less problematic eating patterns (Watson et al., 2013). As a result, stress and unpleasant life experiences encountered because of common sociocultural group status, as well as cultural ideas and values, may have a role in understanding and treating binge-eating disorder among African American women (Scott et al., 2019).

Trauma

Eating disorders often begin as an attempt to address underlying issues. For example, binge-eating has been discovered to be a coping technique for the impacts of trauma (Lewis et al., 2013; Sutherland, 2013). Trauma and distress are linked to an increased risk of binge-eating disorder and a worsening of symptoms in African American women (Adamus-Leach et al., 2013; Wilson et al., 2012). When compared to European American women, African American women with binge-eating disorders indicate much greater rates of trauma exposure. PTSD is also frequent among African American women with binge-eating disorder and is linked to more severe binge-eating disorder symptoms (Grilo et al., 2012; Scott et al., 2019). Eating disorders such as anorexia, bulimia, compulsive overeating, and dieting are frequent across a wide range of women, owing to their origins as logical "survival tactics" that utilize food to cope with oppression, trauma, and poverty (Godbolt et al., 2022).

Ross (2019) discussed a participant's personal battle with emotional eating. The participant claimed that a split with her first boyfriend sparked recollections of her past sexual assault trauma. This resulted in excessive yo-yo dieting, which eventually led to anorexia and bulimia. She starved herself for weeks during her anorexic stage. During her bulimic period, after overeating, the participant used laxatives and exercise to try to reduce the calories. She kept her struggle hidden for years. Even though the previous experience is consistent with research demonstrating that binge-eating, or emotional overeating is frequently used to cope with challenging feelings produced by prior trauma, clinicians seldom presume that eating disorders affect African American women. Furthermore, there are various other issues that influence African American females in terms of trauma and coping that are often neglected or ignored yet have a significant impact on their health (Ross, 2019). Common ideals among African American women, such as the "strong Black woman" and the need to always display outward strength, may guide coping methods for stress and trauma. Internalization of the ideal of the "strong Black woman" has been found to moderate the association between trauma exposure and binge-eating by impacting both emotional control and eating for psychological reasons (Scott et al. 2019).

Obesity

Historically, eating disorders have been known as disorders affecting individuals who are underweight. However, research shows that this is not so (Ralph et al., 2022). Eating disorders prevalence is growing especially in individuals with higher weight (Ralph et al., 2022). Obesity is related to binge-eating disorder and may be the consequence of relentless binge-eating (Assari, 2018; Franko et al., 2012). Obesity and binge-eating research has repeatedly shown that food has been utilized as a harmful coping method for individuals of all races. Few research has looked at binge-eating among African American women and how it relates to addressing the repercussions of social inequity, which leads to racism and sexism (Godbolt et al., 2022; Mowatt et al., 2013). About 50-80% of African American females with binge-eating disorders are obese in comparison to 30-50% European American females. This is important, obese females have a higher risk for various health issues such as high blood pressure, heart disease, stroke, Type 2 diabetes, certain cancers, respiratory dysfunction, osteoarthritis, infertility, liver disease, and gallbladder disease (Scott et al., 2019). Moreover, obese African American females with binge-eating disorder have similar rates as Latina females and higher rates than European American females experiencing coexisting psychiatric issues (Grilo et al., 2013).

Although binge-eating disorder is more common among African Americans, they are less likely to be diagnosed with eating disorders and more likely to be advised about obesity related to overeating. Obesity is a significant health risk for health issues including diabetes, heart disease, and hypertension in African Americans. Obesity is often reported as the presenting cause of depression, another significant health issue among African Americans. Research suggests that obesity is more prevalent in minority females than in European American females and is increasing among African Americans and Hispanics (Franko et al., 2012). Obesity is more prevalent in African American women than any other race. African Americans are at a 50% increased risk of obesity compared to European Americans. The risk for African American women is 80% with four of five being overweight or obese (Assari, 2018). Compared with European American females, current research shows comparable or higher rates of binge-eating in African American females (Lydecker & Grilo, 2016; Udo et al., 2016). One study found that the prevalence of binge-eating in African American females was almost 5% compared to 2.5% in European American females. More than 30% of females with obesity also reported binge-eating (Goode et al., 2019).

Some studies suggest that binge-eating disorder is more prevalent in females compared to males and binge-eating disorder is a more noticeable cause of obesity for females than males. Moreover, binge-eating disorder is related to obesity in African American females of low socioeconomic status (Assari, 2018). African American females report higher rates of binge incidents and higher frequency of co-existing mood disorders than European American females. Approximately 23% of African American females engage in some type of binge-eating. Binge-eating disorders can have serious effects on the health and well-being of African American females. Binge-eating disorders and obesity are co-occurring conditions, especially for African American females (Scott et al., 2019). Binge-eating disorders in African American females is also related to psychological issues. Approximately 50% of African American females with binge-eating disorders also fit the criteria of coexisting mood disorder, with major depression, social phobia, and dysthymia as the most reported. Furthermore, more than 80% of African American females with binge-eating disorders have mood disorders during their lifetime (Scott, 2019).

Sociocultural Factors

Eating habits in African American women are also impacted by eating behaviors in the context of social activities, as well as the experience of both good and negative emotions, such as eating for both celebrations and sorrow. Moreover, eating may be regarded as a spiritual experience with deep significance. African American members indicate that the process of preparing and sharing food is holy, and that the technique of cooking and seasoning food follows cultural standards and honors African American cultural traditions. As a result, any intervention aiming to target eating behaviors and practices must recognize the importance of eating in this culture (Scott et al., 2019). African American females may be at risk for eating disorders due to sociocultural variables in addition to more conventional risk factors. Sociocultural factors that go beyond the typical risk factors for eating disorders appear to be risk factors for African American females. That is, acculturation, racism, and socioeconomic status (SES) may influence the causes of, and the way African American females display certain eating attitudes and practices. Due to their SES, African American females may have little access to healthy food options, making them more likely to engage in unhealthy, weight-gaining eating habits (Talleyrand, 2011). Furthermore, eating habits among African Americans are impacted by their social environment, which includes romantic partners and children. Addressing linkages between sociocultural variables and food may improve binge-eating disorder treatments. These societal effects are certainly crucial factors to examine when studying binge-eating in African American women (Scott et al., 2019). Kelly et al. (2018) is one of the few studies to directly examine the link between discrimination and eating disorders. Research suggested that the reported discrimination after the 2016 U.S. election was related to higher loss of control eating frequency among African American men. Researchers should continue to identify how discrimination and oppression may increase the risk of eating disorders in African Americans. Clinicians should be conscious that discrimination might intensify eating disorders. Munn-Chernoff et al. (2015) investigated whether genetic and environmental effects on eating disorders varied among African American and European American women in the U.S. The findings revealed that the overall genetic and environmental impacts on eating disorders were similar across races (with the stipulation that the most significant environmental influences may change depending on race) (Munn-Chernoff et al., 2015).

AFRICAN AMERICANS VIEWS ON MENTAL HEALTH

Participants discussed mental health in terms of perception: ''if you think you have problems, then you have problems, if you think you don't, then you don't" (Samuel, 2015, p. 36). In Ward et al. (2013) study, participants were hesitant to admit to having psychological issues, and were worried about the stigma attached to mental health disorders but were willing to seek mental health care. Older African Americans exhibit a variety of mental health information-seeking behaviors. Research shows that African American elders consider doctors and preachers as the main sources of mental health information (Stanbury et al., 2013). African American women also have different feelings and beliefs about binge-eating. Specifically, when compared to European American women, African American women with binge-eating disorders exhibit less anxiety about their weight and form, less dietary control, and less overall concern about their binge-eating episodes. Although there is discomfort, it is lesser in African American females than in European American females (Scott et al., 2019). Many of these young people appeared to view mental health issues as insignificant or unworthy of much attention and many appeared to believe that they were immune to such problems. (Samuel, 2015).

Spirituality and Religion

According to one survey, nearly 40% of African Americans believe clergy to be their main source of support when depressed. Clergy members are respected members of the community who speak for their religious institutions, sharing institutional and denominational perspectives on mental illness (Campbell, 2021). Campbell & Winchester (2020), found that most participants thought that churches, including their own, were ready to recognize and respond to the mental health needs of African American and Christian communities. The church's capacity to recognize and resolve the lack of mental health services in African American communities, where members experience higher rates of mental health issues, was stressed the greatest. Many African Americans avoid standard mental health services because they think the physicians are untrustworthy or cannot relate to them. In the past, the Black Church served as a refuge for African Americans and met a range of needs in the neighborhood. Most participants thought that the church could build on these assets and traditions to get above the social and cultural constraints that conventional practitioners face. Respondents predicted that more people would seek out programs that could heal and restore individuals, families, and communities as the Black Church delivers services in a more culturally sensitive manner and offers a secure, trusted space for community members (Campbell & Winchester, 2020). The majority of the African American clergy respondents talked about how the Black community had different perspectives on mental health (Campbell, 2021). Diverse cultural perspectives, attitudes, or experiences are feeding binge-eating disorders and associated behaviors in African American women (Scott et al., 2019).

African Americans retain culture-specific ideas concerning mental health concerns. These include denials of mental health issues, which are frequently cloaked in myths or folklore, and the use of religion and spiritual abilities to cope with mental health issues (Samuel, 2015). African Americans believed the church should be more engaged in promoting mental health and well-being, as well as assisting African American and Christian communities in understanding the significance of sustaining good mental health in total well-being and spiritual health. Because churches are considered the center of Black communities, the significance they place on issues has a significant impact on how seriously community members consider such concerns. If the church emphasizes mental health because of its capacity to speak the language of the community, then community members will prioritize it as well, transforming the narrative many Black Americans have about mental health in a more positive, healthy, and healing manner (Campbell & Winchester, 2020).

Stigma

There is already a tremendous taboo in the African American community when it comes to openly discussing mental health issues. Several more people spoke about the stigma related to mental illness, focusing on how prevalent it is in the African American community, particularly the church. One Reverend indicated, "In the Black community, there's not a lot of open discussion about mental health. It gets a bad rap" (Campbell, 2021, p. 6). Many participants held the opinion that environmental factors rather than internal factors are to blame for mental health disorders (Samuel, 2015). Most of the participants agreed that language that is disparaging or shameful, as well as code words for mental illness, are frequently used to convey stigma against mental health. The following remarks made by an African American female Pastor serve as a succinct summation of what many participants, particularly African Americans, suggested. "When I was younger, I could recall codes like "Oh, they're just special or she's just touched." (Campbell, 2021, p. 6). Samuel (2015) study found that most participants stated that the African American community is less accepting of persons with mental health problems than other groups, and that having mental health problems as a 'black person' in a 'black area' is more stigmatizing. One participant stated, ''For me, I don't tell anybody outside my family that I go to counseling. If I do, they would think I am nuts, like my head is not working right, or like I don't" (Samuel, 2015, p. 38). The most frequent causes of mental health issues according to participants were dysfunctional families, racism and discrimination, and the stress of residing in an underprivileged area. One participant said,

No black man in America has good mental health because of the stress of dealing with racism even in some place that you may think it was good place. Sometimes when they look at you and see your color, the rules begin to change. (Samuel 2015, p. 35)

WHY MOST AFRICAN AMERICANS AVOID MENTAL HEALTH TREATMENT

Mental illness stigma is a significant concern to public health and communities in the United States (Casados 2017; Parcesepe & Cabassa 2013), disproportionately affecting racial and ethnic minority populations (Misra et al., 2021). Stigma has several negative consequences for individuals with mental health issues, including evading treatment, remaining silent about one's mental health condition and withdrawing from others (Mayer et al., 2021), and only seeking spiritual interventions from religious leaders rather than mental health professionals (Campbell, 2021). Culture is a legitimate and important aspect to examine when considering the pattern of mental health help-seeking behaviors among African Americans. According to the findings, mental health stigma, poor treatment, peer fear and humiliation, and mistrust of mental health clinicians were significant obstacles to mental health care usage (Samuel, 2015). Goode et al. (2020), emphasize evidence indicating that African American women are much less likely than European American women to seek treatment for binge-eating disorder or an eating disorder, and are notably more likely to withdraw from clinical trials. The findings indicate that more effort is required to improve access to care and adapt treatment for African Americans suffering from binge-eating disorders. Goode et al. (2020), underline the importance of treatment outcome measures that have been validated in African American women, and purposeful examination of outcomes for African Americans to guarantee that treatments are equally effective for individuals of diverse backgrounds. Access to care for eating disorders is less common among African Americans compared to European Americans. Moreover, binge-eating and binge-eating disorders may be more serious in African American females who fail to seek care (Goode et al., 2019). There is a misconception that African American women are safe from eating disorders. However, eating disorders were originally conceived based on the underutilization of treatment for African American women of upper socioeconomic status (Harris, 2015). The literature indicated that many children, adolescents, and youth who meet the criteria for an eating disorder may not get these effective treatments for a variety of reasons including limited treatment seeking behavior (Bohrer et al., 2017; Forrest et al., 2017; McLean et al., 2019), limited access to specialized care, and stigma associated with the illness and treatments. More specifically, a lack of provider training and a restricted capacity to deliver individual and family therapy to meet service demand contribute to limited access to specialized eating disorder treatment (Dufour, 2022). According to Samuel (2015), many individuals did not access mental health care due to the following culturally driven views: (1) Participants denied having any mental health issues. They refused to regard mental health issues on the same level as other curable ailments, and as a result, they saw no need for the treatment service provided and did not contemplate using it. (2) Participants stated that racism, discrimination, and other environmental stresses, such as living conditions in impoverished communities and unpleasant interpersonal connections, promote mental health issues. As a result, they proposed that rather than offering counseling services to individuals suffering from mental health problems, interventions aiming at alleviating human suffering caused by mental health problems should be focused on their fundamental causes—the environment (Samuel, 2015).

African American's have a distrust for healthcare practitioners. Several participants alluded to the Tuskegee Syphilis Study, a 1930s United States Public Health Service research study that unethically recruited African American males to follow the consequences of untreated syphilis. Furthermore, Reverend Shelby adds that some of the skepticism in the mental health system stems from African Americans' attitudes toward psychiatric drugs (Campbell, 2021). Stansbury et al. (2013) found that some participants were unaware of available mental health services, placing them at a higher risk of not receiving critical care. This finding underlines the need to educate African Americans about mental health treatment options (Stansbury et al., 2013). According to research on African Americans, mental health, and help-seeking, African Americans have a higher burden of untreated mental health disorders than any other ethnic group (Cook et al., 2014; Dempsey et al., 2016). African Americans are also less likely than other racial or ethnic groups to seek professional counseling services and instead rely on churches and religious leaders to address their mental health needs (Avent & Cashwell, 2015; Campbell & Winchester, 2020; Jackson, 2015).

African Americans frequently face numerous barriers to traditional counseling services, including a lack of diverse clinicians, stigma within the African American community regarding mental health issues, and the development of cultural mistrust of White society because of historical and current abuses (Avent & Cashwell, 2015; Dempsey et al., 2016; Hays, 2015). Church members may seek out the Black Church for their mental health problems due to a history of church assistance, free programs, and familiar and culturally comparable practitioners (Campbell & Winchester, 2020; Dempsey et al., 2016). Although therapy is recommended, many African American females with binge-eating disorders may not use these services. Moreover, less than 8% of African American females with binge-eating disorders seek treatment for eating disorders compared to more than 20% of European American females. According to research, the few African American women who do obtain treatment may differ dramatically from those who do not seek treatment. African American women who fit the binge-eating disorder criteria and receive therapy are more likely to have a higher BMI, greater dietary constraints, and more anxiety about their shape and eating than those who do not receive treatment. Furthermore, African American women who have undergone binge-eating disorder treatment had fewer pretreatment binge-eating episodes than African American women with binge-eating disorder who did not access care (Scott et al., 2019). Those who do not seek treatment, which is most African American women with binge-eating disorder, appear to have a higher disease burden than those who do. Even African American women with binge-eating disorder who seek treatment may benefit from customized therapies, since African American women are more than twice as likely as European American women to drop out of treatment (Thompson-Brenner et al., 2013).

Another reason for low treatment participation and poor treatment outcomes among African American women with binge-eating disorder might be a lack of treatments that address the specific life events, attitudes, beliefs, and preferences linked with binge-eating. For example, eating disorders among African American women may linked to repressive experiences such as racism, classism, poverty, or abuse (Scott et al., 2019). People of larger weight who have lived with an eating disorder report being misdiagnosed, disregarded by health professionals, and marginalized or excluded from eating disorder treatment options. Except for binge-eating disorder, this demographic is frequently overlooked in eating disorder studies (Ralph et al., 2022). Older African Americans, typically underutilize formal mental health treatments. Older African Americans frequently have favorable opinions regarding mental health services but are unaware of how to access mental health treatment. Even though older African Americans are less likely than European Americans to seek and participate in mental health care, African Americans' use of mental health services was shown to be connected to their belief in treatment effectiveness. As a result, the more African Americans believe in the efficacy of mental health treatments, the more likely they are to seek and participate in treatment. When they seek official mental health care, evidence indicates they prefer to meet with their doctor. Rather than using the official mental health system, older African Americans report using cultural coping mechanisms and contacting informal sources such as family, friends, and pastors to manage mental health concerns (Stansbury et al., 2013). Peer groups can be a double-edged sword. In one case, peers pushed participants to utilize mental health treatment services; in another, they mocked participants for using mental health services. Participants agreed that their social network had a key part in deciding whether to receive mental health services. Many family members encouraged some participants and discouraged others from using mental health care, according to the service usage model. (Samuel, 2015).

POSSIBLE TREATMENT OPTIONS FOR AFRICAN AMERICANS SUFFERING FROM EATING DISORDERS

There are various treatments for binge-eating and binge-eating disorders including behavioral weight loss (BWL), cognitive behavioral therapy (CBT), and interpersonal psychotherapy (IPT) (Goode et al., 2022). Furthermore, evidence-based therapies, such as family-based treatment (FBT) and cognitive behavioral therapy (CBT), have been shown to be effective in lowering ED symptoms and facilitating recovery in adolescents with eating disorders (Linardon et al., 2017; Stiles-Shields et al., 2012). The creation and assessment of evidence-based psychosocial therapies (EBPIs) for eating disorders and other mental health problems is a significant step forward (Kazdin et al., 2017). Typical interventions that focus on food, weight, or form distress as correlates of binge-eating disorder may be unsuitable or require other approaches when treating African American women (Scott et al., 2019).

Food addiction and eating disorders are primarily about emotions rather than food. African American women may develop cultural attitudes that increase their risk of emotional eating and make seeking and accepting treatment for the condition more challenging (Ross, 2019). They may use food to dull their feelings or to divert their attention away from challenges in their life. Repressed emotions, like a beach ball held underwater, might erupt with a fury, typically in another form, such as overeating. When it comes to recovering from eating disorders, integrative medicine has a lot to offer all women, particularly African American women. Binge-eating, emotional eating, anorexia and bulimia, and compulsive overeating all occur in the context of complex, interwoven circumstances; therefore, an integrated approach to therapy makes sense. When working with African American clients, it is critical to investigate their trauma history, as indicated in the Adverse Childhood Experiences research. A terrible history cannot be changed, but the client may adjust how they care for themselves considering their experiences. Similarly, they cannot alter their physique but can change the connection with it. Eating, unlike other compulsive activities, is not something that can be avoided. A new, healthy connection with eating must be created (Ross, 2019).

The Role of the Black Church

Black churches are geographically situated to provide mental health services to African Americans, removing structural impediments and other difficulties with accessibility that frequently hinder many African Americans from utilizing existing resources. Furthermore, because churches provide guidance on matters of a religious and spiritual nature, their settings are already conducive to quiet, personal dialogues (Campbell & Winchester, 2020). One may also assume that churches may not have as many difficulties in creating rapport or trust since they have frequently demonstrated their ability to recognize and handle the concerns of African American communities. They also have a better understanding of their communities' needs and the socio-cultural and historical aspects connected to those challenges. Because of this, they may be better equipped to provide a solution-oriented approach to the mental health concerns that African Americans frequently seek. Participants also commented extensively about the church being more active in efforts to reduce the stigma associated with mental health help-seeking and service use among African Americans in general and specifically African American Christians (Hankerson & Weissman, 2012; Neely-Fairbanks et al., 2018). According to Stansbury et al. (2013) older African Americans support intervention strategies that include family, friends, faith, exercise, doctors, and clergy. Participants viewed unofficial help as crucial for managing and recovering from mental health disorders. A rising amount of study has highlighted the critical significance of spirituality and African American clergy in African Americans' mental health help-seeking behavior (Stansbury et al., 2013). Churches could collaborate with established organizations, hire private practitioners, or rely on the ministerial work of licensed clinicians to provide a greater range of treatments at a wider price range (Campbell & Winchester, 2020).

CONCLUSION

Despite the seriousness of disordered eating symptoms and risk factors, research into racial disparities in eating disorder symptomatology has been sparse (Howard et al., 2019). In addition, despite increasing awareness of the importance of including people from diverse racial and ethnic backgrounds (Kazdin et al., 2017), African Americans, continue to be underrepresented in eating disorder research, intervention, and prevention efforts (Wiley, 2020). Research indicates that disadvantage (Becker et al., 2017, 2019; Coffino, Grilo, & Udo, 2020; Lydecker, & Grilo, 2019) and discrimination (Kelly et al., 2018; Kelly et al., 2020; Mason et al., 2017) are crucial factors associated with eating disorders. To understand and validate the experiences of African Americans with eating disorders, these socioeconomic determinants of health must be included in research, case conceptualization, and therapy. A clinician, for example, may want to talk with a client about how prejudice, discrimination, and institutional racism have affected their mood and eating habits. Clinicians can also help clients establish a positive racial/ethnic identity and coping strategies for dealing with racism as well as tools for participating in larger social justice and advocacy activities (French et al., 2020). In addition, recent multicultural guidelines for psychologists, social workers, and other healthcare practitioners (AAMFT, 2015; Clauss-Ehlers et al., 2019; NASW, 2015) encourage advocacy and systemic interventions that may address the underlying environmental causes of psychological distress. Wiley (2020) suggests that the eating disorder field investigates how systemic intervention might help to reduce eating disorders in diverse communities. There have been few publications on the possible link between discrimination and eating disorders, therefore, further research on the influence of discrimination and eating disorders among African Americans is important. The impacts of racism in the past and present, as well as the trauma connected with racism, may play a major part in the health of African American women. When addressing eating disorders in African American women, historical portrayals and the pain linked with racism must be recognized (Ross, 2019).

It is critical that clinicians take a holistic approach and seek to comprehend the entire experiences of African American clients, which involves not only their physical health but also their emotional lives and the numerous ways in which racism, discrimination, poverty, trauma, and adverse childhood experiences can lead to eating disorders. It is critical to understand the probable causes and symptoms of eating disorders in African American clients, so they do not suffer in silence (Ross, 2019). Culturally responsive care for eating disorders is important. It is also important to recognize the detrimental impact of stereotypes and stigma African Americans experience surrounding eating disorders. Professionals need to collaborate with African American communities to raise awareness of eating disorders and tackle stigma, especially the stereotype that eating disorders only affect European Americans. In addition, more research is necessary to characterize the therapeutic challenges faced by African American males. Cooperation between churches and mental health practitioners and organizations is important and religious leaders should place greater emphasis on the mental health and well-being of the church and community members (Campbell & Winchester, 2020).

REFERENCES

Adamus-Leach, H. J., Wilson, P. L., O'Connor, D. P., Rhode, P. C., Mama, S. K., & Lee, R. E. (2013). Depression, stress and body fat are associated with binge eating in a community sample of African American and Hispanic women. *Eating and Weight Disorders*, *18*(2), 221–227. doi:10.100740519-013-0021-3 PMID:23760851

Almenara, C. A. (2022). 40 years of research on eating disorders in domain-specific journals: Bibliometrics, network analysis, and topic modeling. *PLoS One*, *17*(12), 1–21. doi:10.1371/journal.pone.0278981 PMID:36520823

American Association for Marriage and Family Therapy (AAMFT). (2015). *Code of ethics*. AAMFT. https://www.aamft.org/Legal_Ethics/Code_of_Ethics.aspx

American Psychiatric Association. (2013). *Feeding and eating disorders. In Diagnostic and statistical manual of mental disorders (5th ed.)*. APA. https://doiorg.libproxy.lib.unc.edu/10.1176

Assari, S. (2018). Perceived discrimination and binge eating disorder; gender differences in African Americans. *Journal of Clinical Medicine*, *7*(5), 89. doi:10.3390/jcm7050089 PMID:29695062

Avent, J. R., & Cashwell, C. S. (2015). The Black Church: Theology and implications for counseling African Americans. *The Professional Counselor*, *5*(1), 81–90. doi:10.15241/jra.5.1.81

Awad, G. H., Norwood, C., Taylor, D. S., Martinez, M., McClain, S., Jones, B., Holman, A., & Chapman-Hilliard, C. (2015). Beauty and body image concerns among African American college women. *The Journal of Black Psychology*, *41*(6), 540–564. doi:10.1177/0095798414550864 PMID:26778866

Becker, C. B., Middlemass, K., Taylor, B., Johnson, C., & Gomez, F. (2017). Food insecurity and eating disorder pathology. *International Journal of Eating Disorders*, *50*(9), 1031–1040. doi:10.1002/eat.22735 PMID:28626944

Becker, C. B., Middlemass, K. M., Gomez, F., & Martinez-Abrego, A. (2019). Eating disorder pathology among individuals living with food insecurity: A replication study. *Clinical Psychological Science*, *7*(5), 1144–1158. doi:10.1177/2167702619851811

Bohrer, B. K., Carroll, I. A., Forbush, K. T., & Chen, P. Y. (2017). Treatment seeking for eating disorders: Results from a nationally representative study. *International Journal of Eating Disorders*, *50*(12), 1341–1349. doi:10.1002/eat.22785 PMID:28963793

Campbell, A. D. (2021). Clergy perceptions of mental illness and confronting stigma in congregations. *Religions*, *12*(12), 1–14. doi:10.3390/rel12121110

Campbell, R. D., & Winchester, M. R. (2020). How the Black church can address mental health with Black Americans. *Social Work & Christianity*, *47*(2), 105–122. doi:10.34043wc.v47i2.63

Casados, A. T. (2017). Reducing the Stigma of Mental Illness: Current Approaches and Future Directions. *Clinical Psychology: Science and Practice*, *24*(3), 306–323. doi:10.1111/cpsp.12206

Clauss-Ehlers, C. S., Chiriboga, D. A., Hunter, S. J., Roysircar, G., & Tummala-Narra, P. (2019). APA multicultural guidelines executive summary: Ecological approach to context, identity, and intersectionality. *The American Psychologist*, *74*(2), 232–244. doi:10.1037/amp0000382 PMID:30762387

Coffino, J. A., Grilo, C. M., & Udo, T. (2020). Childhood food neglect and adverse experiences associated with DSM-5 eating disorders in U.S. National Sample. *Journal of Psychiatric Research, 127*, 75–79. doi:10.1016/j.jpsychires.2020.05.011 PMID:32502721

Cook, B. L., Zuvekas, S. H., Carson, N., Ferris, G. F., Vesper, A., & McGuire, T. G. (2014). Assessing racial/ethnic disparities in treatment across episodes of mental health care. *Health Services Research, 49*(1), 206–229. doi:10.1111/1475-6773.12095 PMID:23855750

Dempsey, K., Butler, S. K., & Gaither, L. (2016). Black churches and mental health professionals: Can this collaboration work? *Journal of Black Studies, 47*(1), 73–87. https://www.jstor.org/stable/24572960. doi:10.1177/0021934715613588

Dufour, R., Novack, K., Picard, L., Chadi, N., & Booij, L. (2022). The use of technology in the treatment of youth with eating disorders: A scoping review. *Journal of Eating Disorders, 10*(1), 182. doi:10.118640337-022-00697-5 PMID:36434657

Flowers, K. C., Levesque, M. J., & Fischer, S. (2012). The relationship between maladaptive eating behaviors and racial identity among African American women in college. *The Journal of Black Psychology, 38*(3), 290–312. doi:10.1177/0095798411416459

Forrest, L. N., Smith, A. R., & Swanson, S. A. (2017). Characteristics of seeking treatment among U.S. adolescents with eating disorders. *International Journal of Eating Disorders, 50*(7), 826–833. doi:10.1002/eat.22702 PMID:28323350

Franko, D. L., Thompson, D. R., Forbush, K. T., Bryson, S. W., Crow, S. J., Gorin, A. A., & Wilson, G. T. (2012). Racial/Ethnic differences in adults in randomized clinical trials of binge eating disorder. *Journal of Consulting and Clinical Psychology, 80*(2), 186–195. doi:10.1037/a0026700 PMID:22201327

French, B. H., Lewis, J. A., Mosley, D. V., Adames, H. Y., Chavez-Dueñas, N. Y., Chen, G. A., & Neville, H. A. (2020). Toward a psychological framework of radical healing in communities of color. *The Counseling Psychologist, 48*(1), 14–46. doi:10.1177/0011000019843506

Galmiche, M., Déchelotte, P., Lambert, G., & Tavolacci, M. P. (2019). Prevalence of eating disorders over the 2000–2018 period: A systematic literature review. *The American Journal of Clinical Nutrition, 109*(5), 1402–1413. doi:10.1093/ajcn/nqy342 PMID:31051507

Godbolt, D., Opara, I., & Amutah-Onukagha, N. (2022). Strong Black women: Linking stereotypes, stress, and overeating among a sample of Black female college students. *Journal of Black Studies*, *53*(6), 609–634. doi:10.1177/00219347221087453 PMID:36710718

Goode, R. W., Cowell, M. M., Mazzeo, S. E., Cooper-Lewter, C., Forte, A., Olayia, O., & Bulik, C. M. (2019). Binge eating and binge-eating disorder in Black women: A systematic review. *International Journal of Eating Disorders*, *53*(4), 491–507. doi:10.1002/eat.23217 PMID:31922293

Grilo, C. M., White, M. A., Barnes, R. D., & Masheb, R. M. (2012). Posttraumatic stress disorder in women with binge eating disorder in primary care. *Journal of Psychiatric Practice*, *18*(6), 408–412. doi:10.1097/01.pra.0000422738.49377.5e PMID:23160245

Grilo, C. M., White, M. A., Barnes, R. D., & Masheb, R. M. (2013). Psychiatric disorder co- morbidity and correlates in an ethnically diverse sample of obese patients with binge eating disorder in primary care settings. *Comprehensive Psychiatry*, *54*(3), 209–216. doi:10.1016/j.comppsych.2012.07.012 PMID:22943959

Groesz, L. M., McCoy, S., Carl, J., Saslow, L., Stewart, J., Adler, N., Laraia, B., & Epel, E. (2012). What is eating you? Stress and the drive to eat. *Appetite*, *58*(2), 717–721. doi:10.1016/j.appet.2011.11.028 PMID:22166677

Hambleton, A., Pepin, G., Le, A., Maloney, D., Aouad, P., Barakat, S., Boakes, R., Brennan, L., Bryant, E., Byrne, S., Caldwell, B., Calvert, S., Carroll, B., Castle, D., Caterson, I., Chelius, B., Chiem, L., Clarke, S., Conti, J., & Maguire, S.National Eating Disorder Consortium. (2022). Psychiatric and medical comorbidities of eating disorders: Findings from a rapid review of the literature. *Journal of Eating Disorders*, *10*(132), 1–23. doi:10.118640337-022-00654-2 PMID:36064606

Hankerson, S. H., & Weissman, M. M. (2012). Church-based health programs for mental disorders among African Americans: A review. *Psychiatric Services (Washington, D.C.)*, *63*(3), 243–249. doi:10.1176/appi.ps.201100216 PMID:22388529

Harris, S. M. (2015). Black American female eating dysfunctions and body image: A bioecological perspective. *Negro Educational Review*, *66*(1-4), 27–54. doi:10.13140/RG.2.1.4962.6640

Hays, K. (2015). Black churches' capacity to respond to the mental health needs of African Americans. *Social Work & Christianity*, *42*(3), 293–312.

Howard, L. M., Haislip, B. N., Heron, K. E., & Xiao, X. H. (2019). Associations among social connections, body dissatisfaction, and disordered eating in African American and European American college women. *Psi Chi Journal of Psychological Research*, *24*(1), 33–42. doi:10.24839/2325-7342.JN24.1.33

Jackson, B. K. (2015). Licensed professional counselors' perceptions of pastoral counseling in the African American community. *The Journal of Pastoral Care & Counseling*, *69*(2), 85–101. doi:10.1177/1542305015586773 PMID:26227938

Jahraus, J. (2018). Medical complications of eating disorders. *Psychiatric Annals*, *48*(10), 463–467. doi:10.3928/00485713-20180912-04

Javaras, K. N., Runfola, C. D., Thornton, L. M., Agerbo, E., Birgegård, A., Norring, C., Yao, S., Råstam, M., Larsson, H., Lichtenstein, P., & Bulik, C. M. (2015). Sex- and age-specific incidence of healthcare- register-recorded eating disorders in the complete Swedish 1979–2001 birth cohort. *International Journal of Eating Disorders*, *48*(8), 1070–1081. doi:10.1002/eat.22467 PMID:26769444

Karlstad, J., Moe, C. F., Stokland, R. A., & Brinchmann, B. S. (2022). "Balancing within a closed family system": A grounded theory study of how family life is affected by having a family member with an eating disorder. *Journal of Eating Disorders*, *10*(1), 1–10. doi:10.118640337-022-00669-9 PMID:36217195

Kazdin, A. E., Fitzsimmons-Craft, E. E., & Wilfley, D. E. (2017). Addressing critical gaps in the treatment of eating disorders. *International Journal of Eating Disorders*, *50*(3), 170–189. doi:10.1002/eat.22670 PMID:28102908

Kelly, N. R., Cotter, E. W., Guidinger, C., & Williamson, G. (2020). Perceived discrimination, emotion dysregulation and loss of control eating in young men. *Eating Behaviors*, *37*, 101387. doi:10.1016/j.eatbeh.2020.101387 PMID:32353703

Kelly, N. R., Smith, T. M., Hall, G. C., Guidinger, C., Williamson, G., Budd, E. L., & Giuliani, N. R. (2018). Perceptions of general and postpresidential election discrimination are associated with loss of control eating among racially/ethnically diverse young men. *International Journal of Eating Disorders*, *51*(1), 28–38. doi:10.1002/eat.22803 PMID:29149497

Kessler, R. C., Berglund, P. A., Chiu, W. T., Deitz, A. C., Hudson, J. I., Shahly, V., Aguilar-Gaxiola, S., Alonso, J., Angermeyer, M. C., Benjet, C., Bruffaerts, R., de Girolamo, G., de Graaf, R., Maria Haro, J., Kovess-Masfety, V., O'Neill, S., Posada-Villa, J., Sasu, C., Scott, K, & Xavier, M. (2013). The prevalence and correlates of binge eating disorder in the World Health Organization world mental health surveys. *Biological Psychiatry*, *73*(9), 904–914. doi:10.1016/j.biopsych.2012.11.020 PMID:23290497

Kroon Van Diest, A. M., Tartakovsky, M., Stachon, C., Pettit, J. W., & Perez, M. (2014). The relationship between acculturative stress and eating disorder symptoms: Is it unique from general life stress? *Journal of Behavioral Medicine*, *37*(3), 445–457. doi:10.100710865-013-9498-5 PMID:23456250

Lewis, J. A., Mendenhall, R., Harwood, S. A., & Browne Huntt, M. (2013). Coping with gendered racial microaggressions among Black women college students. *Journal of African American Studies*, *17*(1), 51–73. doi:10.100712111-012-9219-0

Linardon, J., Wade, T. D., de la Piedad Garcia, X., & Brennan, L. (2017). The efficacy of cognitive- behavioral therapy for eating disorders: A systematic review and meta-analysis. *Journal of Consulting and Clinical Psychology*, *85*(11), 1080–1094. doi:10.1037/ccp0000245 PMID:29083223

Lydecker, J. A., & Grilo, C. M. (2016). Different yet similar: Examining race and ethnicity in treatment-seeking adults with binge eating disorder. *Journal of Consulting and Clinical Psychology*, *84*(1), 88–94. [REMOVED HYPERLINK FIELD] doi:10.1037/ccp0000048 PMID:26348841

Lydecker, J. A., & Grilo, C. M. (2019). Food insecurity and bulimia nervosa in the United States. *International Journal of Eating Disorders*. https://doi. doi:org/10.1002/eat.23074

Mason, T. B., Lewis, R. J., & Heron, K. E. (2017). Indirect pathways connecting sexual orientation and weight discrimination to disordered eating among young adult lesbians. *Psychology of Sexual Orientation and Gender Diversity*, *4*(2), 193–204. doi:10.1037gd0000220

Mayer, L., Corrigan, P. W., Eisheuer, D., Oexle, N., & Rüsch, N. (2021). Attitudes towards Disclosing a Mental Illness: Impact on Quality of Life and Recovery. *Social Psychiatry and Psychiatric Epidemiology*, *57*(2), 363–374. doi:10.100700127-021-02081-1 PMID:33895868

Mayes, S. D., Fernandez-Mendoza, J., Baweja, R., Calhoun, S., Mahr, F., Aggarwal, R., & Arnold, M. (2014). Correlates of suicide ideation and attempts in children and adolescents with eating disorders. *Eating Disorders*, *22*(4), 352–366. doi:10.1080/10640266.2014.915694 PMID:24842006

McLean, S. A., Caldwell, B., & Roberton, M. (2019). Reach out and recover: Intentions to seek treatment in individuals using online support for eating disorders. *International Journal of Eating Disorders*, *52*(10), 1137–1149. doi:10.1002/eat.23133 PMID:31298791

Micali, N., Hagberg, K. W., Petersen, I., & Treasure, J. L. (2013). The incidence of eating disorders in the UK in 2000–2009: Findings from the General Practice Research Database. *BMJ Open*, *3*(5), e002646. doi:10.1136/bmjopen-2013-002646 PMID:23793681

Misra, S., Jackson, V. W., Chong, J., Choe, K., Tay, C., Wong, J., & Yang, L. H. (2021). Systematic review of cultural aspects of stigma and mental illness among racial and ethnic minority groups in the United States: Implications for interventions. *American Journal of Community Psychology*, *68*(3-4), 486–512. doi:10.1002/ajcp.12516 PMID:33811676

Mowatt, R. A., French, B. H., & Malebranche, D. A. (2013). Black/female/body hypervisibility and invisibility: A Black feminist augmentation of feminist leisure research. *Journal of Leisure Research*, *45*(5), 644–660. doi:10.18666/jlr-2013-v45-i5-4367

Munn-Chernoff, M. A., Grant, J. D., Agrawal, A., Koren, R., Glowinski, A. L., Bucholz, K. K., Madden, P. A. F., Heath, A. C., & Duncan, A. E. (2015). Are there common familial influences for major depressive disorder and an overeating–binge eating dimension in both European American and African American female twins? *International Journal of Eating Disorders*, *48*(4), 375–382. doi:10.1002/eat.22280 PMID:24659561

National Association of Social Workers (NASW). (2015). *Standards and indicators for cultural competence in social work practice*. NASW. https://www.socialworkers.org/Practice/Practice-Standards-Guidelines

Neely-Fairbanks, S. Y., Rojas-Guyler, L., Nabors, L., & Banjo, O. (2018). Mental illness knowledge, stigma, help-seeking behaviors, spirituality and the African American church. *American Journal of Health Studies*, *33*(4), 162–174. doi:10.47779/ajhs.2018.69

Parcesepe, A. M., & Cabassa, L. J. (2013). Public stigma of mental illness in the United States: A systematic literature review. *Administration and Policy in Mental Health*, *40*(5), 384–399. doi:10.100710488-012-0430-z PMID:22833051

Pike, K. M., Hoek, H. W., & Dunne, P. E. (2014). Cultural trends and eating disorders. *Current Opinion in Psychiatry*, *27*(6), 436–442. doi:10.1097/YCO.0000000000000100 PMID:25211499

Ralph, A. F., Brennan, L., Bryne, S., Caldwell, B., Farmer, J., Hart, L. M., & Hay, P. (2022). Management of eating disorders for people with higher weight: Clinical practice guideline. *Journal of Eating Disorders, 10*(121), 1–42. doi:10.118640337-022-00622-w PMID:35978344

Ross, C. C. (2019). African-American women and eating disorders: Depression, and the strong Black woman archetype. *Eating Disorders Review, 30*(5), 1–1.

Samuel, I. A. (2015). Utilization of mental health services among African American male adolescents released from juvenile detention: Examining reasons for within-group disparities in help-seeking behaviors. *Child & Adolescent Social Work Journal, 32*(1), 33–43. doi:10.100710560-014-0357-1

Sbrocco, T., Osborn, R., Clark, R. D., Hsiao, C. W., & Carter, M. M. (2012). Assessing the stages of change among African American women in a weight management program. *The Journal of Black Psychology, 38*(1), 81–103. doi:10.1177/0095798411403618 PMID:24683280

Scott, T. N., Gil-Rivas, V., & Cachelin, F. M. (2019). The need for cultural adaptations to health interventions for African American women: A qualitative analysis. *Cultural Diversity & Ethnic Minority Psychology, 25*(3), 331–341. doi:10.1037/cdp0000228 PMID:30272472

Sinha, S., & Warfa, N. (2013). Treatment of eating disorders among ethnic minorities in western settings: A systematic review. *Psychiatria Danubina, 25*(Suppl 2), S295–S299. PMID:23995197

Smith, A. R., Zuromski, K. L., & Dodd, D. R. (2018). Eating disorders and suicidality: What we know, what we don't know, and suggestions for future research. *Current Opinion in Psychology, 22*, 63–67. doi:10.1016/j.copsyc.2017.08.023 PMID:28846874

Stansbury, K.L., Peterson, T.L., & Beecher, B. (2013). An exploration of mental health literacy among older African Americans. *Aging & Mental Health, 17*(2), 226.232. doi:10.1080/13607863.2012.724652

Stiles-Shields, C., Hoste, R. R., Doyle, P. M., & Le Grange, D. (2012). A review of family based treatment for adolescents with eating disorders. *Reviews on Recent Clinical Trials, 7*(2), 133–140. doi:10.2174/157488712800100242 PMID:22353196

Sulkowski, M. L., Dempsey, J., & Dempsey, A. G. (2011). Effects of stress and coping on binge eating in female college students. *Eating Behaviors, 12*(3), 188–191. doi:10.1016/j.eatbeh.2011.04.006 PMID:21741016

Sutherland, M. E. (2013). Overweight and obesity among African American women: An examination of predictive and risk factors and weight-reduction recommendations. *Journal of Black Studies*, *44*(8), 846–869. doi:10.1177/0021934713511639

Talleyrand, R. M. (2011). Eating disorders in African American girls: Implications for counselors. *Journal of Counseling and Development*, *88*(3), 319–324. doi:10.1002/j.1556-6678.2010.tb00028.x

Talleyrand, R. M., Gordon, A. D., Daquin, J. V., & Johnson, A. J. (2017). Expanding our understanding of eating practices, body image, and appearance in African American women: A qualitative study. *The Journal of Black Psychology*, *43*(5), 464–492. doi:10.1177/0095798416649086

Thompson, C., & Park, S. (2016). Barriers to access and utilization of eating disorder treatment among women. *Archives of Women's Mental Health*, *19*(5), 753–760. doi:10.100700737-016-0618-4 PMID:26971265

Thompson-Brenner, H., Franko, D. L., Thompson, D. R., Grilo, C. M., Boisseau, C. L., Roehrig, J. P., Richards, L. K., Bryson, S. W., Bulik, C. M., Crow, S. J., Devlin, M. J., Gorin, A. A., Kristeller, J. L., Masheb, R., Mitchell, J. E., Peterson, C. B., Safer, D. L., Striegel, R. H., Wilfley, D. E., & Wilson, G. T. (2013). Race/ethnicity, education, and treatment parameters as moderators and predictors of outcome in binge eating disorder. *Journal of Consulting and Clinical Psychology*, *81*(4), 710–721. doi:10.1037/a0032946 PMID:23647283

Thornton, L. M., Watson, H. J., Jangmo, A., Welch, E., Wiklund, C., von Hausswolff-Juhlin, Y., Norring, C., Herman, B. K., Larsson, H., & Bulik, C. M. (2017). Binge-eating disorder in the Swedish national registers: Somatic comorbidity. *International Journal of Eating Disorders*, *50*(1), 58–65. doi:10.1002/eat.22624 PMID:27642179

Udo, T., & Grilo, C. M. (2018). Prevalence and correlates of DSM-5-defined eating disorders in a nationally representative sample of U.S. adults. *Biological Psychiatry*, *84*(5), 345–354. doi:10.1016/j.biopsych.2018.03.014 PMID:29859631

Udo, T., & Grilo, C. M. (2019). Psychiatric and medical correlates of DSM-5 eating disorders in a nationally representative sample of adults in the United States. *International Journal of Eating Disorders*, *52*(1), 42–50. doi:10.1002/eat.23004 PMID:30756422

Udo, T., White, M. A., Lydecker, J. L., Barnes, R. D., Genao, I., Garcia, R., Masheb, R. M., & Grilo, C. M. (2016). Biopsychosocial correlates of binge eating disorder in European American and African American women with obesity in primary care settings. *European Eating Disorders Review*, *24*(3), 181–186. doi:10.1002/erv.2417 PMID:26640009

Van Alsten, S. C., & Duncan, A. E. (2020). Lifetime patterns of comorbidity in eating disorders: An approach using sequence analysis. *European Eating Disorders Review*, *28*(6), 709–723. doi:10.1002/erv.2767 PMID:32748537

van Hoeken, D., & Hoek, H. W. (2020). Review of the burden of eating disorders: Mortality, disability, costs, quality of life, and family burden. *Current Opinion in Psychiatry*, *33*(6), 521–527. doi:10.1097/YCO.0000000000000641 PMID:32796186

Volpe, U., Tortorella, A., Manchia, M., Monteleone, A. M., Albert, U., & Monteleone, P. (2016). Eating disorders: What age at onset? *Psychiatry Research*, *238*, 225–227. doi:10.1016/j.psychres.2016.02.048 PMID:27086237

Ward, E. C., Wiltshire, J. C., Detry, M. A., & Brown, R. L. (2013). African American men and women's attitude toward mental illness, perceptions of stigma, and preferred coping behaviors. *Nursing Research*, *62*(3), 185–194. doi:10.1097/NNR.0b013e31827bf533 PMID:23328705

Watson, L. B., Ancis, J. R., White, D. N., & Nazari, N. (2013). Racial identity buffers African American women from body image problems and disordered eating. *Psychology of Women Quarterly*, *37*(3), 337–350. doi:10.1177/0361684312474799

Weigel, A., Lowe, B., & Kohlmann, S. (2019). Severity of somatic symptoms in outpatients with anorexia and bulimia nervosa. *European Eating Disorders Review*, *27*(2), 195–204. doi:10.1002/erv.2643 PMID:30318829

Welch, E., Jangmo, A., Thornton, L. M., Norring, C., von Hausswolff-Juhlin, Y., Herman, B. K., Pawaskar, M., Larsson, H., & Bulik, C. M. (2016). Treatment-seeking patients with binge-eating disorder in the Swedish national registers: Clinical course and psychiatric comorbidity. *BMC Psychiatry*, *16*(1), 1–8. doi:10.118612888-016-0840-7 PMID:27230675

Wilson, P. L., O'Connor, D. P., Kaplan, C. D., Bode, S., Mama, S. K., & Lee, R. E. (2012). Relationship of fruit, vegetable, and fat consumption to binge eating symptoms in African American and Hispanic or Latina women. *Eating Behaviors*, *13*(2), 179–182. doi:10.1016/j.eatbeh.2012.01.007 PMID:22365808

Chapter 5
Factitious Disorder Among the African-American Population

LaVelle Hendricks
Texas A&M University, Commerce, USA

Dimitra Smith
Texas A&M University, Commerce, USA

Karl Mitchell
Texas A&M University, Commerce, USA

Elizabeth Hudson
Texas A&M University, Commerce, USA

Jovaria Baig
Texas A&M University, Commerce, USA

ABSTRACT

Factitious disorder, also known as Munchausen syndrome, is a mental health condition in which a person intentionally exaggerates physical or psychological symptoms in themselves or in someone else. The rationale behind this behavior is to assume the role of a sick person and receive attention, sympathy, or emotional support from others. People with factitious disorder may go to great lengths to produce or falsify symptoms, such as taking medication, inducing vomiting, tampering with medical devices, or lying about their medical history. They may also seek out medical procedures, hospitalizations, or surgeries that are not necessary or that pose a significant risk to their health.

DOI: 10.4018/978-1-6684-8918-5.ch005

INTRODUCTION

Factitious disorder, also known as Munchausen syndrome, is a mental health condition in which a person intentionally exaggerates physical or psychological symptoms in themselves or in someone else. The rationale behind this behavior is to assume the role of a sick person and receive attention, sympathy, or emotional support from others. People with factitious disorder may go to great lengths to produce or falsify symptoms, such as taking medication, inducing vomiting, tampering with medical devices, or lying about their medical history. They may also seek out medical procedures, hospitalizations, or surgeries that are not necessary or that pose a significant risk to their health (Carnahan & Anupam, 2023). Factitious disorder is unlike malingering, which involves faking symptoms for some external gain, such as financial compensation or avoiding work. In contrast, people with factitious disorder regularly seek attention and care from medical professionals (Mayo Clinic, 2023).

The cause of factitious disorder is not fully understood, but it is believed to be related to a history of trauma or abuse, a need for control, and a desire for attention or emotional support. It is a severe illness that can lead to significant harm and even death in extreme cases. The treatment of factitious disorder typically involves psychotherapy, such as cognitive-behavioral therapy (CBT) or psychodynamic therapy, to address underlying psychological issues and improve coping skills. Treatment with CBT targets the identification of distorted thoughts and beliefs that contribute to the individual's behavior. CBT can also help the person develop healthier coping strategies, improve problem-solving skills, and address underlying emotional issues. In several cases, medication may also be used to manage underlying mental health conditions (Baig, Levin, Lichetnthal, & Breitbart, 2015).

Treatments for factitious disorders can also include family therapy. Family therapy is essential because it can help individuals with a factitious disorder by involving family members in therapy, as they can provide support, gain a better understanding of the condition, and learn how to effectively communicate and respond to the individual's needs. Family therapy can also address any family dynamics or conflicts that may be contributing to the disorder. Along with individuals with factitious disorders can benefit from family therapy, group therapy, and support groups. These resources can provide helpful assistance.as well. Group therapy or support groups involve participating in group therapy or support groups with individuals who have similar experiences that can provide a sense of validation, reduce isolation, and offer opportunities for shared learning and support (Lawlor & Kirakowski, 2014). Treating factitious disorder can also be challenging because the individuals with this condition cultivate resistance to acknowledging or accepting their behaviors. However, the combination of therapeutic approaches and medications can be beneficial.

It is important to note that treatment for factitious disorder can be challenging due to the individual's resistance to change, denial of the problem, and potential lack of trust in healthcare professionals. Thus, building a therapeutic alliance, providing a supportive environment, and working collaboratively with the individual are essential components of treatment. It is also important for healthcare professionals to ensure the safety and well-being of the person with a factitious disorder, as well as to establish appropriate boundaries and avoid reinforcing the behavior. Ideally, the treatment of factitious disorder should focus on addressing underlying psychological issues and promoting healthier coping strategies (McCullumsmith & Ford, 2011). The establishment of a multidisciplinary team of mental health and medical professionals can also be essential to ensuring quality and substantive treatment.

While causes and treatments for the disorder should be understood by healthcare professionals, culturally competent care must also be prioritized for any clinician or treatment team. Factitious disorder can affect individuals from any racial or ethnic background, including African Americans. The prevalence of factitious disorder across different racial and ethnic groups is not well-documented, as it is an underdiagnosed and often undisclosed condition. However, it is important to recognize that factitious disorder can appear in individuals from diverse backgrounds. In the context of African Americans and factitious disorder, it is essential to approach the topic with cultural sensitivity and awareness of the unique experiences and challenges faced by this community. Factors such as historical mistrust of the healthcare system, disparities in access to quality healthcare, and cultural beliefs and attitudes toward illness and seeking help may influence how factitious disorder is understood and addressed within the African American community (Jaghab, Skodnek, & Padder, 2006).

It is crucial for healthcare professionals to provide culturally competent care and establish trustful relationships when working with individuals from any background, including African Americans, who could be experiencing factitious disorder. This involves understanding and respecting cultural beliefs and practices, addressing potential barriers to treatment, and considering the broader sociocultural context in which the individual lives (Willenberg, 1994). Regardless of one's racial or ethnic background, open and non-judgmental communication, patient education, and collaborative treatment planning are important components of supporting individuals with factitious disorders. Engaging family members or trusted community members in the treatment process can also be valuable in providing support and promoting understanding (Geneva, 1992). In essence, recognizing the diversity within the experience of factitious disorder and tailoring treatment approaches to meet the unique needs and cultural contexts of individuals, including African Americans, is necessary for effective care (Mohammad, Khalid, McDonald, & Shelley, 2018).

Factitious disorder can appear alongside other mental health conditions, including but not limited to depression, anxiety, or personality disorders. The presence of these co-occurring conditions can influence the overall presentation and treatment approach for everyone (Sutherland & Rodin, 1990). It is important to approach each case of factitious disorder with a comprehensive and individualized assessment to understand the specific patterns, motivations, and underlying factors contributing to the behavior. This allows for tailored treatment plans and interventions that address the unique needs of each person.

Treatments should also be specific to the populations healthcare professionals work with and include evidence-based practices. For example, individuals with substance abuse disorders may require many of the relevant treatments discussed (e.g., individual, group, and/or family therapy). Additionally, while the prevalence and particular manifestations of factitious disorder among African American drug users is not well-documented due to limited research, it is important to recognize that factitious disorder can potentially occur in individuals with substance use disorders, including African Americans (Carnahan & Jha, 2022). Factitious disorder in the context of drug use may involve the fabrication or exaggeration of physical or psychological symptoms to manipulate medical professionals or obtain certain medications. Individuals with substance use disorders may engage in factitious behavior to maintain their drug use, access prescription medications, or fulfill their addiction-related needs (Boegner & Bauer, 1996).

There are several factors that can influence how factitious disorder is expressed and addressed within the African American community of drug users, including access to healthcare, experiences of discrimination, socioeconomic status, and cultural beliefs (Sinha & Smolik, 2021). Healthcare professionals working with African American drug users should be aware of the potential for factitious disorder and exercise vigilance in recognizing signs of inconsistent symptoms, frequent emergency room visits, or a pattern of seeking precise medications without legitimate medical reasons (Mailis-Gagnon, Blumberger, Nicholson, & Zurowski, 2008).

Treatments for college students must also be specific to the population and provide culturally competent care. For example, college students may face various pressures and stressors related to academic performance, social interactions, and transitioning to adulthood. These pressures, coupled with individual psychological factors, can contribute to the development of factitious disorder behaviors. In the context of African American college students, cultural beliefs, experiences of racism and discrimination, and the pursuit of academic and professional success could influence the manifestation of factitious disorder. The desire for attention, sympathy, or perceived advantages within the college environment may also contribute to the development of factitious behaviors (Frye & Feldman, 2012). Hence, healthcare professionals, college counselors, and university staff should be vigilant in recognizing potential signs of factitious disorder among African American college students. Signs can include inconsistencies in reported symptoms, frequent medical visits or emergency room visits, or a pattern of seeking specific medications without authentic medical reasons (Frye & Feldman, 2012).

Cultural competency is fundamental when addressing factitious disorder among African American college students. Healthcare professionals, university counseling centers, and staff should be culturally sensitive to the potential barriers to care, and the unique challenges faced by African American students. Building trust, encouraging open communication, and providing additional support through counseling services or referrals to mental health professionals can be beneficial in the treatment process. (Cornelis, C., 2002).

In the African American religious communities, the prevalence and specific manifestations of factitious disorder are inadequately documented due to limited research specifically focused on this population. However, it is important to recognize that factitious disorder can potentially impact any individual within any religious or cultural community, including the African American religious community. Often, religious communities offer support during challenging times with emotional problems, psychological distress, family issues, or personal issues. The African American religious community can play a significant role in providing support, guidance, and a sense of belonging to its members. However, individuals within these communities may still experience psychological challenges and engage in factitious behavior for various reasons. (Reich, P., Gottfried, M., 1983).

Within the African American religious community, factors such as faith, spirituality, cultural beliefs, and the importance of seeking direction from religious leaders can influence the perception of factitious disorder. Individuals could engage in factitious behavior to seek attention, sympathy, or perceived spiritual rewards within their religious community. (Gatison, A, 2012).

It is also important for religious leaders and healthcare professionals within the African American religious community, to be cognizant of the potential signs of factitious disorder, such as unpredictable symptoms, repeated medical or emergency appointments, and a behavioral pattern of seeking medications without valid medical reasons. (Reich, J., Hanno, P., 1997). Cultural competency is vital when addressing factitious disorder within the African American religious community. Healthcare professionals and religious leaders should approach the issue with sensitivity, respect, and an understanding of the cultural and religious context. It is beneficial and recommended to collaborate with trusted community members, involve religious leaders in the treatment process, and provide support through counseling or referrals to mental health professionals. (Jacobs, E., Rolle, I., Ferrans, 2006).

African Americans enlisted in the military experience unique challenges and stressors associated with military service that contribute to developing or expressing factitious disorder behaviors. These unique factors can include the demands of military life, deployment experiences, exposure to trauma, and the desire for attention or perceived advantages within the military environment. (Lande, R., Williams, L., 2013). In providing mental health care to African American service members, healthcare professionals, and leadership must recognize potential signs of factitious disorders among this population. It is critical that healthcare professionals and leadership pay close attention to key indicators that may include inconsistencies in reported symptoms, patterns of seeking unnecessary medical care or claiming medical conditions, and a history of unexplained medical emergencies (Lande, R., Willimas, L., 2013).

Culturally competent care among African American military community is needed when addressing factitious disorder within this population. African American service members often face unique experiences, cultural dynamics, and challenges. It is important that healthcare professionals and military leaders practice sensitivity when working with African American service members. In addressing factitious disorders among African Americans in the military, culturally appropriate interventions, such as building trust, providing support through military healthcare resources and mental health programs, and ensuring access to culturally appropriate interventions, are crucial in addressing factitious disorders within this population.

To better understand these specific factors among African Americans in the military, it is important to state that more research is needed to address the factors, experiences, and treatment outcomes of factitious disorders. Conducting more research studies regarding factitious disorder faced by African American military service personnel will be informative when addressing culturally responsive interventions to address the complexities between factitious disorder and military service within this population. (Lewis, H., 2021). It is important to recognize that individuals with factitious disorders can face challenges regardless of their racial or ethnic background. However, it is crucial to acknowledge that experiences may vary based on individual circumstances, cultural factors, and the availability of resources within specific communities. Among the African American community, these conditions may be less well-known or misunderstood, which often leads to the Stigma and misunderstanding faced by individuals with factitious disorders, as they may encounter judgment and lack of understanding from family, friends, and healthcare providers. (Middlesex Health, 2023).

RESOURCES

It is important to note that these resources are meant to provide information and support, but they should not replace professional medical advice or therapy. If you or someone you know is experiencing a factitious disorder or any mental health condition, it is recommended to consult with a qualified healthcare professional for an accurate diagnosis and appropriate treatment.

Visit https://www.psychforums.com/factitious-disorder-imposed-on-self.

National Alliance on Mental Illness (NAMI): NAMI is a reputable organization that offers resources and support for individuals with mental health conditions and their families. They provide education, advocacy, and various support programs. Visit their website: https://www.nami.org/

Mayo Clinic: Mayo Clinic offers comprehensive information on factitious disorder, including symptoms, causes, diagnosis, and treatment options. Their website provides reliable and easy-to-understand resources for individuals seeking information about the condition. Visit: https://www.mayoclinic.org/

MedlinePlus: MedlinePlus, a service of the U.S. National Library of Medicine, provides reliable and up-to-date information on factitious disorders. Their website offers overviews, treatment options, and links to relevant research articles. Visit: https://medlineplus.gov/

WebMD provides a comprehensive overview of factitious disorders, including symptoms, causes, diagnosis, and treatment. Their website offers articles, expert advice, and a community forum where individuals can share their experiences and seek support. Visit: https://www.webmd.com/

Mental Health America (MHA): MHA is a leading nonprofit organization dedicated to addressing mental health issues. Their website provides resources on various mental health conditions, including factitious disorder. Visit: https://www.mhanational.org/

The TLC Foundation for Body-Focused Repetitive Behaviors: While primarily focused on body-focused repetitive behaviors, this foundation provides resources and support for individuals with factitious disorder as well. Their website offers information, treatment referrals, and a community forum. Visit: https://www.bfrb.org/

Factitious Disorder on Reddit: The Factitious Disorder subreddit provides a platform for individuals to discuss and share experiences related to factitious disorder. It can serve as a supportive online community. Visit: https://www.reddit.com/r/FactitiousDisorder/

REFERENCES

Ackermann, G., Haugke, C., Schaumann, R., von Salis-Soglio, G., & Rodloff, A. C. (2000). Chronic factitious illness presenting as Munchausen's gonarthritis. *European Journal of Clinical Microbiology & Infectious Diseases*, *19*(1), 70–71. doi:10.1007100960050016 PMID:10706187

APA. (2019). *Acta Dermatovenerologica Alpina, Pannonica, et Adriatica*, 13-15.

Addison, T. E., & Talan, K. H. (1974). Letter: Jet-set Münchausen syndrome. *The New England Journal of Medicine, 291*(22), 1195. doi:10.1056/NEJM197411282912225 PMID:4419976

Aduan, R. P., Fauci, A. S., Dale, D. C., Herzberg, J. C., & Wolff, S. M. (1979). Factitious fever and self-induced infection: A report of 32 cases and review of the literature. *Annals of Internal Medicine, 90*(2), 230–242. doi:10.7326/0003-4819-90-2-230 PMID:443658

Alicandri-Ciufelli, M., Moretti, V., Ruberto, M., Monzani, D., Chiarini, L., & Presutti, L. (2012). Otolaryngology fantastica: The ear, nose, and throat manifestations of Munchausen's syndrome. *The Laryngoscope, 122*(1), 51–57. doi:10.1002/lary.22373 PMID:22095880

Ameh, V., & Speak, N. (2008). Factitious hypoglycaemia in a nondiabetic patient. *European Journal of Emergency Medicine, 15*(1), 59–60. doi:10.1097/MEJ.0b013e3282aa3f70 PMID:18180671

American Psychiatric Association. (1994). *Diagnostic and Statistical Manual of Mental Disorders: DSM-4*. American Psychiatric Association.

American Psychiatric Association. (2000). *Diagnostic and Statistical Manual of Mental Disorders Text Revision: DSM-4-TR*. American Psychiatric Association.

Ando, T., Nomura, T., Sejiyama, S. Y., Shin, T., Mori, K. I., Sumino, Y., Sato, F., & Mimata, H. (2014). Munchausen syndrome in the act of creating and enacting macroscopic hematuria. *Urologia Internationalis, 93*(3), 371–372. doi:10.1159/000357919 PMID:24576852

Ando, T., Nomura, T., Sejiyama, S. Y., Shin, T., Mori, K. I., Sumino, Y., Sato, F., & Mimata, H. (2014). Munchausen syndrome in the act of creating and enacting macroscopic hematuria. *Urologia Internationalis, 93*(3), 371–372. doi:10.1159/000357919 PMID:24576852

Arnulf, I., Zeitzer, J. M., File, J., Farber, N., & Mignot, E. (2005). Kleine–Levin syndrome: A systematic review of 186 cases in the literature. *Brain, 128*(12), 2763–2776. doi:10.1093/brain/awh620 PMID:16230322

Bahna, S. L., & Oldham, J. (2014). Munchausen stridor — A strong false alarm of anaphylaxis. *Allergy, Asthma & Immunology Research, 6*(6), 577–579. doi:10.4168/aair.2014.6.6.577 PMID:25374759

Baig, M. R., Levin, T. T., Lichtenthal, W. G., Boland, P. J., & Breitbart, W. S. (2015). Facitious Disorder (Munchausen's Syndrome) in Oncology: Case Report and Literature Review. *Psycho-Oncology*, *25*(6), 707–711. doi:10.1002/pon.3906 PMID:26179957

Baig, M. R., Levin, T. T., Lichtenthal, W. G., Boland, P. J., & Breitbart, W. S. (2015). Factitious disorder (Munchausen's syndrome) in oncology: Case report and literature review. *Psycho-Oncology*, 1. PMID:26179957

Ballas, S. K. (1996). Factitious sickle cell acute painful episodes: A secondary type of Munchausen syndrome. *American Journal of Hematology*, *53*(4), 254–258. doi:10.1002/(SICI)1096-8652(199612)53:4<254::AID-AJH10>3.0.CO;2-C PMID:8948666

Barkin, J. A., Biagini, T. M., & Barkin, J. S. (2013). Factitious disorder as a cause of gastrointestinal bleeding: Use of a gastroenterologist's "secondary survey". *The American Journal of Gastroenterology*, *108*(3), 456–458. doi:10.1038/ajg.2012.420 PMID:23459058

Bass, C., & Halligan, P. (2014). Factitious disorders and malingering: Challenges for clinical assessment and management. *Lancet*, *383*(9926), 1422–1432. doi:10.1016/S0140-6736(13)62186-8 PMID:24612861

Bauer, M., & Boegner, F. (1996). Neurological syndromes in factitious disorder. *The Journal of Nervous and Mental Disease*, *184*(5), 281–288. doi:10.1097/00005053-199605000-00003 PMID:8627273

Baweja, R., Baweja, R., & Hameed, A. (2014). Munchausen's syndrome with rare hematological disorder, systemic mastocytosis: A case report, J Neuropsychiatry Clin Neurosci Bhargava, D., Al-Abri, R., Rizvi, SG, Okbi, MH AL, Bhargava, K. and Al Adawi, S. (2007). Phenomenology and outcome of factitious disorders in otolaryngology clinic in Oman. *International Journal of Psychiatry in Medicine*, *37*(2), 229–240.

Biarge, M. M., García-Alix, A., Hoyo, M., Alarcón, A., Pipaón, M., & Hernández, F. (2014). Intussusception in a preterm neonate; a very rare, major intestinal problem — Systematic review of cases. *Journal of Perinatal Medicine*, *32*(2), 190–194.

Biarge, M. M., García-Alix, A., Hoyo, M. L., Alarcón, A., Pipaón, M. S., Hernández, F., Pérez, J., & Quero, J. (2004). Intussusception in a preterm neonate; a very rare, major intestinal problem — Systematic review of cases. *Journal of Perinatal Medicine*, *32*(2), 190–194. doi:10.1515/JPM.2004.036 PMID:15085900

Boden, J. M., & Fergusson, D. M. (2011). Alcohol and depression. *Addiction (Abingdon, England)*, *106*(5), 906–914. doi:10.1111/j.1360-0443.2010.03351.x PMID:21382111

Bovasso, G. B. (2014). Cannabis abuse as a risk factor for depressive symptoms. *The American Journal of Psychiatry*, 9. PMID:11729021

Boyd, A. S., Ritchie, C., & Likhari, S. (2014). Munchausen syndrome and Munchausen syndrome by proxy in dermatology. *Journal of the American Academy of Dermatology*, *71*(2), 376–381. doi:10.1016/j.jaad.2013.12.028 PMID:24613506

Briere, J., & Gil, E. (1998). Self-mutilation in clinical and general population samples: Prevalence, correlates, and functions. *The American Journal of Orthopsychiatry*, *68*(4), 609–620. doi:10.1037/h0080369 PMID:9809120

Bright, R., Damon, L., & Eisendrath, S. (2001). A case of factitious aplastic anemia. *International Journal of Psychiatry in Medicine*, *31*(4), 433–441. doi:10.2190/TUJB-B2M7-6UPV-XPLV PMID:11949741

Carnahan, K. T. (2023). *Factitious Disorder*. StatPearls Publishing.

Carney, M. W., & Brown, J. P. (1983). Clinical features and motives among 42 artifactual illness patients. *The British Journal of Medical Psychology*, *56*(1), 57–66. doi:10.1111/j.2044-8341.1983.tb01532.x PMID:6838782

Chambers, E., Yager, J., Apfeldorf, W., & Camps-Romero, E. (2007). Factitious aortic dissection leading to thoracotomy in a 20-year-old man. *Psychosomatics*, *48*(4), 355–358. doi:10.1176/appi.psy.48.4.355 PMID:17600175

Chen, L. P., Murad, M. H., Paras, M. L., Colbenson, K. M., Sattler, A. L., Goranson, E. N., Elamin, M. B., Seime, R. J., Shinozaki, G., Prokop, L. J., & Zirakzadeh, A. (2010). Sexual abuse and lifetime diagnosis of psychiatric disorders: Systematic review and meta-analysis. *Mayo Clinic Proceedings*, *85*(7), 618–629. doi:10.4065/mcp.2009.0583 PMID:20458101

Chen, L. P., Murad, M. H., Paras, M. L., Colbenson, K. M., Sattler, A. L., Goranson, E. N., Elamin, M. B., Seime, R. J., Shinozaki, G., Prokop, L. J., & Zirakzadeh, A. (2010). Sexual abuse and lifetime diagnosis of psychiatric disorders: Systematic review and meta-analysis. *Mayo Clinic Proceedings*, *85*(7), 618–629. doi:10.4065/mcp.2009.0583 PMID:20458101

Chew, B. H., Pace, K. T., & Honey, R. J. (2002). Munchausen syndrome presenting as gross hematuria in two women. *Urology*, *59*(4), 601. doi:10.1016/S0090-4295(01)01608-9 PMID:11927327

Conner, K. R., Pinquart, M., & Duberstein, P. R. (2008). Meta-analysis of depression and substance use and impairment among intravenous drug users (IDUs). *Addiction (Abingdon, England), 103*(4), 524–534. doi:10.1111/j.1360-0443.2007.02118.x PMID:18261192

Crawford, S. M., Jeyasanger, G., & Wright, M. (2005). A visitor with Munchausen's syndrome. *Clinical Medicine (London, England), 5*(4), 400–401. doi:10.7861/clinmedicine.5-4-400 PMID:16138498

Dahale, A. B., Hatti, S., Thippeswamy, H., & Chaturvedi, S. K. (2014). Factitious disorder — Experience at a neuropsychiatric center in southern India. *Indian Journal of Psychological Medicine, 36*(1), 62–65. doi:10.4103/0253-7176.127253 PMID:24701013

DeWitt, D. E., Ward, S. A., Prabhu, S., & Warton, B. (2009). Patient privacy versus protecting the patient and the health system from harm: A case study. *The Medical Journal of Australia, 191*(4), 213–216. doi:10.5694/j.1326-5377.2009.tb02755.x PMID:19705982

Dhir, V., Arya, V., Chandra Malav, I., Gupta, R., & Dey, A. B. (2007). Idiopathic systemic capillary leak syndrome (SCLS): Case report and systematic review of cases reported in the last 16 years. *Internal Medicine (Tokyo, Japan), 46*(12), 899–904. doi:10.2169/internalmedicine.46.6129 PMID:17575386

Donegan, D., Hickey, D. P., & Smith, D. (2012). Hypoglycemia after simultaneous pancreas-kidney transplant: Fact or factitious? *Pancreas, 41*(6), 974–976. doi:10.1097/MPA.0b013e31823fb6ff PMID:22781913

Eastwood, S., & Bisson, J. L. (2008). Management of factitious disorders: A systematic review. *Psychotherapy and Psychosomatics, 77*(4), 209–218. doi:10.1159/000126072 PMID:18418027

Edi-Osagie, E. C., Hopkins, R. E., & Edi-Osagie, N. E. (1998). Munchausen's syndrome in obstetrics and gynecology: A review. *Obstetrical & Gynecological Survey, 53*(1), 45–49. doi:10.1097/00006254-199801000-00023 PMID:9440129

Farrier, J. N., & Mansel, R. E. (2002). Dermatitis artefacta of the breast: A series of case reports. *European Journal of Surgical Oncology, 28*(2), 189–192. doi:10.1053/ejso.2001.1214 PMID:11884056

Feldman, M. D., & Eisendrath, S. J. (1996). The spectrum of factitious disorders, American Psychiatric Publishing

Feldman, M. D. Phillips (Ed.), K.A. (2008). Factitious disorder, in somatoform and factitious disorders, American Psychiatric Publishing

Feldman, M. D., & Brown, R. M. (2002). Munchausen by proxy in an international context. *ChildAbuse & Neglect*, *26*(5), 509–524. doi:10.1016/S0145-2134(02)00327-7 PMID:12079087

Feldman, M. D., & Brown, R. M. (2002). Munchausen by proxy in an international context. *ChildAbuse & Neglect*, *26*(5), 509–524. doi:10.1016/S0145-2134(02)00327-7 PMID:12079087

Fliege, H., Grimm, A., Eckhardt-Henn, A., Gieler, U., Martin, K., & Klapp, B. K. (2007). Frequency of ICD-10 factitious disorder: Survey of senior hospital consultants and physicians in private practice. *Psychosomatics*, *48*(1), 60–64. doi:10.1176/appi.psy.48.1.60 PMID:17209151

Fliege, H., Scholler, G., Rose, M., Willenberg, H., & Klapp, B. F. (2002). Factitious disorders and pathological self-harm in a hospital population: An interdisciplinary challenge. *General Hospital Psychiatry*, *24*(3), 164–171. doi:10.1016/S0163-8343(02)00171-8 PMID:12062141

Ford, C. V. (1973). The Munchausen syndrome: A report of four new cases and a review of psychodynamic considerations. *International Journal of Psychiatry in Medicine*, *4*(1), 31–45. PMID:4709440

Ford, C. V. (1973). The Munchausen syndrome: A report of four new cases and a review of psychodynamic considerations. *International Journal of Psychiatry in Medicine*, *4*(1), 31–45. PMID:4709440

Ford, C. V., Friedmann, C. T., & Faguet, R. A. (Eds.), (1982). Munchausen syndrome, in extraordinary disorders of human behaviour. Springer US

Frye, E. M., & Feldman, M. D. (2012). Factitious Disorder by Proxy in Educational Settings: A Review. *Educational Psychology Review*, *24*(1), 47–61. doi:10.100710648-011-9180-9

Fujiwara, T., Kubo, T., Yano, K., & Hosokawa, K. (2008). A case of intractable recurrent abdominal cutaneous ulceration caused by self-injection of menstrual blood. *European Journal of Plastic Surgery*, *30*(6), 303–304. doi:10.100700238-007-0199-6

Gao, J., Li, Y., Cai, Y., Chen, J., Shen, Y., Ni, S., Wei, Y., Qiu, Y., Zhu, X., Liu, Y., Lu, C., Chen, C., Niu, Q., Tang, C., Yang, Y., Wang, Q., Cui, W., Xia, J., Liu, T., & Tao, M. (2012). Perceived parenting and risk for major depression in Chinese women. *Psychological Medicine*, *42*(05), 921–930. doi:10.1017/S0033291711001942 PMID:21943491

Gatison, Annette Madlock, PhD. (2021). A Woman Approach to Caring for Patients With Empirically Unverifiable Symptoms. *AMA Journal of Ethics*. PMID:34351260

Gavin, H., On the feigned and factitious diseases of soldiers and seamen; with hints for the examination, and rules for the detection of impostors, 1843

Giuliodori, K., Campanati, A., Rosa, L., Marconi, B., Cellini, A., & Brandozzi, G. (2014). Factitious disorders in adults: Two cases of unusual skin ulcers. *Acta Dermatovenerologica Alpina, Panonica, et Adriatica*, *23*(1), 13–15. PMID:24638866

Giuliodori, K., Campanati, A., Rosa, L., Marconi, B., Cellini, A., & Brandozzi, G. (2014). *Factitious disorders in adults: two cases of unusual skin ulcers.*

Gordon, D. K., & Sansone, R. A. (2013). A relationship between factitious disorder and borderline personality disorder. *Innovations in Clinical Neuroscience*, *10*(11–12), 11. PMID:24563814

Gregurek-Novak, T., Novak-Bilić, G., & Vučić, M. (2005). Dermatitis artefacta: Unusual appearance in an older woman. *Journal of the European Academy of Dermatology and Venereology*, *19*(2), 223–225. doi:10.1111/j.1468-3083.2005.01022.x PMID:15752297

Griffiths, E. J., Kampa, R., Pearce, C., Sakellariou, A., & Solan, M. C. (2009). Munchausen's syndrome by Google©. *Annals of the Royal College of Surgeons of England*, *91*(2), 159–160. doi:10.1308/003588409X391938 PMID:19317939

Haddad, S. A., Winer, K. K., Gupta, A., Chakrabarti, S., Noel, P., & Klein, H. G. S. A. (2002). A puzzling case of anemia. *Transfusion*, *42*(12), 1610–1613. doi:10.1046/j.1537-2995.2002.00269.x PMID:12473143

Hammen, C. (2005). Stress and depression. *Annual Review of Clinical Psychology*, *1*(1), 293–319. doi:10.1146/annurev.clinpsy.1.102803.143938 PMID:17716090

Hariharasubramony, A., Chankramath, S., & Srinivasa, S. (2012). Munchausen syndrome as dermatitis simulate. *Indian Journal of Psychological Medicine*, *34*(1), 94–96. doi:10.4103/0253-7176.96171 PMID:22661819

Hariharasubramony, A., Chankramath, S., & Srinivasa, S. (2012). Munchausen syndrome as dermatitis simulate. *Indian Journal of Psychological Medicine, 34*(1), 94–96. doi:10.4103/0253-7176.96171 PMID:22661819

Harper, J. I., & Copeman, P. W. (1983). Dermatitis artefacta presenting as a "vasculitis". *Journal of the Royal Society of Medicine, 76*(11), 970–971. doi:10.1177/014107688307601118 PMID:6631880

Haw, C., Hawton, K., Houston, K., & Townsend, E. (2001). Psychiatric and personality disorders in deliberate self-harm patients. *The British Journal of Psychiatry, 178*(1), 48–54. doi:10.1192/bjp.178.1.48 PMID:11136210

Highland, K. B., & Flume, P. A. (2002). A "story" of a woman with cystic fibrosis. *Chest, 121*(5), 1704–1707. doi:10.1378/chest.121.5.1704 PMID:12006467

Hirayama, Y., Sakamaki, S., Tsuji, Y., Sagawa, T., Takayanagi, N., Chiba, H., Matsunaga, T., Kato, J., & Niitsu, Y. (2003). Fatality caused by self-bloodletting in a patient with factitious anemia. *International Journal of Hematology, 78*(2), 146–148. doi:10.1007/BF02983383 PMID:12953809

Jacobs, M. D., Rolle, I., Ferrans, C. E., Whitaker, E. E., & Warnecke, R. B. (2006). Understanding African Americans' View of the Trushworthiness of Physicians. *Journal of General Internal Medicine, 21*(6), 642–647. doi:10.1111/j.1525-1497.2006.00485.x PMID:16808750

Jafferany, M. D., & Mohammad, F. A. P. A. (2018). The Primary Care Companion for CNS Disorders.

Jaghab, K. (2006). Munchausen's Syndrome and Other Factitous Disorder in Children. *Psychiatry (Edgmont, Pa.), 3*(3), 46–55.

Johnson, B. R., & Harrison, J. A. (2000). Suspected Munchausen's syndrome and civil commitment. *The Journal of the American Academy of Psychiatry and the Law, 28*(1), 74–76. PMID:10774844

Kahn, A., Boroff, E. S., Martin, K. A., Northfelt, D. W., & Heigh, R. I. (2015). Factitious disorder in Crohn's disease: Recurrent pancytopenia caused by surreptitious ingestion of 6-Mercaptopurine. *Case Reports in Gastroenterology, 9*(2), 137–141. doi:10.1159/000382073 PMID:26078732

Kanaan, R. A., & Wessely, S. C. (2010). Factitious disorders in neurology: An analysis of reported cases. *Psychosomatics, 51*(1), 47–54. doi:10.1016/S0033-3182(10)70658-7 PMID:20118440

Kapfhammer, H. P., Rothenhäusler, H. B., Dietrich, E., Dobmeier, P., & Mayer, C. (1998). Artifactual disorders–between deception and self-mutilation. Experiences in consultation psychiatry at a university clinic. *Der Nervenarzt*, *69*(5), 401–409. doi:10.1007001150050289 PMID:9629556

Kendler, K. S., Thornton, L. M., & Gardner, C. O. (2000). Stressful life events and previous episodes in the etiology of major depression in women: An evaluation of the "kindling" hypothesis. *The American Journal of Psychiatry*, *157*(8), 1. doi:10.1176/appi.ajp.157.8.1243 PMID:10910786

Kenedi, C. A., Shirey, K. G., Hoffa, M., Zanga, J., Lee, J. C., & Harrison, J. D. (2011). Laboratory diagnosis of factitious disorder: A systematic review of tools useful in the diagnosis of Munchausen's syndrome. *The New Zealand Medical Journal*, *124*(1342), 66–81. PMID:21963927

King, T. F., Shea, P. O., Sullivan, E. P., Srinivasan, R., Griffin, A., Fitzgerald, R., Tormey, W., & Smith, D. (2008). An apparent phaeochromocytoma and abnormal thyroid function tests. *Annals of Clinical Biochemistry*, *45*(2), 215–217. doi:10.1258/acb.2007.007106 PMID:18325190

King, T. F., Shea, P. O., Sullivan, E. P., Srinivasan, R., Griffin, A., Fitzgerald, R., Tormey, W., & Smith, D. (2008). An apparent phaeochromocytoma and abnormal thyroid function tests. *Annals of Clinical Biochemistry*, *45*(2), 215–217. doi:10.1258/acb.2007.007106 PMID:18325190

Kinns, H., Housley, D., & Freedman, D. B. (2013). Munchausen syndrome and factitious disorder: The role of the laboratory in its detection and diagnosis. *Annals of Clinical Biochemistry*, *50*(3), 194–203. doi:10.1177/0004563212473280 PMID:23592802

Klonsky, E. D., Oltmanns, T. F., & Turkheimer, E. (2014). Deliberate self-harm in a nonclinical population: Prevalence and psychological correlates. *The American Journal of Psychiatry*, 9. PMID:12900314

Koufagued, K., Chafry, B., Benyass, Y., Abissegue, Y., Benchebba, D., Bouabid, S., & Belkacem, C. (2015). Munchausen syndrome revealed by subcutaneous limb emphysema: A case report. *Journal of Medical Case Reports*, *9*(1), 1–4. doi:10.118613256-015-0649-x PMID:26282124

Koufagued, K., Chafry, B., Benyass, Y., Abissegue, Y., Benchebba, D., Bouabid, S., & Belkacem, C. (2015). Munchausen syndrome revealed by subcutaneous limb emphysema: A case report. *Journal of Medical Case Reports*, *9*(1), 1–4. doi:10.118613256-015-0649-x PMID:26282124

Krahn, L., Li, H., & O'Connor, M.K. (2014). Patients who strive to be ill: factitious disorder with physical symptoms. *Am J Psychiatry, 9*.

Lande, R. Gregory, Williams, MC USA (Ret), Lisa Banks, MSN, APRN-BC. (2013). Prevalence and Characteristics of Military Malingering. *Oxford Academic Journal Article*, *178*(1), 50–54. PMID:23356119

Lawlor, A., & Kirakowski, J. (2014). When the lie is the truth: Grounded theory analysis of an online support group for factitious disorder. *Psychiatry Research*, *218*(1), 209–218. doi:10.1016/j.psychres.2014.03.034 PMID:24745468

Levenson, J. L., Chafe, W., & Flanagan, P. (2007, January). (207). Factitious ovarian cancer: Feigning via resources on the internet. *Psychosomatics*, *48*(1), 71–73. doi:10.1176/appi.psy.48.1.71 PMID:17209154

Libow, J. A. (2000). Child and adolescent illness falsification. *Pediatrics*, *105*(2), 336–342. doi:10.1542/peds.105.2.336 PMID:10654952

Lin, J. L., Servat, J. J., Bernardino, C. R., Goldberg, R. A., & Levin, F. (2012). Bilateral corneal perforations and autoproptosis as self-induced manifestations of ocular Munchausen's syndrome. *Orbit (Amsterdam, Netherlands)*, *31*(4), 252–255. doi:10.3109/01676830.2012.669013 PMID:22571651

Livaoğlu, M., Kerimoğlu, S., Hocaoğlu, C., Arvas, L., & Karacal, N. (2008). Munchausen's syndrome: A rare self-mutilation syndrome. *Dermatologic Surgery*, *34*(9), 1288–1291. doi:10.1097/00042728-200809000-00024 PMID:18616542

Mailis-Gagnon, A., Nicholson, K., Blumberger, D., & Zurowski, M. (2008). Characteristics and period prevalence of self-induced disorder in patients referred to a pain clinic with the diagnosis of complex regional pain syndrome. *The Clinical Journal of Pain*, *24*(2), 176–185. doi:10.1097/AJP.0b013e31815ca278 PMID:18209524

Maur, K. V., Wasson, K. R., DeFord, J. W., & Caranasos, G. J. (1973). Munchausen's syndrome: A thirty-year history of peregrination par excellence. *Southern Medical Journal*, *66*(6), 629. doi:10.1097/00007611-197306000-00001 PMID:4733204

Mayo Clinic. (2019). *Factitious Discorder*. Middlesex Heatlth.

McEwen, D. R. (1998). Recognizing Munchausen's syndrome. *J Assoc Perioper Regist Nurs*, *67*(2), 440–442. PMID:9505125

Mehta, N. J., & Khan, I. A. (2002). Cardiac Munchausen syndrome. *Chest*, *122*(5), 1649–1653. doi:10.1378/chest.122.5.1649 PMID:12426266

Muacevic, A., Adler, J. R., Sinha, A., & Smolik, T. (2021). Striving to Die: Medical, Legal, and Ethical Dilemmas Behind Factitous Disorder. *Cureus Publishing Beyond Open Access, 13*(2), e13243.

Nichols, G. R. II, Davis, G. J., & Corey, T. S. (1990). In the shadow of the baron: Sudden death due to Munchausen syndrome. *The American Journal of Emergency Medicine, 8*(3), 216–219. doi:10.1016/0735-6757(90)90326-U PMID:2184806

Nishimura, K., Kobayashi, S., Sugawara, H., Nakajima, I., Ishida, H., Fuchinoue, S., Tanabe, K., & Ishigooka, J. (2012). Psychiatric consultation after kidney transplantation: A 10-year single-center study including outpatients in Japan. *International Journal of Psychiatry in Medicine, 43*(3), 197–209. doi:10.2190/PM.43.3.a PMID:22978079

Nishimura, K., Kobayashi, S., Sugawara, H., Nakajima, I., Ishida, H., Fuchinoue, S., Tanabe, K., & Ishigooka, J. (2012). Psychiatric consultation after kidney transplantation: A 10-year single-center study including outpatients in Japan. *International Journal of Psychiatry in Medicine, 43*(3), 197–209. doi:10.2190/PM.43.3.a PMID:22978079

Norcliffe-Kaufmann, L., Gonzalez-Duarte, A., Martinez, J., & Kaufmann, H. (2010). Tachyarrythmias with elevated cardiac enzymes in Münchausen syndrome. *Clinical Autonomic Research, 20*(4), 259–261. doi:10.100710286-010-0066-6 PMID:20424883

Norman, R.E., Byambaa, M., Butchart, J., Scott, T., & Vos. (2012). *The long-term health consequences of child physical abuse, emotional abuse, and neglect.* NIH.

O'Reilly, R. A., & Aggeler, P. M. (1976). Covert anticoagulant ingestion: Study of 25 patients and review of world literature. *Medicine, 55*(5), 389–399. doi:10.1097/00005792-197609000-00003 PMID:957998

Ogbonmwan, S. E., & Abidogun, K. (2008). A variant of Munchausen syndrome presenting as a gynaecological emergency. *British Journal of Hospital Medicine (London, England), 69*(7), 414–415. doi:10.12968/hmed.2008.69.7.30421 PMID:18833980

Oner, E., Unlu, M., Solgun, B., Kocyigit, H., & Cimen, P. (2015). Munchausen's syndrome: Hemoptysis, hematochezia, hematuria. *Journal of Evolution of Medical and Dental Sciences*, 8091.

Otowa, T., Gardner, C. O., Kendler, K. S., & Hettema, J. M. (2013). Parenting and risk for mood, anxiety and substance use disorders: A study in population-based male twins. *Social Psychiatry and Psychiatric Epidemiology*, *48*(11), 1841–1849. doi:10.100700127-013-0656-4 PMID:23344783

Parent, D. J., Krafft, T., Noel, J. C., Askenasi, R., Goldschmidt, D., Heenen, M., & Linkowski, P. (1994). Cutaneous Münchausen syndrome with presentation simulating pyoderma gangrenosum. *Journal of the American Academy of Dermatology*, *31*(6), 1072–1074. doi:10.1016/S0190-9622(09)80093-5 PMID:7962767

Pascual, A., Miguélez, A., Vanaclocha, F., Rubio, G., & Iglesias, L. (2001). Periocular and perioral artefactual dermatitis: Dermatological and psychiatric management in a hospital setting. *Dermatol Psychosom*, *2*(4), 200–202. doi:10.1159/000049672

Patenaude, B., Zitsch, R. III, & Hirschi, S. D. (2006). Blood — but not bleeding — at a tracheotomy site: A case of Munchausen's syndrome. *Ear, Nose, and Throat Journal*, *85*(10), 677–679. doi:10.1177/014556130608501020 PMID:17124944

Petersdorf, R. G., & Beeson, P. B. (1961). Fever of unexplained origin: Report on 100 cases. *Medicine*, *40*(1), 1–30. doi:10.1097/00005792-196102000-00001 PMID:13734791

Plassmann, R. (1994). Münchhausen syndromes and factitious diseases. *Psychotherapy and Psychosomatics*, *62*(1–2), 7–26. doi:10.1159/000288899 PMID:7984770

Reich, J. D. &, Hanno, P. (1997). Factitious Renal Colic. *Science Direct*, *50*(6), 858–862. PMID:9426714

Reich, P., & Gottfried, L. A. (1983). Factitious Disorder in a Teaching Hospital. *Clinical Review*.

Reich, P., & Gottfried, L. A. (1983). Factitious disorders in a teaching hospital. *Annals of Internal Medicine*, *99*(2), 240–247. doi:10.7326/0003-4819-99-2-240 PMID:6881779

Released, S. I. (2015). *SPSS statistics for windows, version 23.0*. SPSS Inc.

Robertson, M. M., & Hossain, G. (1997). Munchausen's syndrome coexisting with other disorders. *British Journal of Hospital Medicine*, *58*(4), 154–155. PMID:9373405

Rodríguez-Pichardo, A., Hoffner, M. V., García-Bravo, B., & Camacho, F. M. (2010). (19976-2006) Dermatitis artefacta of the breast: A retrospective analysis of 27 patients. Eur. *J. Acad Dermatol Venereol*, *24*(3), 270–274. doi:10.1111/j.1468-3083.2009.03403.x PMID:19694893

Rodríguez-Pichardo, A., Hoffner, M. V., García-Bravo, B., & Camacho, F. M. (2010). Dermatitis artefacta of the breast: A retrospective analysis of 27 patients (1976–2006). *Journal of the European Academy of Dermatology and Venereology, 24*(3), 270–274. doi:10.1111/j.1468-3083.2009.03403.x PMID:19694893

Romano, A., Alqahtani, S., Griffith, J., & Koubeissi, M. Z. (2014). Factitious psychogenic nonepileptic paroxysmal episodes. *Epilepsy & Behavior Case Reports, 2*, 184–185. doi:10.1016/j.ebcr.2014.08.006 PMID:25667902

Rotton, J., Foos, P. W., Van Meek, L., & Levitt, M. (1995). Publication practices and the file drawer problem: A survey of published authors. *Journal of Social Behavior and Personality*.

Rumans, L. W., & Vosti, K. L. (1978). Factitious and fraudulent fever. *The American Journal of Medicine, 65*(5), 745–755. doi:10.1016/0002-9343(78)90792-1 PMID:707533

Saiyasombat, M. I., & Satyanarayan, M. (2012). Pancytopenia secondary to cyclophosphamide in a case of factitious breast cancer. *The Primary Care Companion for CNS Disorders, 14*(2). doi:10.4088/PCC.11l01301 PMID:22943027

Sakado, K., Kuwabara, H., Sato, T., Uehara, T., Sakado, T., & Someya, T. (2000). The relationship between personality, dysfunctional parenting in childhood, and lifetime depression in a sample of employed Japanese adults. *Journal of Affective Disorders, 60*(1), 47–51. doi:10.1016/S0165-0327(99)00150-0 PMID:10940447

Savino, A. C., & Fordtran, J. S. (2006). Factitious disease: Clinical lessons from case studies at Baylor University Medical Center. *Proceedings - Baylor University. Medical Center, 19*(3), 195–208. doi:10.1080/08998280.2006.11928162 PMID:17252033

Schmidt, F., Strutz, F., Quellhorst, E., & Müller, G. A. (1996). Nephrectomy and solitary kidney biopsy in a patient with Munchausen's syndrome. *Nephrology, Dialysis, Transplantation, 11*(5), 890–892. doi:10.1093/oxfordjournals.ndt.a027424 PMID:8671920

Schulz, B., & Strauch, R. J. (2008). A case of factitious subfascial emphysema. *Orthopedics, 31*(5), 495. doi:10.3928/01477447-20080501-26 PMID:19292308

Sheridan, M. S. (2003). The deceit continues: An updated literature review of Munchausen syndrome by proxy. *Child Abuse & Neglect, 27*(4), 431–451. doi:10.1016/S0145-2134(03)00030-9 PMID:12686328

Sowislo, J. F., & Orth, U. (2013). Does low self-esteem predict depression and anxiety? A meta-analysis of longitudinal studies. *Psychological Bulletin, 139*(1), 213–240. doi:10.1037/a0028931 PMID:22730921

Steel, R. M. (2009). Factitious disorder (Munchausen's syndrome). *Journal of the Royal College of Physicians of Edinburgh, 39*(4), 343–347. doi:10.4997/JRCPE.2009.412 PMID:21152477

Stiles, A., Mitrirattanakul, S., & Sanders, B. (2001). Munchausen syndrome presenting in a patient who has undergone temporomandibular joint surgery. Oral surgery, oral medicine, oral pathology, oral radiology, and. *Endodontology, 91*(1), 20–22.

Stroud, C. B., Davila, J., & Moyer, A. (2008). The relationship between stress and depression in first onsets versus recurrences: A meta-analytic review. *Journal of Abnormal Psychology, 117*(1), 206–213. doi:10.1037/0021-843X.117.1.206 PMID:18266498

Sutherland, Amanda J., & Rodin, G. (1990). Factitous Disorder in a General Hospital Setting: Clinical Features and a Review of the Literature. *Psychosomatics, 31*(4), 392–399. doi:10.1016/S0033-3182(90)72133-0 PMID:2247566

Svirsky, J. A., & Sawyer, D. R. (1987). Dermatitis artefacta of the paraoral region. *Oral Surgery, Oral Medicine, and Oral Pathology, 64*(2), 259–263. doi:10.1016/0030-4220(87)90101-0 PMID:3476905

Thynne, T., White, G. H., & Burt, M. G. (2014). Factitious Cushing's syndrome masquerading as Cushing's disease. *Clinical Endocrinology, 80*(3), 328–332. doi:10.1111/cen.12343 PMID:24111609

Vaduganathan, M., McCullough, S. A., Fraser, T. N., & Stern, T. A. (2014). Death due to Munchausen syndrome: A case of idiopathic recurrent right ventricular failure and a review of the literature. *Psychosomatics, 6*(55), 668–672. doi:10.1016/j.psym.2014.05.013 PMID:25262044

van der Feltz-Cornelis, C. M. (2002). The Impact of Factitous Disorder on the Physician-Patient Relationship. An Epistemological Model, Medicine, Heatlth. *Care and Philosophy, 5*, 253–261. PMID:12517033

Whisman, M. A., Sheldon, C., & Goering, P. (2000). Psychiatric disorders and dissatisfaction with social relationships: Does type of relationship matter? *Journal of Abnormal Psychology, 109*(4), 803–808. doi:10.1037/0021-843X.109.4.803 PMID:11196008

Wojewoda, K., Brenner, J., Kąkol, M., Naesström, M., Cubała, W. J., Kozicka, D., Nowicki, R., Sokołowska-Wojdyło, M., & Barańska-Rybak, W. (2012). A cry for help, do not omit the signs. Dermatitis artefacta — Psychiatric problems in dermatological diseases (a review of 5 cases). *Medical Science Monitor, 18*(10), CS85–CS89. doi:10.12659/MSM.883474 PMID:23018360

Wojewoda, K., Brenner, J., Kąkol, M., Naesström, M., Cubała, W. J., Kozicka, D., Nowicki, R., Sokołowska-Wojdyło, M., & Barańska-Rybak, W. (2012). A cry for help, do not omit the signs. Dermatitis artefacta — Psychiatric problems in dermatological diseases (a review of 5 cases). *Medical Science Monitor, 18*(10), CS85–CS89. doi:10.12659/MSM.883474 PMID:23018360

World Health Organization. (1948). The sixth revision of the International Statistical Classification of diseases, injuries and causes of death (ICD-6),

World Health Organization. (1992). *The ICD-10 classification of mental and behavioural disorders: clinical descriptions and diagnostic guidelines.* World Health Organization.

Zamir, E., Read, R. W., & Rao, N. A. (2001). Self-inflicted anterior scleritis. *Ophthalmology, 108*(1), 192–195. doi:10.1016/S0161-6420(00)00480-2 PMID:11150288

Chapter 6
Obsessive-Compulsive Disorder and the African-American Experience

Marian Edwards Ellis
Clarksville Independent School District, USA

ABSTRACT

The purpose of this chapter is to examine obsessive-compulsive disorder (OCD) and its debilitating effects on millions of people world-wide, specifically, African Americans. OCD is often times comorbid and affects various ages, genders, races, ethnicities, in the areas of one's mental health, physical health, social life, family relationships, and employment. Findings include causation and contributory factors such as but not limited to discrimination, racism, environment, lack of knowledge, mistrust in healthcare, mistrust in research studies, bias curriculum, and/or neurological impairments. Another purpose of this study is to awaken the need for mental health services in the African American culture and reduce the stigma attached.

OBSESSIVE-COMPULSIVE DISORDER

What is Obsessive-Compulsive Disorder?

Obsessive-compulsive disorder (OCD) got its definition in the 1990s when the diagnostic manual used by mental health professionals, the Diagnostic and Statistical Manual of Mental Disorders, fourth edition, text revision (DSM-IV-TR), listed OCD as a "severe anxiety disorder" (Davis, 2008, p.5), which is "characterized by uncontrollable intrusive thoughts and action that can only be alleviated by patterns

DOI: 10.4018/978-1-6684-8918-5.ch006

of rigid and ceremonial behavior" (p. 8). The symptoms caused by OCD could be so debilitating that the individual afflicted can no longer function with day-to-day commonalities. Individuals who suffer from OCD are often prone to anxiety and devote significant time to challenges associated with their condition which negatively impacts their relationships and daily routines (p. 8).

Margolis (Ed.) (2002) stated that OCD is the "recurrent, repetitive thoughts (obsessions), behaviors (compulsions), or both that a person recognizes as unreasonable, unnecessary, or foolish yet are intrusive and cannot be resisted" (p. 99). People with OCD do not necessarily have both obsessions and compulsions. They may have one or the other. Obsessions are recurring thoughts of fear of germs or mistakes and/or harming oneself or others. Compulsions differ from obsessions in that they are repetitive actions of rechecking the same things over and over such as windows, doors, locks, refrigerators, appliances, washing of hands, and so on. The largest percentage of people diagnosed with OCD are those in their early adulthood (p. 99). Although this disorder may be hidden using other nonproductive agents like addictions to alcohol or drugs, it can lead to depression.

Because various research and data proved the differences between anxiety disorders and OCD, the DSM-V removed OCD from anxiety disorders and placed it in its own category as 'Obsessive-Compulsive and Related Disorders' (Ameringen, Patterson, & Simpson, 2014, p. 487). For example, Marker and Aylward (2012) found that OCD and Generalized Anxiety Disorder (GAD) were not synonymous because OCD has more negative outcomes. GAD is generally anxiety and worry about everyday situations, whereas the thoughts and worries, that come with OCD, are more detrimental to one's health such as incongruities about one's life. In contrast, people diagnosed with GAD generally do not use compulsions to rid their continuous thoughts (p. 6). Thus, the decision was made to give OCD "its own chapter" (Ameringen, Patterson, & Simpson, 2014, p. 487).

With OCD becoming OCRD, various other disorders with similarities have been grouped into the category such as "body dysmorphic disorder (BDD), trichotillomania (TTM-hair-pulling disorder), excoriation (skin-picking) disorder, hoarding disorder, substance/medication-induced OCRD, OCRD due to another condition, and other specified OCRDs" (Ameringen et al. 2014, p. 487). The researchers concluded that having one of these diagnoses does not rule out all others and that practitioners should recognize that these are related disorders and not "subtypes" (p. 492).

A REVIEW OF THE LITERATURE

Historical Overview

Before (OCD) was classified as a disease or disorder, the focus was on obsessions. These obsessions were most often linked to sexual behaviors or thoughts of dangerous love (Davis, 2008, p. 9). Researchers also studied compulsions which fell into various categories such as "cleaning, checking, and counting" (p.9). Another extension of the disorder explored was Obsessive-Compulsive Personality Disorder (OCPD), which is not a disorder but a personality. The International OCD Foundation defined OCDP as the following:

OCPD is a type of "personality disorder" with these characteristics:

- Rigid adherence to rules and regulations
- An overwhelming need for order
- Unwillingness to yield or give responsibilities to others
- A sense of righteousness about the way things 'should be.' ("What is OCPD?", para. 1)

People diagnosed with OCPD do not realize that their obsessions are obsessive or erroneous.

Davis (2008) compared three different views of past research on OCD and the many problems that occur: medical, psychological, or physiological. Although the researcher does not agree with all three of these angles, he asserted that the phenomena has been "understood in different ways at different times" (p. 24). Additionally, it was once thought that obsessive thoughts only happened to demon-possessed persons because "patients [experienced] horrific, repugnant, threatening, dangerous [thoughts which were]…immoral, sinful disgusting, revealing, dangerous, threatening, alarming, predictive, insane, bewildering, and criminal" (Davis, 2008, p. 15; Krochmalik & Menzies, 2003). Although not the first to theorize this disorder, Freud (1896) posited that obsessional ideas were related to childhood sexual pleasures (as cited in Krochmalik & Menzies, 2003, pp. 4-5; Davis, 2008). Davis devoted an entire chapter to Freud and his obsession with psychoanalysis (p. 127) and obsessional neurosis (p. 132). One might hypothesize that Freud (1893) was correct in his analysis that "no efforts have yet succeeded in making a coherent synthesis of all its variations" regarding OCD (as cited in Davis, 1983, p. 142).

Calle-Ramirez et al. (2022) posited "during the COVID-19 pandemic, the health crisis caused some people to be more susceptible to OCD ("Introduction," para. 2). Thus, Calle-Ramirez et al. reviewed the number of OCD published articles internationally during the COVID-19 pandemic. Due to the restraints of mobility during the pandemic, studies have shown an increase in "anxiety-related disorders, including OCD" ("Introduction," para. 2). Using the *SCOPUS* database, one of the largest databases with approximately 40,804 journals, Calle-Ramirez et al. found 391 articles published which were connected to a higher education or research institution and focusing on OCD during the pandemic. The most published papers were produced by Eric Storch of Baylor College of Medicine in the United States during the COVID-19 pandemic ("Table 5"). Although other countries produced papers that were cited in Calle-Ramirez et al., for the purpose of this chapter, the focus is on primarily the United States, OCD, and African Americans; nevertheless, the researchers did find that the United States had "the highest scientific production on OCD, accounting [for] 24.6%" during COVID-19 ("Results," para. 2).

OCD AND THE AFRICAN AMERICAN EXPERIENCE

Misdiagnosis Amongst African American Adults

Not all diagnostic instruments are created equal, nor do they produce equivalent results when it pertains to African Americans. Williams, La Torre, and Sharif (2020) also addressed issues with various diagnostic instruments, such as the Maudsley Obsessional Compulsive Inventory (MOCI), Padua Inventory, and the Structured DSM-IV Clinical Interview Axis I Disorders. Researchers have not agreed on the accuracy of these diagnostics when it comes to outcomes for African Americans' accurate diagnoses. However, most researchers agreed that the Yale-Brown Obsessive Compulsive Scale (Y-BOCS) was found to be the most effective (Williams et al., 2020, p. 9).

Chasson, Williams, Davis, and Combs (2017) conducted a study analyzing structured interviews using the results of the DSM-IV Axis I disorders (SCID-I) and African Americans' misdiagnosis. Seventy-four African American adults with OCD were recruited by the University of Pennsylvania School of Medicine at the Center for the Treatment and Study of Anxiety ("Methods," paras. 1-2). Participants' educational levels varied from 7-12 years of high school through graduate or professional school. The assessment was given by "trained master and doctoral-level community clinicians and doctoral-level expert OCD interviewers" ("Measures," para. 1). Participants were given the following scales: Y-BOCS, Brown assessment of beliefs scale (BABS), Obsessive beliefs questionnaire-brief version (OBQ-44), Obsessive-compulsive inventory-revised (OCI-R), Beck depression inventory-II (BDI-II), Global assessment of functioning (GAF), Clinical global impression (CGI), and Clinical global impression (CGI) (paras. 6-12). Since clinicians in this study were not employees of the university, community therapists "attended reliability meetings and...training" ("Procedures," para. 2). As predicted, the Y-BOCS was more accurate in its diagnosis of OCD versus the SCID-OCD with African Americans. Chasson et al. (2017) suggested a need for questions to be added to the SCID-OCD regarding symptoms "common" to African Americans to improve its efficacy ("Discussion," para. 5).

OCD and Alcoholism

Over a six-month frame, Cobb and Assari (2019) sought correlations between alcoholism and gender differences among low-income African Americans living in the South Los Angeles area. The researchers cross-referenced comorbid psychiatric disorders. One hundred and fifty classified participants were ages 45 and up with at least one psychiatric disorder, including OCD. Because the focus of this study was on substance disorder (SUD) with alcoholism versus a non-substance disorder (non-SUD) cooccurrence ("Background," para. 1), specificities with regard to the various mental illnesses were not discussed. This study revealed that low-income African American men with at least one psychiatric disorder had a higher use of alcohol than low-income African American women; even though the women outnumbered the men in this study 2:1.

Racism and Mistrust

Research on men's health shows African Americans who experience racism may have a higher rate of mental health issues (Wong & Wester, 2016, p. 738; Williams et al., 2021). Additionally, English (1983) noted that "Black men proportionately [had] the highest rate of mental disorders as compared to other age and racial groups, especially for those between the ages 18 and 34" and were admitted to mental institutions at far greater rates than Whites and "suffer[ed] fatalities from psychoses and neuroses" (p. 10). Thus, African Americans were less likely to receive accurate diagnoses or selected for specialized therapies. Another finding was that "racism, discrimination, poverty, migration, urbanization, and similar factors [were all] related to mental health" (English, 1983, p.15). English firmly believed that considering minorities' cultures were important when establishing healthcare practices and stated the following:

In order to strengthen healthcare practices to produce better outcomes for ethnic minorities, their culture must be taken into account. Practices must be relevant and responsive and considerate of minority/ethnic worldviews. Four categories: 1) bicultural/multicultural, 2) acculturated/assimilated, 3) native-oriented/traditional, 4) transitional/marginal. (p. 18)

From the review of the literature, many researchers are echoing the sentiment of needed change when it comes to training and educating practitioners.

As with other researchers, Williams, LaTorre, and Sharif (2020) agreed that practitioners should approach ethnic clients with a "multiculturalist and anti-racist" lens (p. 2). Williams et al. added that the stigma, stereotypes, or "traumatic experiences" (p. 6) that haunt ethnic minorities, particularly African Americans, maybe the cause of OCD such as images of police brutality during the Civil Rights Movement or the contamination theory of Black people being unclean (p. 6). These negative images could produce self-identity issues within the African American population. Self-perception and positive ethnic identity may be a solution to OCD because "strong positive ethnic identity can provide resilience in the face of discrimination" (p. 2). African Americans adults who are afflicted with OCD and parents of children with OCD may fear the threat of discrimination when searching for treatment options, which "evoke feelings of shame, fear, or stigma" (Kolvenbach et al., 2018; Williams et al., 2020, p. 7).

Researchers found that the first instance of an African American OCD diagnosis was found during a dermatology experiment in New York where African Americans were seeking treatment for skin issues due to excessive washing (Williams et al., 2020, p. 6). These instances brought the contamination theory to the forefront with African Americans experiencing "contamination symptoms at twice the rate of European Americans" (Wheaton et al., 2013; Williams et al., 2020, p. 6).

Williams (2007) conducted a qualitative study on the racial differences in OCD. Using an exploratory factor analysis (EFA) with a mixture of Padua and additional cleanliness items, Williams discovered that "there was a substantial racial difference on almost all items in the direction of Blacks expressing more concern regarding contamination on the Padua items and expressing greater concern about cleanliness and personal appearance on the attitude items" (p. 49). Through Williams' (2007) four-study analysis, it can be concluded that cleanliness may be an African American tradition versus an OCD symptom and that finding valid instruments to measure OCD with regard to cultural differences is important to receiving reliable outcomes. Interesting findings were things such as Blacks being less likely to desire a pet or touch an animal without feeling dirty or having the need to wash hands due to concerns about germs (p. 49).

Wheaton, Berman, Berman, Fabricant, and Abramowitz (2013) assessed obsessive-compulsive group differences between symptoms and beliefs across various populations, such as Whites, African Americans, Latinos, and Asians. However, for the purpose of this review, the focus is on the comparison between the dominant culture and that of African Americans. Over 1600 hundred university students from "Introductory Psychology" participated in self-report measures, with approximately 75% White and 13% African Americans participating (p. 11). The students completed the Dimensional Obsessive – Compulsive Scale (DOCS), rating "five items…a) time occupied by obsessions and rituals, b) avoiding behavior, c) associated distress, d) functional interference, and e) difficulty disregarding the obsessions and …compulsions" (p. 12). During the data analysis using a one-way ANOVA, Cronbach's alpha revealed African Americans were slightly higher on the scale than Whites or European Americans for overall DOCS total, contamination, and unacceptable thoughts (p. 13). African American group means (SDs) were slightly higher in all areas using the DOCS: total score, contamination, responsibility for harm, unacceptable thoughts, and symmetry (p. 13). However, the group means on the OBQ were slightly higher only in the areas of total score, responsibility/threat, and importance/control of thoughts (p. 13). The findings of this study suggested that there was no significance in contamination for African Americans even though their DOCS scale was higher; however, it may not have been detected on the OBQ. Additionally, the group membership was a predictor "between obsessive beliefs and unacceptable thoughts" (p. 18).

Regarding the consequences of racism and the African American experience, Walker (2020) emphasized that people of color should be involved in research studies that involve Black cultural phenomena. Walker stated that "if people of African descent are not involved in generating the hypothesis or question that forms the basis of research, the study could be ill-informed from the outset" (p. 68). She explored the various deceitful studies of the past such as the Tuskegee syphilis experiment, J. Marion Sims' gynecological experiment, and the African Holocaust (p. 69). For reasons such as these, Walker concluded that it is difficult for African Americans to trust experiments and the world of research.

Regarding the Tuskegee Experiment and its lasting effects, Ruffins (1998) explored the development of conspiracy theories amongst the Black community. Ruffins noted the work of Gorelick and colleagues who studied the extent to which African Americans were in fear of being used as a "guinea pig" ("Bad for Black Health," para. 9). Ruffins reported the shortage of bone marrow transplants for African Americans versus Whites due to the lack of the African American participants as bone marrow donors and being able to find a possible match in their time of need (paras. 12-13). Ruffins did note that between 1993-1996, the number of African American donors increased from 22% to 42% (para. 15).

Bazargan, Cobb, and Assari (2021) questioned "How do we move from mistrust to a state of trust?" (p. 11). The researchers suggested addressing bias and prejudices within medical practices as the key, suggesting extensive training, and "implementing strategies that increase power-sharing and trust-building mechanisms" (p. 11). Their focus was on discovering ways to reach those patients who are generally overlooked and undervalued. They reviewed a study of 4,389 where 30% of their participants were African American, and the outcome was the belief that outside factors affect medical participation such as police brutality, and discrimination based on race, income, and language spoken (p. 11).

Walker (2020) agreed with other experts that "racial discrimination is psychologically and physically harmful to Black people" (p. 70). A study of 343 Black women in Detroit, Michigan, revealed that those who were exposed to discrimination more often were poorer in health and had more instances of depression. Walker also found that these individuals were linked to more diagnoses of atherosclerosis, a health condition caused by smoking and having high cholesterol (p. 71).

Walker's (2020) intent in writing about the unequal mental health system towards African Americans was to provide an open and honest conversation on the past, present, and future and bring awareness to the importance of psychological fortitude (PF), the ability to reason, control one's feelings, and problem solve. Some people might describe PF as mental toughness or mental fortitude. Walker stated that "good research that is developed with [Black people] in mind can facilitate higher PF" (p. 78).

Another point Walker (2020) made was the danger of assimilation and the "alien-self disorder" (p. 91). The fear of not fitting in with the dominant culture has caused many African Americans to lose a sense of self-identity and their culture. This is the alien-self disorder, coined by Akbar (1991), which is when the individual no longer fits in with his own culture, denies racism, and mostly relates to the dominant culture (as cited in Walker). Walker pointed out that the person of African descent does not want to bring any negative attention to himself that would be different from what is considered acceptable to the White race (p. 91).

Orem (2017) analyzed OCD within the main character within the TV series, *Grey's Anatomy*. Although Dr. Bailey is a fictionalized character on this show, the obsessions, and compulsions she faced are real to many people of color in America. Orem (2017) recognized the hypocritical nature of economic and political systems and the stereotypical discourse regarding Black women with OCD in America as compared to White men. Bailey's character was portrayed as someone whose OCD interfered with her work as a surgeon and therefore could potentially lead to disastrous ends; however, the characters of White men such as "*Monk's* Adrian Monk, *Scrubs'* Kevin Casey, or Melvin Udall of *As Good as It Gets*...bestows nearly superhuman talents that render them highly intelligent and capable of excelling in their careers.... [indicating] genius and career excellence" (p. 173). Orem also observed the easy access Bailey had to mental health treatment in this parody however contrary that may be to the average African American (p. 181).

African American Children Studies

Harris and Graham (2007) asserted that African American children were often identified with mental health issues far more so than their White counterparts (p. 66). Dawson (1991) stated that "African-American children who live in families with a history of mental illness, who experience multiple moves, experience homelessness, and live in violent neighborhoods, are at high risk for the adverse mental health outcomes discussed in the Insiders' Voice (as cited in Harris and Graham, 2007, p. 66). Harris and Graham implied that controversy over using the proper diagnostic tools has been a focus for years. They argued that tools such as the DSM-IV do not consider important factors that could influence the results of the assessment such as "cultural, socio-political, and environmental" (p. 70). An important argument is that African American children were more often misdiagnosed due to mental health professionals "lack of knowledge and subsequent inaccurate assessments or diagnoses" (p.80).

According to Kolvenbach, Fernández de la Cruz, Mataix-Cols, Patel, and Jassi (2018), the incidence of OCD is seen in comparable numbers within all ethnic groups. The researchers noted that despite these similarities, treatment access has not been equal, and barriers have been present for ethnic minorities (p. 99). Possible reasons provided included treatment costs, limited healthcare knowledge, health belief system variations, and not having local access to clinical services. The purpose of the study was to assess the barriers that may hinder access to OCD specialist services for children belonging to different ethnic backgrounds (p. 100). A qualitative study, consisting of "20 transcribed interviews" was conducted by interviewing parents of children from white and ethnic minority backgrounds (p. 100). The subjects "were recruited from the National and Specialist OCD, BDD, and Related Disorders Clinic for Young People... [located in] London, United Kingdom" (p. 100). The interviews included questions that assessed their opinions related to treatment access based on their personal experience. The information was analyzed using a thematic approach to interpret the meaning or themes present (p. 100).

Kolvenbach et al.'s (2018) sample participants were 20 parents whose backgrounds were White and people of color across the UK. Common barriers were deemed present for both respondent groups such as "lack of knowledge...regarding mental health issues" and resources. The limitations may have been negative prior encounters, limited health resources, time and financial constraints, and trust challenges concerning the mental health system (p. 101). The researchers recommended that policymakers consider these factors when devising healthcare and other policies for all minority populations, even those outside of the United States.

Additionally, Latzman et al. (2011) found a significant difference between African American girls across three cohorts of school-age children (elementary, middle, and high school) with symptoms of anxiety which included OCD; however, they did not find significance between boys as compared to their White counterparts. Students were given the Revised Child Anxiety and Depression Scale (RCADS), a DSM-based scale. This study was conducted through the University of Mississippi's and the Mississippi Children's Home Services" (p. 337).

Recruitment Efforts

The research presented by Coles, Heimberg, Barry, and Weiss (2013) was an examination of the factors that contributed to the underdiagnosis of,and limited service utilized by African Americans with OCD. They found that out of "20 clinical trials...only 1.3% of participants were African American" (p. 779). The authors proposed that despite the widespread availability of effective treatment options for this type of mental health condition, there may be barriers to treatment access for certain groups of people, facilitated by insufficient mental health literacy (MHL). The researchers assessed the relationships between public knowledge and perception, in addition to other influential factors that may impact MHL on a broad scale to advance the understanding of what leads to substantial rates of incorrect or underdiagnosed OCD cases (Coles et al., 2013).

Coles et al. (2013) utilized a survey method in which 577 adults, who were each selected by the Institute of Survey Research from an initial pool of 10,546 phone numbers within the United States, were asked via telephone to provide input following the verbal description of a scenario involving a person exhibiting OCD symptoms (p. 779). The participants were ruled out if they were not White or Black. The survey was designed to measure the participants' level of OCD recognition, understanding of options available to help those who suffer from the condition, and stigmatization associated with openly discussing related symptoms with others in professional as well as nonprofessional settings (p. 781). The research findings included 90 percent of survey respondents reporting that their recommendation would be to seek professional help for the person whose symptoms were described in the scenario presented to them (p. 782). African Americans were less likely to identify OCD symptoms but could identify symptoms as mental illness. Whites from this study were more likely to seek help from their family physician, and African Americans were less likely to discuss symptoms (p. 782). The authors recommended additional research would be required to address the disparity between this percentage and the significantly lower percentage of individuals who seek professional help for OCD.

Recruitment efforts to gain African American participants in mental health research studies have been challenging. However, studies have shown that African Americans will seek religious advice when faced with adversities. Michalopoulou, Falzarano, and Rosenberg (2009) conducted an OCD study recruiting African Americans to participate (p. 72). Two sets of literature "brochures" were created, one of which contained multicultural images (p. 73). Not even this technique enticed African American participants in this study. As other researchers have pointed out, there have been small numbers of Blacks participating in most studies. Michalopoulou et al. (2009) attempted to alleviate these issues by soliciting the help of a Black Detroit pastor and other Black church leaders, using multicultural literature, and specifically targeting the African American community (pp. 78-79). Nevertheless, out of "200 packets," only one was returned from an African American (p. 77). Additionally, Shavers et al. (2001) reported that "sixty-four percent of African American participants [in a separate study within this same geographic location] indicated that they did believe that all racial/ethnic groups share the risks of medical research equally" (Michalopoulou, 2009, p.77). Using a non-standardized assessment instrument and only having one response mode, "standardized mail" were the limitations in this study (p. 79).

Black Caribbeans vs. African Americans

Taylor, Ngugyen, Sinkewicz, Joe, and Chatters (2013) conducted a study in the United States regarding Black Caribbeans in comparison to African Americans and various mental illnesses such as comorbid mood and anxiety disorders since Acosta and de la Cruz (2011) found that Caribbean Americans represent "18% of the foreign-born [U. S. population and] makeup 49% of the immigrant population in New York, 45% in Rhode Island, and 43% in Massachusetts" (as cited in Taylor et al., 2012, p.410). Taylor et al. reported that Caribbean men were more likely to have a psychiatric illness and MDD than U. S. born Black men.

Woodard et al (2008) found that almost half of Black Caribbeans would eventually suffer from a psychiatric disorder (as cited in Tayor et al., 2013, p. 411). The method used in the Taylor et al. study was gleaning information from the National Survey of American Life: Coping with Stress in the 21st Century (NSAL). Over half of the 6,082 participants were African American and 1,621 Black Caribbeans (p. 413). Each person in these two categories classified themselves as black. Male and female participants were equally divided as well.

Taylor et al. (2013) sought correlations in three areas: anxiety disorders, suicide behavior, and substance abuse. Participants were asked what type of medical treatments sought such as "specialty mental health…general medical…and any services… [such as]...religious and spiritual advisors, counselors, and social workers" (pp. 414-415). Interestingly, Black Caribbeans with a comorbid "mood and anxiety" condition had higher use of mental treatment services (p. 418); however, African Americans had a higher percentage of mood and/or anxiety disorders than Black Caribbeans. Of the Black Caribbean sample, only "7.19% had comorbid mood and anxiety disorder, 8.66%...mood disorder only, and 11.46% had an anxiety disorder only" (p. 415). African American percentages almost doubled with 15.19% having a mood disorder only and 17.74% having an anxiety disorder only. Older Black Caribbean men with comorbid disorders were more likely to have higher suicidal thoughts and behaviors and substance abuse than Black Caribbean women (p. 417). Taylor et al. (2013)helped fill a gap in the literature regarding Black Caribbeans within the United States who classify their race as Black.

Williams et al. (2021) explored the mental health of Black Caribbeans as well, specifically pertaining to OCD because "people with OCD have heightened rates of other mental disorders" (p. 54). Their study was a comparison of African American and Black Caribbeans' OCD symptoms with a hypothesis that the lower SES and "self-rated physical and mental health" participants would be more likely to experience increased OCD symptoms (pp. 56-57). The NSAL was also used to glean information for their study. They "assessed...contamination [obsessions]... and unacceptable thoughts.... [along with] four types of compulsive behaviors" (p. 58). The multivariate relationships were analyzed with SAS 9.13. Black Caribbeans and African Americans had similar results regarding obsessions, compulsions, and symptom types; however, the younger generation of Black Caribbeans had a higher rate of OCD symptoms. Moreover, Black Caribbeans were more likely to seek treatment than African Americans. Furthermore, Williams et al. (2021) found a correlation with socioeconomic status as stated in the hypothesis and that psychiatric disorders may make people more "at risk for downward social mobility" (p. 69). This study has added to the body of literature for Black Caribbeans as Williams et al. reported that they were even less likely to be included in research studies than African Americans or grouped together.

Curriculum Development

King, Moody, Thompson, and Bennett (1983) wrote a chapter on moving curriculum development forward focusing on African American culture and including them within the constructs of significant figures in society rather than low-level stereotypes. They asserted the following:

Curriculum development must first address the attempt of existing curricula to render Black people 'outcasts of evolution.' The various curricula do not allow Black people, in any fundamental way, to represent themselves as being in the world, as part of the world and in unity with it....Second, curriculum development must address existing curricula that are designed to render Black people 'powerless'.... Third, curriculum development must attend to curricula that do not allow Black people to bring about change in their human condition....These three elements form the core of the problem. pp. 4

King et al.'s (1983) purpose was to awaken higher education to change its curricula in psychology to aim at representing Black people in a more positive role and one that would move future African Americans to higher social mobility.

Bell, Bland, Houston, and Jones (1983) produced a study on the need to update Black curricula in psychiatry programs. The purpose of their research was to prove that curricula changes needed to be made to enhance or improve the treatment of Black people in residential facilities. They argued that Freudian principles of psychiatry were grounded in Anglo-middle-class concepts that are not consistent with or relevant to all racial and ethnic groups. Bell et al. (1983)claimed that "significant progress will occur only when the core curriculum content of psychiatric education in our training institutions changes" (p. 207). Additionally, myths and stereotypes from the early nineteenth and twentieth centuries have made it even more difficult for Black people to receive equal and ethical mental health treatments. In exploring the racist untruths of these centuries, Blacks were thought to be inferior to Whites, especially Black men with smaller brains and the inability to reason. Ray (1856) found that Black people were thought to have the inability to have mental illness because they were an "uncivilized race" (as cited in Bell et al., 1983, p. 213). Current research must continue to eradicate these myths and stereotypes.

OTHER RELATED DISORDERS

Trichotillomania (TTM): Hair Pulling Disorder

Falkenstein, Rogers, Malloy, and Haaga (2015) provided an overview of treatment outcomes for a related OCRD, trichotillomania (TTM), known as hair-pulling disorder. Because OCD research is limited, especially regarding African Americans, their work echoes that of other researchers identifying minorities as being "underrepresented" in this subject area, regardless of "socioeconomic status" and being "less likely to receive empirically supported treatments" (p. 642). Although mixed reviews on the effectiveness of Cognitive Behavioral Therapy (CBT) for African Americans have been recorded, with regard to OCRDs, the research is limited (p. 642). Falkenstein et al. found that African Americans most often sought remedies for TTM through their hair care professional rather than a mental health professional. Yet again, the researchers stressed the lack of research on African Americans and minorities' treatment outcomes.

In Falkenstein et al.'s (2015) study of 60 participants, nine were African American and 38 were White. Varied measurements were used to test the efficacy of treatments such as the *Massachusetts General Hospital Hairpulling Scale* (MGH-HPS), *Trichotillomania Diagnostic Interview-Revised* (TDI-R), *Psychiatric Institute Trichotillomania Scale* (PITS), *Trichotillomania Course and Treatment Interview* ("unpublished measure"), *Structured Clinical Interview for DSM-IV-TR Axis I Disorders-Patient Edition* (SCID-I/P), *World Health Organization Quality of Life-Brief Version* (WHOQOL-BREF), *Sheehan Disability Scale* (SDS), and the *Client Satisfaction Questionnaire* (CSQ-8). The data were analyzed using SPSS version 19. Falkenstein et al. found that there was no significance between Whites and African Americans when comparing clinical significance or predicting remission. However, there was significance with regard to reliable change (p. 647). Whites benefited more from self-help online therapy than their African American counterparts, but with face-to-face therapy, no significance was found. There were limitations to this study such as "the small sample size of minorities" (p. 649).

Neal-Barnett, Statom, and Stadulis (2011) through a qualitative study sought to incorporate "cultural factors into [their] TTM research" because of the lack thereof (p. 208). Their focus was on African-American women only. These women were more likely to pull from their scalp, eyelashes, and eyebrows as revealed through other studies; however, Neal-Barnett et al. (2011)posited that "hair texture, grade, and length can influence an African American female's perception of attractiveness, self-esteem, and self-worth" (p. 208). They discovered that the higher the anxiety score, the more correlations were found between TTM and OCD symptoms. Females who were deemed "chronic hair pullers" (p. 209) were solicited through the Internet via www.trich.org, and an online support group for African American female chronic hair pullers. Eighty-four participants were employed, with education ranging from high school graduates to graduate degree recipients with a median income ranging from $40,000 to $55,000. The categorical age ranges were from 18-55, and the majority claimed a religious affiliation. The measures used were the *Hair Pulling Survey (HPS)*, *NIMH Trichotillomania Symptom Severity (TSS) Scale, Trichotillomania Impairment Scale (TIS)*, and *The Symptom Checklist Revised (SCL-90R)*. The White women participants have used the TSS and TIS with a reliability range from 0.71 to 0.81 in the past; however, Neal-Barnett et al. were the first to use the scales with an all African American population (p. 209). Of the four highest reported hair-pulling areas for African American women, the scalp, 85.4%; the eyebrows, 39.0%; the pubic area, 29.3%; and the eyebrows, 24.4% (p. 210). A positive correlation between TTM and OC symptoms was found in this study in addition to "higher levels of severity [being] associated with higher OC scores" (p. 211).

Tic-Related Obsessive-Compulsive Disorder

Stein (2000) noted "that OCD is phenotypically and genetically heterogeneous in nature" (as cited in Mukai, 2021, p. 191). Tic-related OCD is a new diagnostic within the DSM-V as a subtype of OCRD. Anyone with a history of TD or presently diagnosed with TD, falls into this subtype with a comorbid diagnosis with OCD. Mukai et al. explained the need for such a study since there is a lack of "a valid diagnosis of tic-related [TD] OCD" (p. 192). Therefore, the researchers evaluated 29 Japanese patients who were diagnosed with OCD and had received treatment with SSRIs along with 15 "healthy controls" who had never had any type of head trauma or a "neurological disease" among other factors (p. 192). Interviews, scales, including Y-BOCS and the Dimensional Yale-Brown Obsessive-Compulsive Scale (DY-BOCS). Studies have shown that "oxygenated hemoglobin (oxy-Hb) increases and deoxygenated hemoglobin (deoxy-Hb) decreases" (p. 194) have direct correlations to brain activity. Near-infrared spectroscopy (NIRS) studies confirmed that people with "[OCD have fewer] prefrontal cortex (PFC) activation" (p. 192). The purpose of their study was to analyze TD related OCD and hemodynamic changes. This study also found significant correlations suggesting that TD related OCD had "lower activation in a wide range of PFC" (p. 195). This type of study should be conducted within the African American community.

Neurology

Zai (2004) wrote a Master of Science thesis on the biochemical and neurological influence and overlap of OCD and schizophrenia on the brain which could be caused by an autoimmune disease. Although the focus of this research was on the similarities of the two diseases. The exactness of the development of OCD has not been agreed upon by all clinicians; however, the neurotransmitter serotonin has been prescribed to ease the symptoms. When this method is unsuccessful, surgery may be an option. Zai contended that "medications targeted at the abnormal region of the brain will more likely improve symptom severity due to their specificity to concentrate on a specific area of interest and the limit the number of adverse effects" (p. 6). Additional medical approaches and equipment have been used to discover neurobiological factors of OCD such as magnetic-reasoning imaging (MRI) and positron emission tomography (PET) scans. Baxter et al. (1987) stated that "MRI studies of untreated OCD patients have shown loss of tissue in the caudate nuclei, an important part of the basal ganglia…[and] increased glucose metabolic rates… in the left orbital gyrus" (as cited in Zai, 2004, p. 6). Zai also cited additional morphological abnormalities such as a hyperfunctional fronto-striatal, enlarged thalamus, and impaired prefrontal cortex (p. 8).

Zai (2004) hypothesized that genetic markers in the HLA would correlate with an overactive immune response such as an autoimmune disorder in people with OCD (p. 29). This study was carried out in Toronto, Canada, with 150 participants and their parents, interviewed with DSM-IV and given Y-BOCS. In order to qualify for this study, participants had to be affected by OCD or OCRD within the family such as "either a clinical or subclinical OC behaviour [*sic*] level, or for an OCD spectrum disorder, which …included body dysmorphic disorder, trichotillomania, skin picking, Gilles de la Tourette's syndrome (TS), or chronic/motor vocal tics" (p. 48). Different studies have linked Myelin Oligodendrocyte Glycoprotein (MOG), a protein that is attributed to autoimmune diseases such as multiple sclerosis and affecting the nervous system, to OCD. Zai, with the assistance of Dr. Bezchibnyk, sought to explore this phenomenon. Zai found a significance between OCD and the MOG gene, specifically regarding children and further explained other neurological possibilities:

OCD might be considered as an immune-mediated basal ganglia disorder with consequent movement abnormalities in some cases and manifestation of psychiatric symptoms similar to PANDAS….immunotherapies might be indicated in common psychiatric disorders to induce automatic remission and therefore system remediation….positive streptococcal serology alone is inadequate for such a diagnosis, as GABHS is so prevalent in the pediatric community. pp. 110-111

Zai (2004) cautioned readers on the possibility of false negatives within research and urged others who may replicate this study to explore multiple comparisons.

TREATMENT FOR OCD

According to Margolis (2002), treatment for OCD is very similar to that of other panic disorders (p. 100). In addition to "cognitive and behavioral psychotherapy," (p. 100) medications such as "SSRs…(citalopram (Celexa), fluoxetine (Prozac), fluvoxamine (Luvox), paroxetine, and sertraline)" have been prescribed by either psychiatrists or medical doctors (p. 100). Studies have shown that these drugs may be more beneficial to those who have compulsions.

In addition to medications, neurological operations have been performed. The report of neurological surgeries began in 1947 according to Lai et al. (2020), and neurological ablation has also been an option among others (pp. 356-357). Despite these interventions, some patients have not been successful. For example, Davis (2008) shared the story of his own mother-in-law, who was diagnosed with OCD and tried various treatment options during the 1950s, one of which was topectomy and later, psychosurgery. Neither operation was successful, and both are no longer performed. Davis (2008) also criticized pharmaceutical companies and the media for promoting means which have known failures or were ambiguous. Davis pushes for a biocultural approach just as some of the others like Walker (2020) and Williams et al. (2020).

Lai et al. (2020) sought out the effectiveness of neurosurgical ablation and found that some procedures do have positive outcomes, but several patients had to have repeat procedures such as "repeated cingulotomy and/or an additional subcaudate tractotomy" (p. 358). These researchers only recommend these procedures for the most severe cases.

IMPLICATIONS FOR FUTURE STUDIES

Gadelkarim et al. (2019) sought to find a correlation between OCD, OCPD, and autism-spectrum disorder (ASD). Wikramanayake et al. (2018) posited that "ASD is a common though often overlooked comorbidity in treatment-seeking OCD patients" (as cited in Gadelkarim et al., p. 298). The 106 patients in this study diagnosed with OCD were from the United Kingdom and race was not used as a variable. Scales and assessments used were Compulsive Personality Assessment Scale (CPAS), Y-BOCS, Autism Spectrum Quotient (AQ), BABS, along with clinical notes. Fifty percent of the participants revealed a correlation between OCPD and ASD traits. Furthermore, the researchers hinted that patients diagnosed with OCD who carry OCPD and ASD traits were less likely to be employed. This study could be replicated within the African American community in the United States.

Research has shown that children of parents with OCD or more likely to develop the disorder (Black, Gaffney, Scholosser, & Gabel, 2003). Unfortunately, of the 21 participants with OCD and having at least one child under the age of 18, only one African American participated. This type of study could not only add to the literature on OCD and the Black community but would help practitioners and parents with educating their children and recognizing the warning signs.

Storch et al. (2014) posited that most literature surrounding OCD is that of adults and thus decided to add to the field of research by discovering correlations between OCD symptom insight and children. Using the Child Assessment of Beliefs Scale (CABS), Storch et al. (2014) assessed 110 participants between the ages of 6 to 17 years old who had a first diagnosis of OCD. Of the 110 participants, two were African American. Parents and their children were rated regarding perceptions and beliefs and a total score was used to determine "insight in the presentation and treatment of OCD in youth" (pp. 614-615). Additionally, other assessments were used such as *CY-BOCS, Clinician Global Impression-Severity (CGI-Severity),*

Obsessive-Compulsive Inventory-Child Version (OCI-CV), Children's Depression Inventory-Short Form (CDI-SF), and Child Behavior Checklist (CBCL) (p. 615). After careful analyses and reliability measures were taken, a series of computations were completed:

All correlations were estimated using full-information maximum likelihood (FIML) estimation in Mplus, where all study variables were included in the estimation model. This correlation matrix was also to compute the PCA; factor scores were then computed by the regression method, and all correlations with the factor scores were estimated by FIML estimation where all study variables and these computed factor scores were included in the estimation model (with the exception of the original CABS scores…). p. 616

As a result, CABS showed a correlation between youth insight and OCD; however, results were not valid regarding "overall model fit" (Storch et al., 2014, p. 617). At least 38.2% of the youth assessed revealed poor insight, and no significance was found "between insight and hoarding" (p. 618). In conclusion, Storch et al. felt it important for children and their parents to recognize the symptoms of OCD and recognize it as a psychological or mental illness, thus being able to recognize false beliefs such as "[I have to put my crayons in a certain order otherwise mommy will die" (p. 618). Due to the limitation of very few African Americans participating in this study, a correlation based on race cannot be obtained; therefore, this type of study could add to the Black Studies and mental illness literature.

A study of a Muslim practicing Pakistan community and the correlations between religious beliefs, self-esteem, and OCD was conducted by Ghafoor, Schulz, and Mohsin (2018). The 200-person sample was from various government hospitals consisting of a mixture of male and female participants, ages 18 years and older (p. 174). Using SPSS 21, *t*-tests and Chi-tests were conducted. Additionally, "mediation analysis was carried out using PROCESS (add-on for SPSS for mediation and moderation analyses" (p. 174). The researchers found that high Muslim religious practices correlated with low self-esteem in people with OCD in their community, and those without OCD had higher self-esteem. Shafran, Watkins, and Charman (1996) concluded that "OCD could lead to low self-esteem" due to the "so-called guilt presumption" (as cited in Ghafoor, Schulz, & Mohsin, 2018, pp. 175-177).

Researchers have hinted at a significance between religion and OCD symptoms. Berman et al. (2020) posited in one of their hypotheses that "spirituality [would] moderate the relationship between nationality and OCD symptom dimensions" (p. 445) within their population of Latinx or Hispanic private university students in Northeast Mexico. The other participants in this research were White students from a public university in the Southeast United States. Using the *Dimensional*

Obsessive Compulsive Scale (DOCS) and the *Spirituality Experiences Index* (SEI), "five hierarchical linear regression analyses" were used to examine OC symptoms with regard to spirituality and nationality (p. 446). Berman et al. (2020) found that in the Mexican population, the extent of religious or spiritual beliefs correlated with the level of OC symptoms. These researchers sought to fill a void in the literature with regard to "nationality (USA vs. Mexico), spirituality, and the severity of OC symptom dimensions" (p. 448). Although Berman et al. warned about the validity of their conclusions due to the Mexican sample, this type of study could benefit the African American community as well.

CONCLUSION

Obsessive-Compulsive Disorder has become one of the top four mental disorders in the United States (Davis, 2008, p. 210), affecting "1 to 2 percent of the population" ("Obsessive"). For accuracy in OCD diagnosis, mental health professionals must use "a bicultural approach" and not exclude the "social, historical, and cultural elements [of their patients]...[and]...examine their own methods, biases, and premises" (p. 210). Additionally, CBT, a therapy to change one's thoughts, may not be effective across all cultures and ethnicities with regard to OCD; however, Williams et al. (2020) suggested that clinicians can adjust their own practices and familiarize themselves with their clients' cultures, religious practices, worldviews, and various healing practices (Williams et al., 2020).

Medical mistrust among the Black community is yet a barrier within the 2020's. This mistrust can be detrimental not only to physical health but mental as well. Continued research in the areas of African Americans and mental health issues is needed, especially in the area of OCD, which is still limited. Furthermore, therapists, psychologists, psychiatrists, clinicians, and the like, should consider using more appropriate instruments for diagnosing OCD, such as Y-BOCS, DOCS, and OCI-R rather than the SCID-OCD, especially for people of color (Chasson et al., 2017). Bazargan et al. (2021) suggested a collaboration between "healthcare clinicians on existing barriers of stigma and health inequalities developed outside of medicine" (p. 11).

REFERENCES

Ameringen, M., Patterson, B., & Simpson, W. (2014). Dsm-5 Obsessive-compulsive and related disorders: Clinical implications of new criteria. *Depression & Anxiety (1091-4269), 31*(6), 487–493. doi:10.1002/da.22259

Bazargan, M., Cobb, S., & Assari, S. (2021). Discrimination and medical mistrust in a racially and ethnically diverse sample of California adults. *Annals of Family Medicine*, *19*(1), 4–15. doi:10.1370/afm.2632 PMID:33431385

Bell, C. C., Bland, I. J., Houston, E., & Jones, B. E. (1983). Curriculum development implementation: Enhancement of knowledge and skills for the psychiatric treatment of black populations. In J. C. Chunn II, P. J. Dunston, & F. Ross-Sheriff (Eds.), *Mental health & people of color: Curriculum development and change* (pp. 205–238). Howard University Press.

Berman, N. C., Gallegos-Guajardo, J., Reuman, L., Ramirez, M., Valdez, G., & Abramowitz, J. S. (2020). Cross-cultural differences in obsessive-compulsive symptom dimensions across young adults in Mexico and USA. *Mental Health, Religion & Culture*, *23*(5), 443–454. doi:10.1080/13674676.2020.1793309

Black, D. W., Gaffney, G. R., Schlosser, S., & Gabel, J. (2003). Children of parents with obsessive-compulsive disorder – a 2-year follow-up study. *Acta Psychiatrica Scandinavica*, *107*(4), 305–313. doi:10.1034/j.1600-0447.2003.02182.x PMID:12662254

Calle-Ramirez, X. M., Hernandez, R. M., Saavedra-Lopez, M. A., Esteban, R. F. C., Chaperro, J. E. T., Mamani-Benito, O., & Campos-Ugaz, W. A. (2022). Worldwide scientific production on obsessive-compulsive disorders in time of COVID-19 pandemic. *AVFT, 41*(9), 679-683.

Chasson, G. S., Williams, M. T., Davis, D. M., & Combs, J. Y. (2017). Missed diagnoses in African Americans with obsessive-compulsive disorder: The structured clinical interview for DSM-IV Axis I disorders (SCID-I). *BMC Psychiatry*, *17*(1), 1–10. doi:10.118612888-017-1422-z PMID:28716021

Cobb, S., & Assari, S. (2019). Psychiatric disorders and alcohol consumption among low-income African Americans: Gender differences. *Brain Sciences (2076-3425)*, *9*(4), 86. doi:10.3390/brainsci9040086

Davis, L. J. (2008). *Obsession: A history*. The University of Chicago Press. doi:10.7208/chicago/9780226137797.001.0001

English, R. A. (1983, November). The challenge for mental health minorities and their world views. *Second Annual Robert L. Sutherland Lecture*. University of Texas at Austin.

Falkenstein, M. J., Rogers, K., Malloy, E. J., & Haaga, D. A. F. (2015). Race/Ethnicity and treatment outcome in a randomized controlled trial for trichotillomania (hair-pulling disorder). *Journal of Clinical Psychology, 71*(7), 641–652. doi:10.1002/jclp.22171 PMID:25846982

Gadelkarim, W., Shahper, S., Reid, J., Wikramanayake, M., Kaur, S., Kolli, S., Osman, S., & Fineberg, N. A. (2019). Overlap of obsessive–compulsive personality disorder and autism spectrum disorder traits among OCD outpatients: An exploratory study. *International Journal of Psychiatry in Clinical Practice, 23*(4), 297–306. doi:10.1080/13651501.2019.1638939 PMID:31375037

Ghafoor, H., Schulz, S. M., & Mohsin, H. (2018). Does religiosity ameliorate the negative impact of obsessive-compulsive disorder on self-esteem? *Mental Health, Religion & Culture, 21*(2), 171–179. doi:10.1080/13674676.2018.1458082

Harris, Y. R., & Graham, J. A. (2014). In the African American child: Development and challenges (pp. 65–80). Springer Publishing Company.

International O. C. D. Foundation. (2010). Obsessive Compulsive Personality Disorder (OCPD). IOCD. https://iocdf.org/wp-content/uploads/2014/10/OCPD-Fact-Sheet.pdf

King, L. M., Moody, S., Thompson, O., & Bennett, M. (1983). Black psychology reconsidered: Notes toward curriculum development. In J. C. Chunn II, P. J. Dunston, & F. Ross-Sheriff (Eds.), *Mental health & people of color: Curriculum development and change* (pp. 3–22). Howard University Press.

Kolvenbach, S., Fernández de la Cruz, L., Mataix, C. D., Patel, N., & Jassi, A. (2018). Perceived treatment barriers and experiences in the use of services for obsessive–compulsive disorder across different ethnic groups: A thematic analysis. *Child and Adolescent Mental Health, 23*(2), 99–106. doi:10.1111/camh.12197 PMID:32677337

Krochmalik, A., & Menzies, R. G. (2003). The classification and diagnosis of obsessive- compulsive disorder. In R. G. Menzies & P. de Silva (Eds.), *Obsessive-compulsive disorder: Theory, research and treatment* (pp. 3–20). Wiley & Sons.

Lai, Y., Wang, T., Zhang, C., Lin, G., Voon, V., Chang, J., & Sun, B. (2020). Effectiveness of and safety of neuroablation for severe and treatment-resistant obsessive-compulsive disorder: A systematic review and meta-analysis. *Journal of Psychiatry & Neuroscience, 45*(5), 356–368. doi:10.1503/jpn.190079 PMID:32549057

Latzman, R. D., Naifeh, J. A., Watson, D., Vaidya, J. G., Heiden, L. J., Damon, J. D., Hight, T. L., & Young, J. (2011). Racial differences in symptoms of anxiety and depression among three cohorts of students in the southern United States. *Psychiatry*, *74*(4), 332–348. doi:10.1521/psyc.2011.74.4.332 PMID:22168294

Margolis, S. (2002). *The Johns Hopkins medical guide to health after 50*. Medlette Associates, Inc.

Marker, C. D., & Aylward, A. G. (2012). Description. In D. Wedding, L. Beutler, K. E. Freedland, L. C. Sobell, & D. A. Wolfe (Eds.), *Generalized Anxiety Disorder* (pp. 6–7). Hogrefe.

Menzies, R. G., & de Silva, P. (Eds.). (2003). Obsessive-compulsive disorder: Theory, research and treatment. Hoboken, NJ: Wiley & Sons. –175. https://doi.org/. 2020.1817554 doi:10.1080/08039488

Michalopoulou, G., Falzarano, P., & Rosenberg, D. (2009). Recruitment of African Americans for obsessive compulsive disorder treatment research. *Journal of Health Disparities Research and Practice*, *3*(1), 71–82.

Mukai, K., Matsuura, N., Miyauchi, M., Hashimoto, T., Yamanishi, K., Maebayashi, K., Hayashida, K., & Matsunaga, H. (2021). Evaluation of hemodynamic changes using near-infrared spectroscopy in patients with tic-related obsessive–compulsive disorder. *Psychiatry and Clinical Neurosciences*, *75*(6), 191–199. doi:10.1111/pcn.13207 PMID:33543818

Neal-Barnett, A., Statom, D., & Stadulis, R. (2011). Trichotillomania symptoms in African American women: Are they related to anxiety and culture? *CNS Neuroscience & Therapeutics*, *17*(4), 207–213. doi:10.1111/j.1755-5949.2010.00138.x PMID:20406247

Orem, S. (2017). (Un)necessary procedures: Black women, disability, and work in Grey's Anatomy. *African American Review*, *50*(2), 169–183. doi:10.1353/afa.2017.0020

Ruffins, P. (1998). The Tuskegee experiment's long shadow. *Black Issues in Higher Education*, 26. https://link.gale.com/apps/doc/A53257761/ITOF?u=txshrpub100292&sid= bookmark-ITOF&xid=e83e0d32

Storch, E. A., De Nadai, A. S., Jacob, M. L., Lewin, A. B., Muroff, J., Eisen, J., & Murphy, T. K. (2014). Phenomenology and correlates of insight in pediatric obsessive-compulsive disorder. *Science Direct, 55*, 613-620. http://dx.doi.org/. 2013.09.014 doi:10.1016/j.comppsych

Taylor, R., Nguyen, A., Sinkewicz, M., Joe, S., & Chatters, L. (2013). Comorbid mood and anxiety disorders, suicidal behavior, and substance abuse among Black Caribbeans in the U.S.A. *Journal of African American Studies, 17*(4), 409–425. doi:10.100712111-012-9237-y

Walker, R. (2020). *The unapologetic guide to Black mental health : Navigate an unequal system, learn tools for emotional wellness, and get the help you deserve.* EBSCO Host. https://search.ebscohost.com/login.aspx?direct=true&db=nlebk&AN=2267576&site=ehost-live

Wheaton, M., Berman, N., Fabricant, L., & Abramowitz, J. (2013). Differences in obsessive–compulsive symptoms and obsessive beliefs: A comparison between African Americans, Asian Americans, Latino Americans, and European Americans. *Cognitive Behaviour Therapy, 42*(1), 9–20. doi:10.1080/16506073.2012.701663 PMID:23134374

Williams, M. T. (2007). *Racial differences in the assessment of obsessive-compulsive disorder* (Publication No. 3294804). [Doctoral dissertation, University of Virginia] Proquest Dissertations and Thesis.

Williams, M. T., La Torre, J. T., & Sharif, N. (2020). Cultural competency in the treatment of obsessive-compulsive disorder: Practitioner guidelines. *Cognitive Behaviour Therapist, 13*(e48), 1–25. doi:10.1017/S1754470X20000501

Williams, M. T., Taylor, R. J., George, J. R., Schlaudt, V. A., Ifatunji, M. A., & Chatters, L. M. (2021). Correlates of obsessive-compulsive symptoms among Black Caribbean Americans. *International Journal of Mental Health, 40*(1), 53–77. doi:10.1080/00207411.2020.1826261 PMID:33840831

Wong, Y. J., & Wester, S. R. (2016). *APA Handbook of Men and Masculinities.* American Psychological Association. doi:10.1037/14594-000

Zai, G. C. M. (2016). *Genetics of obsessive-compulsive disorder: From phenotypes to pharmacogenetics* (Order No. 10140946). Sci Tech Premium Collection.

Chapter 7
Paranoia Disorder and the African-American Community

Dimitra Smith
Texas A&M University, Commerce, USA

LaVelle Hendricks
Texas A&M University, Commerce, USA

John Kuykendall
University of Indianapolis, USA

David Tolliver
Texas A&M University, Commerce, USA

ABSTRACT

African Americans have experienced grave inequities in healthcare. These inequities have extended to mental health and continue to be a concern for African Americans. Paranoia is a mental health challenge that exists among African Americans, for varying reasons, including impacts from slavery, trauma, and current systematic discrimination. Due to low representation of healthcare providers among the African American community and African American distrust in the medical community, African Americans often turn to their church and the spiritual community for healing and support.

DOI: 10.4018/978-1-6684-8918-5.ch007

AFRICAN AMERICANS AND MENTAL HEALTH CHALLENGES: AN OVERVIEW

This chapter will discuss information related to paranoia in the African American community. In this chapter, information about African Americans' overall mental health will be included, followed by specific information regarding paranoia and the impact of paranoia among African Americans. It must be noted that African American and Black will be used interchangeably throughout this chapter.

Mental health is essential to the overall well-being of all populations, particularly African Americans, and is influential in developing healthy and fulfilling life outcomes. Even with the increased awareness and expressed the importance of taking care of your mental health, African Americans have historically faced challenges in accessing quality mental healthcare due to social, economic, and cultural barriers (Salami, Denga, Taylor, Ajayi, Jackson, Aswfaw, Salma, 2021). These challenges are even more significant regarding conditions such as paranoia and schizophrenia, which disproportionately affect African Americans (Wolny, Moussa-Tooks, Bailey, & O'Donnell, 2023). African Americans' difficulties with mental health conditions, specifically paranoia and schizophrenia, continue to contribute to how these challenges have affected their mental health outcomes.

Throughout history, the challenges faced by African Americans in accessing quality mental healthcare can be traced back to slavery. During slavery, African Americans were subjected to inhumane treatment and extreme stress, which had severe psychological consequences and are still prevalent today (Burroughs, 2022). However, mental health treatment was not a priority for enslavers, and enslaved individuals were denied access to any form of mental healthcare. Furthermore, after slavery, African Americans faced social and economic barriers that hindered their access to quality mental healthcare. For instance, they were denied access to mental health hospitals and other healthcare facilities segregated by race (Stern & Nellis, 2017).

Moreover, during the Jim Crow era, African Americans were subjected to systemic racism, further hindering their access to quality healthcare. The Civil Rights movement led to significant progress in addressing systemic racism, but disparities in healthcare access persisted. A 2019 National Alliance on Mental Illness (NAMI) report found that African Americans are 20% more likely to experience mental health problems than the general population (Harris, McKinney, & Fripp, 2019). Yet, they are less likely to receive treatment. Often going untreated, these mental health challenges are passed down generationally and impact decades of family lineages.

AFRICAN AMERICANS AND MENTAL HEALTH

As we delve deeper into the experiences of African Americans and mental health, the stance on mental health incorporates many aspects of the African American experience. Historically, mental health and working with mental health among the African American community have stayed among informal support systems and have remained the duty of the family and the church. The importance of the Black church has been documented in 4 areas of community medicine: primary care delivery, community mental health, health promotion and disease prevention, and health policy (Levin, 1984).

Family is an essential component of the African American experience, and for African Americans, family is at the core of what it means to be African American. Given the tight bond among the community, family beliefs and cultural norms indicate that the family is there to assist with many issues, including mental health. The protective nature of the African American community may come from the challenge of being Black in America. To seek mental health treatment would allow for an added label or stigma. For this reason, African Americans rely on their family to cope with mental health issues because the mental illness label is shameful, and knowledge of the diagnosis outside of the family could cause adverse reactions and a double stigma, which could lead to further discrimination (Newhill & Harris, 2007).

Speaking of discrimination, the medical field has not always been kind to African Americans. African Americans risk being misdiagnosed and not taken as seriously as their Caucasian counterparts (Kranke, Guada, Kranke, & Floersch (2012). Aligning with misdiagnoses and the lack of concern towards African Americans by medical professionals, African Americans fear the use of medications will cause people to be dependent on them; they also worry about safety issues of medicines and the belief that it might make people "crazy" (Mathews et al., 2006). In addition, the racial disparities that continue to exist in mental health service utilization have motivated African Americans to seek mental health services significantly less than their white counterparts (Conner, K. O., Lee, B., Mayers, V., Robinson, D., Reynolds III, C. F., Albert, S., & Brown, C., 2010). In short, African Americans mostly do not want to be associated with mental illness because of the discrimination and related public stigma. Ultimately, the disassociation with mental illness can negatively impact an individual's engagement and use of services (Corrigan & Kleinlein, 2005).

The Role of the Church in the Mental Health of African Americans

Church has always been viewed as providing a source and strength to many African Americans' issues. According to Bolden & Wicks (2005) and Kranke, Guada,

Kranke, & Floersch (2012), "many African Americans seek mental health counseling from church ministers and clergy because it is believed that prayer can solve all problems" (p. 67). The Black church has always played a vital role in the overall development of the Black community. This support by the church is not limited to just spiritual matters but includes economic, financial, social, and mental well-being. The American Psychiatric Association reports only one in three Black Americans in need of mental health care receives it (Metraux, 2022). Thus, the Black church must continue supporting the Black community as Black Americans struggle with substance use disorders, paranoia, schizophrenia, bipolar, and other psychoses, and mental healing issues. Bipolar disorders, schizophrenia, and other psychoses chatters

(Dempsey, Butler & Gaither, 2016). Historically, African Americans have relied on their faith in dealing with mental health issues. There has always been a connection between religion and the hardships African Americans have faced. A belief remains at the forefront for many African Americans that prayer is the key to unresolved life situations, including mental health (Chatters, Taylor, Jackson, Lincoln, 2008).

WHY DO MOST AFRICAN AMERICANS AVOID MENTAL HEALTH TREATMENT OPTIONS?

The underutilization of mental health services and resources among the African American community may be due, in part, to what researchers coined "cultural mistrust" (Caldwell & Obasi, 2010). Cultural mistrust, in short, is the lack of trust among certain cultures toward a certain thing. For this chapter, cultural mistrust is the African American population's mistrust of mental health services and resources. The hesitation among African Americans dates to the medical experiments on Black men around the 1970s. The Tuskegee Syphilis Study is so much a part of the African American community that these events and acts of disservice to the African American community has and continues to cause deep suspicion of the medical profession (Duster, 2006). Additionally, acts such as misdiagnosed and overrepresentation among involuntary hospital admissions (Garb, 1997, 1998; Lindsey & Paul, 1989; Neighbors, Jackson, Campbell, & Williams, 1989; Whaley, 2001a); and bias in the provision of mental health services (Whaley, 2001a) are additional reasons for the mistrust of African American regarding mental health treatment.

Those African Americans that utilize the mental health system may have pessimistic views toward treatment because of negative experiences. In particular, one study (Mathews et al., 2006) illustrated how African Americans believed their concerns and mental health needs were not adequately addressed within the medical establishment. In addition, participants reported that mental health providers were not competent enough to work effectively with them. African American parents felt they were being blamed and interrogated for their child's illness rather than assisted, which led to concerns about a lack of Black professionals in mental health. For this reason, among the African Americans who do seek mental health treatment, they attend fewer sessions and are more likely to discontinue therapy before the recommended termination timeline (Miranda & Cooper 2004).

Early theorists argued that White service providers had limited ability to help Black consumers because of their lack of understanding of Black culture, history, and the experiences of Blacks living in a primarily White society (Banks, Grambs, 1971). This position implied that Blacks are less likely to trust White therapists and to seek their services, and thus, it is in the best interest of Black consumers to receive benefits from Black therapists.

One study confirmed that most Black clients preferred Black Therapists (Blank, Mahmood, Fox, Guterbock, 2002). Many participants felt that such young men might respond best to talk with other young Black men who have been successfully treated for mental health problems, adding that such individuals would be viewed as credible role models for seeking treatment.

WHAT IS PARANOIA?

Paranoia Personality Disorder (PPD) is a condition in which "mistrust of other people is the cardinal feature" (Carroll, 2009, p. 40). In addition, "PPD has a close relationship with childhood trauma and social stress" (Lee, 2017, p. 152). The importance of childhood trauma as a predictor of PPD symptoms indicates that social learning and relationship history may play a causal role in the development of the disorder. It was once theorized to be associated with schizophrenia due to the phenomenological similarity of suspiciousness to paranoid delusion, but the evidence for this association is not strong (Lee, 2017, p. 160). The most likely differential diagnoses of PPD are normality; other personality disorders such as schizoid, schizotypal, avoidant, narcissistic, antisocial, and comorbidity; anxiety disorders such as social phobia, social anxiety, panic disorder; depression; delusional disorder; and other psychotic illnesses such as schizophrenia, chronic organic psychoses, substance-induced psychoses, and brief reactive psychoses (Wolny, Moussa-Tooks, Bailey O'Donnell, & Hetrick, 2023). Historically, *Paranoid personality* is characterized by mistrust, interest in secret motives, irritability, discontent, fault-finding, feelings of being treated unjustly and oppressed, and excessive self-evaluation (Kraepelin, 1921).

THE IMPACTS OF PARANOIA ON AFRICAN AMERICANS

Given the limited amount of research on paranoia and the history of late diagnosis among elderly patients, the urgency to consider social and cultural impacts and influences among the African American community is paramount. Paranoia and schizophrenia disproportionately affect African Americans. According to NAMI (2019), African Americans are 1.5 to 2 times more likely to develop schizophrenia than the general population. Additionally, paranoia is a common symptom among African Americans with schizophrenia, which is thought to result from their experiences with systemic racism and discrimination. Several empirical research studies have led researchers to conclude that the frequent exposure to racism toward African Americans (and other individuals of color) can have "adverse health consequences" (Greer, Brondolo, & Brown, 2014; Greer & Spalding, 2017, p. 588). It is well documented that systematic racism and discrimination exist in areas of housing and employment (May 2018). These same structures are evident in education (Greer & Spalding, 2017) and public entities, such as restaurants, hotels, and movie theaters (May, 2018). Given the above, it is not alarming that a large percentage of the African American population is impacted by paranoia. At just about every turn in life, African Americans are met with some sort of situation and circumstance that has the potential to lead to paranoia systems.

Studies have shown that African Americans with schizophrenia and paranoia are less likely to receive appropriate treatment than other racial groups (Satcher, 2013; Williams & Mohammad, 2009). They are also more likely to be misdiagnosed with substance abuse, leading to inadequate treatment (Jordan, 2021). African Americans are also more likely to be hospitalized involuntarily and receive more restrictive treatments than other racial groups, such as seclusion and restraint (Williams & Mohammad, 2009).

African Americans have faced historical challenges in accessing quality mental healthcare, significantly affecting their mental health outcomes. For example, paranoia and schizophrenia are two mental health conditions that disproportionately affect African Americans, and they are less likely to receive appropriate treatment. Therefore, it is essential to address the historical and systemic barriers that have hindered African Americans' access to quality mental healthcare to ensure they receive the care they need to improve their mental health outcomes.

An exploratory study of 1,114 elderly African American elderly patients (62 years and older) was conducted to understand paranoid symptomatology among the population. The study considered "The impact of demographics, social support, cognitive deficit, ad health status self-ratings on health, vision, hearing, memory, and personal characteristics on paranoid symptoms" (Bazargan, Bazargan, King, 2001, p. 366). The researchers were alarmed by the findings. Ten percent (10%) of the participants had symptoms of paranoia. This finding was alarming because the study sample included African Americans who might have received greater social support. For the researchers, this implied that if elderly African Americans with substantial social support from the community, in addition to receiving support from a senior service facility, would reveal symptoms of paranoia, then there may be a significant increase in paranoia symptoms among African American elderly patients not receiving such support. In addition, among this population, depression was identified "as the strongest correlate of paranoid ideation symptoms" (Bazargan, Bazargan, King, 2001).

POSSIBLE TREATMENT OPTIONS FOR AFRICAN AMERICANS SUFFERING FROM PARANOIA

Untreated mental illness among older adults is one of the most significant challenges facing the mental health service delivery system (President's New Freedom Commission on Mental Health, 2003). This is, in part, to the idea that untreated mental health conditions indicate a significant number of untreated mental health concerns among the younger population.

African Americans have developed what is referred to as *healthy cultural paranoia* (Whaley, 2001b). This term is used "to describe an African American cultural response style resulting from experiences with racism and oppression in White American society" (Grier & Cobbs, 1968; Ridley, 1984; Terrell & Terrell, 1981; Whaley, 2001b, p. 514) and the "apprehension experienced by African Americans during interracial clinical situations" (Grier & Cobbs, 1968; Ridley, 1984, p. 514). The term *healthy cultural paranoia* has caused controversy in the research and medical communities. Many believe that the term paranoia should not be used so loosely and should be reserved for the intended use of medical diagnosis. The term *cultural mistrust* is more representative of the attitudes and beliefs of African Americans.

Even with the healthy cultural paranoia, it does not negate the idea that mental health and paranoia are real experiences for African Americans and health treatment options are needed.

CONCLUSION

In conclusion, paranoia is a common mental illness among the African American community, brought on by many external forces, including systematic racism and trauma. While most cases go undiagnosed due to many occurrences, such as mistrust of the medical profession, African Americans have found faith in churches and their pastors. African Americans must be able to find the needed help and treatment regarding mental illness. Undiagnosed and untreated illnesses can lead to long-term impacts. It is the responsibility of everyone to ensure to the well-being of all.

REFERENCES

Banks, J. A. & Grambs, J. D. (). Black Self-Concept: Implications for Education and Social Science. McGraw-Hill.

Bartels, S. J. (2003). Improving the United States' system of care for older adults with mental illness: Findings and recommendations for the President's New Freedom Commission on Mental Health. *The American Journal of Geriatric Psychiatry, 11*(5), 486–497. doi:10.1097/00019442-200309000-00003 PMID:14506082

Bazargan, M., Bazargan, S., & King, L. (2001). Paranoid ideation among elderly African American persons. *The Gerontologist, 41*(3), 366–373. doi:10.1093/geront/41.3.366 PMID:11405434

Blank, M. B., Mahmood, M., Fox, J. C., & Guterbock, T. (2002). Alternative mental health services: The role of the Black church in the South. *American Journal of Public Health, 92*(10), 1668–1672. doi:10.2105/AJPH.92.10.1668 PMID:12356619

Bolden, L., & Wicks, M. (2005). Length of stay, admission types, psychiatric diagnoses, and the implications of stigma in African Americans in the nationwide inpatient sample. *Issues in Mental Health Nursing, 26*(10), 1043–1059. doi:10.1080/01612840500280703 PMID:16283998

Burroughs, A. D. (2022). Black Market: An Exploration of Black Mental Health in America. *Psychology from the Margins, 4*(1), 1.

Carroll, A. (2009). Are you looking at me? Understanding and managing paranoid personality disorder. *Advances in Psychiatric Treatment, 15*(1), 40–48. doi:10.1192/apt.bp.107.005421

Chatters, L. M., Taylor, R. J., Jackson, J. S., & Lincoln, K. D. (2008). Religious coping among african americans, caribbean blacks and non-hispanic whites. *Journal of Community Psychology, 36*(3), 371–386. doi:10.1002/jcop.20202 PMID:21048887

Conner, K. O., Lee, B., Mayers, V., Robinson, D., Reynolds, C. F. III, Albert, S., & Brown, C. (2010). Attitudes and beliefs about mental health among African American older adults suffering from depression. *Journal of Aging Studies, 24*(4), 266–277. doi:10.1016/j.jaging.2010.05.007 PMID:21423819

Corrigan, P., & Kleinlein, P. (2005). The impact of mental illness stigma. In P. Corrigan (Ed.), *On the stigma of mental illness: Practical strategies for research and social change* (pp. 11–44). American Psychological Association. doi:10.1037/10887-001

Dempsey, K., Butler, S. K., & Gaither, L. (2016). Black churches and mental health professionals: Can this collaboration work? *Journal of Black Studies*, *47*(1), 73–87. doi:10.1177/0021934715613588

Duster, T. (2006). Explaining differential trust of DNA forensic technology: Grounded assessment or inexplicable paranoia? *The Journal of Law, Medicine & Ethics*, *34*(2), 293–300. doi:10.1111/j.1748-720X.2006.00034.x PMID:16789950

Floersch, J., Kranke, B., & Munson, M. R. (2011). A qualitative investigation of self-stigma among adolescents taking psychiatric medication. *Psychiatric Services (Washington, D.C.)*, *62*(8), 893–899. doi:10.1176/ps.62.8.pss6208_0893 PMID:21807828

Garb, H. N. (1997). Race bias, social class bias, and gender bias in clinical judgment. *Clinical Psychology: Science and Practice*, *4*(2), 99–120. doi:10.1111/j.1468-2850.1997.tb00104.x

Garb, H. N. (1998). *Studying the clinician.* American Psychological Association.

Greer, T. M., & Spalding, A. (2017). The Role of age in understanding the psychological effects of racism for African Americans. *Cultural Diversity & Ethnic Minority Psychology*, *23*(4), 588–594. doi:10.1037/cdp0000148 PMID:28301183

Grier, W. H., & Cobbs, P. M. (1968). *Black rage.* Basic Books.

Harris, J. R. A., McKinney, J. L. G., & Fripp, J. (2019). "God Is a Keeper": A Phenomenological Investigation of Christian African American Women's Experiences With Religious Coping. *The Professional Counselor*, *9*(3), 171–184. doi:10.15241/jrah.9.3.171

Jackson, J. S., Campbell, L., & Williams, D. (1989). The influence of racial factors on psychiatric diagnosis: A review and suggestions for research. *Community Mental Health Journal*, *25*(4), 301–311. doi:10.1007/BF00755677 PMID:2697490

Jordan, S. (2021). Neurodiversity in children and the struggles of being misdiagnosed. *Black Wall Street Media.* https://blackwallst.media/neurodiversity-in-children-and-the-struggles-of-being-misdiagnosed

Kraepelin, E. (1921). Manic Depressive Insanity and Paranoia. Arno Press. doi:10.1097/00005053-192104000-00057

Kranke, D., Guada, J., Kranke, B., & Floersch, J. (2012). What do African American youth with a mental illness think about help-seeking and psychiatric medication?: Origins of stigmatizing attitudes. *Social Work in Mental Health, 10*(1), 53–71. doi:10.1080/15332985.2011.618076

Lee, R. J. (2017). Mistrustful and misunderstood: A review of paranoid personality disorder. *Current Behavioral Neuroscience Reports, 4*(2), 151–165. doi:10.100740473-017-0116-7 PMID:29399432

Levin, J. S. (1984). The Role of the black church in community medicine. *Journal of the National Medical Association, 76*, 477–483. PMID:6737505

Lindsey, K. P., & Paul, G. L. (1989). Involuntary commitment to public mental institutions: Issues involving the overrepresentation of Blacks and assessment of relevant functioning. *Psychological Bulletin, 106*(2), 171–183. doi:10.1037/0033-2909.106.2.171 PMID:2678200

Mathews, A., Corrigan, P., Smith, B., & Aranda, F. (2006). A qualitative exploration of African Americans' attitudes toward mental illness and mental illness treatment seeking. *Rehabilitation Education, 20*(4), 253–268. doi:10.1891/088970106805065331

May, R. A. B. (2018). Velvet rope racism, racial paranoia, and cultural scripts: Alleged dress code discrimination in urban nightlife, 2000–2014. *City & Community, 17*(1), 44–64. doi:10.1111/cico.12286

Miranda, J., & Cooper, L. A. (2004). Disparities in care for depression among primary care patients. *Journal of General Internal Medicine, 19*(2), 120–126. doi:10.1111/j.1525-1497.2004.30272.x PMID:15009791

National Alliance on Mental Illness. (2019). *African American Mental Health.* NAMI. https://www.nami.org/Your-Journey/Identity-and-Cultural-Dimensions/Black-African- American

Newhill, C., & Harris, D. (2007). African American consumers' perceptions of racial disparities in mental health services. *Social Work in Public Health, 23*(2/3), 107–124. doi:10.1080/19371910802151861 PMID:19306590

Ridley, C. R. (1984). Clinical treatment of the nondisclosing Black client: A therapeutic paradox. *The American Psychologist, 39*(11), 1234–1244. doi:10.1037/0003-066X.39.11.1234 PMID:6507987

Salami, B., Denga, B., Taylor, R., Ajayi, N., Jackson, M., Asefaw, M., & Salma, J. (2021). Original qualitative research-Access to mental health for Black youths in Alberta. *Health Promotion and Chronic Disease Prevention in Canada: Research. Policy & Practice*, *41*(9), 245.

Satcher, D. (2013). Addressing racial and ethnic disparities in health: The need for a national agenda. *Journal of the National Medical Association*, *105*(2, Suppl), 1S–2S.

Stern, E., & Nellis, M. (2017). The intersection of race and diagnosis among individuals with severe mental illness: A review. *Journal of Clinical Psychology*, *73*(12), 1671–1682.

Terrell, F., & Terrell, S. L. (1981). An inventory to measure cultural mistrust among Blacks. *The Western Journal of Black Studies*, *5*, 180–184.

Whaley, A. L. (2001a). Cultural mistrust and the clinical diagnosis of paranoid schizophrenia in African American patients. *Journal of Psychopathology and Behavioral Assessment*, *23*(2), 93–100. doi:10.1023/A:1010911608102

Whaley, A. L. (2001b). Cultural mistrust: An important psychological construct for diagnosis and treatment of African Americans. *Professional Psychology, Research and Practice*, *32*(6), 555–562. doi:10.1037/0735-7028.32.6.555

Williams, M. T., & Mohammed, S. A. (2009). Discrimination and racial health disparities: Evidence and needed research. *Journal of Behavioral Medicine*, *32*(1), 20–47. doi:10.100710865-008-9185-0 PMID:19030981

Wolny, J., Moussa-Tooks, A. B., Bailey, A. J., O'Donnell, B. F., & Hetrick, W. P. (2023). Race and self-reported paranoia: Increased item endorsement on subscales of the SPQ. *Schizophrenia Research*, *253*, 30–39. doi:10.1016/j.schres.2021.11.034 PMID:34895794

Chapter 8
Narcissistic Personality Disorder and the African-American Culture

James M. Devlin
Texas A&M University, Commerce, USA

Marvin Dale Bellows
Texas A&M University, Commerce, USA

Samone Donald
Texas A&M University, Commerce, USA

ABSTRACT

The present chapter covers the diagnostic criteria related the Narcissistic Personality Disorder (NPD) and takes into consideration the African American culture. The chapter presents specific information related to NPD and its elements as presented in the Diagnostic Statistical Manual V-Text Revisions (DSM-V-TR, American Psychology Association [APA]). Furthermore, the authors of this chapter present historically and contemporary issues of the African American Culture into the scope of diagnostic measures and specifically NPD. The authors also present alternative to diagnostic classifications as it relates to the African American culture and community.

DOI: 10.4018/978-1-6684-8918-5.ch008

"Most mental illness goes untreated, especially in communities of color. Fifty-two percent of Whites with Any Mental Illness (AMI) received mental health services in 2020, compared to 37.1% of Blacks and 35% of Hispanics."

According to SAMHSA, "service cost or lack of insurance coverage was the most frequently cited reason for not using mental health services across all racial/ethnic groups." A 2021 report by HHS cites "persistent systemic social inequities and discrimination" that worsen stress and associated mental health concerns for POC during the COVID-19 pandemic when 40.3% of Hispanics experienced current depression, and 36.9% had an increase or initiation of substance use, compared to 25.3% depression and 14.3% substance use in Whites." (National Institute of Mental Health, 2020)."

INTRODUCTION

Narcissistic Personality Disorder (NPD) is a personality disorder found and described in the Diagnostic Statistical Manual-Text Revision (DSM-V-TR; American Psychiatric Association [APA], 2022). The DSM-V-TR provides diagnostic criteria, symptoms, prevalence rates, presence of symptoms, duration, and differential diagnostic considerations. It categorizes 10 specific personality disorders, which the American Psychiatric Association (APA, 2022, pp. 733-734) describes as "an enduring pattern of the individual's inner experience and behavior that deviates markedly from the norms and expectations of the individual's culture, is pervasive and inflexible, has an onset in adolescence or early adulthood, is stable over time, and leads to distress or impairment." Nosologically, these conditions are separated into three groups, referred to as Cluster A, Cluster B, and Cluster C. Cluster A describes personality features that are odd or eccentric. Cluster B describes features that are dramatic in affect, cognition, and behavior. Cluster C describes features that are anxious and avoidant.

NPD CRITERIA

NPD is summarized in the DSM-V-TR (APA, 2022, p.760) as "a pattern of grandiosity, need for admiration, and lack of empathy" and is categorized within Cluster B. The following criteria for the diagnosis of Narcissistic Personality Disorder:

A pervasive pattern of grandiosity (in fantasy or behavior), need for admiration, and lack of empathy beginning by early adulthood and present in a variety of contexts, as indicated by five (or more) of the following:

1. Has a grandiose sense of self-importance (e.g., exaggerates achievements and talents, expects to be recognized as superior with commensurate achievements).
2. Is preoccupied with fantasies of unlimited success, power, brilliance, beauty, or ideal love.
3. Believes that he or she is "special" and unique and can only be understood by, or should associate with, other special or high-status people (or institutions).
4. Requires excessive admiration.
5. Has a sense of entitlement (i.e., unreasonable expectations of especially favorable treatment or automatic compliance with his or her expectations).
6. Is interpersonally exploitative (i.e., takes advantage of others to achieve his or her own ends).
7. Lacks empathy: is unwilling to recognize or identify with the feelings and needs of others.
8. Is often envious of others or believes that others are envious of him or her.
9. Shows arrogant, haughty behaviors or attitudes.

NPD Symptoms

In addition to the diagnostic criterion, there are other experiences common among those with NPD. Individuals with NPD tend to be very sensitive to criticism and do not handle the perceived loss of competition well and they may respond to these things with extreme behaviors such as social withdraw and experience distressing feelings of emptiness and depression (APA, 2022). Additionally, individuals with NPD shift between two narcissistic states: grandiose narcissism and vulnerable narcissism (Jauk et al., 2021). When in a grandiose state, those with NPD are extraverted, arrogant, charismatic, risk-taking, see life as win-or-lose, and show high self-esteem (Miller et al., 2021). When in a vulnerable state, those with NPD are more withdrawn, distrustful, emotionally reactive, and neurotic (Jauk et al, 2021; Miller et al., 2021). These states can co-occur or shift due to situational and contextual factors. Overlap between these two states exists in the form of antagonism, which is expressed through arrogant, callous, and exploitive behaviors (Miller et al., 2021).

Due to the dramatic nature of the thoughts, feelings, and behaviors experienced by those with NPD, there is significant risk for suicide as a result of stress associated with perceived failures, and suicide attempts in this population tend to be more lethal than those from people diagnosed with other personality disorders (APA, 2022;

Nelson, et al., 2022). In addition to suicide, when faced with a threat to their ego, those with NPD are at an increased risk for aggressive behavior (Miller et al, 2021).

While NPD may be diagnosed in individuals younger than 18 years of age (APA, 2022), symptoms must be significant and well established for at least one year. Additionally, non-pathological narcissism is generally higher among adolescents as a factor of their development. While non-pathological narcissism is evidenced to reduce with age, adults with NPD typically have a stable presentation of narcissistic traits over time (APA, 2022). However, life circumstances including clinical and non-clinical healthy relationships and the development of skills for both achieving success and tolerating failure may reduce the impact of living with this condition.

NDP Demographics

Epidemiological data presented within the DSM-V-TR indicates a range of prevalence rates from less than 0.05% to 6.2% and that between half and three-quarters of those with NPD are male (APA, 2022). One of the epidemiological studies cited in the DSM provided additional data on demographics, indicating that while an overall prevalence rate was 6.2%, the rate among Black Americans was 12.5% and that NPD was negatively correlated with age (Stinson et al., 2008). However, Males (2018) criticizes the conclusions of Stinson et al. (2008) by citing a strong correlation between socioeconomic status and NPD scores in the study and noting that authors have a tendency to reflect cultural bias by explaining African Americans as more pathological rather than linking NPD to the challenges of developing an environment with fewer resources.

Social Impact of NPD

In addition to the personal impact on the individuals experiencing NPD, there is considerable impact on those close to them with individuals in close relation to those with NPD reporting higher levels of burden and grief associated with their relationships than those who have reported on relationships with individuals with other personality disorders, neurotic disorders, mood disorders, and psychotic disorders (Day et al., 2019). If the demographics from Stinson et al. (2008) are accurate and even one African American family member or other person close to those diagnosed with NPD is significantly impacted, then 25% of African Americans are either negatively impacted directly or indirectly by the condition. While we were not able to locate research on the total economic impact this may have on African American communities through loss of working due to mental health, injury, or suicide, costs of treatment, and other factors, we expect the economic impact to be considerable.

Differential Diagnostic Options

In differential diagnosis for NPD, other personality disorders are often the first consideration due to the common general features of personality disorders (APA, 2022, pp). 763-764). Other Category B personality disorders may be particularly likely to be mistaken for NPD given their similarities. Obsessive-compulsive personality disorder (OCPD) may also be considered due to the presence of perfectionism across both disorders and "Category A" personality disorders may be considered due to similarities in dismissive relational styles and grandiosity.

Non-personality disorders may also be considered. Grandiosity is also a symptom of manic or hypomanic phases in bipolar spectrum disorders. Sensitivity to criticism and the presence of deep self-criticism and insecurity are often features of persistent depressive disorder (APA, 2022, pp 763-764).

While all of these conditions may be considered for differential diagnosis, they may also co-occur with NPD. Additionally, those with NPD experience higher rates of depressive disorders, anorexia nervosa, and substance use disorders (APA, 2022, 763-764). These co-occurring disorders increase the clinical complexity and decrease the functional capacity of those with NPD.

NPD Treatment Options

Treatment options for NPD are limited. Complicating matters, therapists tend to avoid working with clients with pathological narcissism as they present unique clinical challenges that are difficult for many therapists to manage (Caligor et al., 2015, Campbell & Miller, 2011). Further, complicating matters, there are limited resources for many with NPD as it has an increased frequency in those with lower socio-economic status (Males, 2018). With limited resources, those with NPD may be forced to receive services from community mental health agencies that often employ early-career therapists, most of whom have little or no training in the assessment and treatment of personality disorders and whose limited experience may make the unique and antagonistic challenges from patients with NPD particularly difficult to withstand.

When treatment is available for individuals with NPD, there is little quality guidance for clinicians. The standards set by the American Psychological Association for evidence-based practices in psychology (EBPP) rely on multiple randomly assigned controlled experiments and ideally meta-analyses of those experiments (Tolin et al, 2015). Research on the treatment of NPD, due to the relatively rare nature of the condition and the fact that narcissistic symptomology itself creates a barrier to help-seeking behaviors, is limited (Caligor et al., 2015).

As it stands, most published information on the treatment of NPD is done in the form of case studies. These case studies sometimes appear in peer-reviewed articles, but also frequently occur in the form of un-reviewed books and treatment guides (King et al, 2020) which represent among the lowest levels of evidentiary support (Tolin et al, 2015).

From the available evidence, endorsed treatments for NPD include psychodynamic models of therapy and cognitive behavioral models of therapy. Psychodynamic models of therapy for NPD focus on two areas – the first being on developing insight into behaviors based on experiences from the past present in interpersonal relationships and the second being focused on the transference between the therapist and the client. Specific approaches include Mentalization-Based Treatment (Drozek & Unruh, 2020) and Transference-Focused Psychotherapy (Diamond & Hersh, 2020). Cognitive-behavioral approaches to treating NPD include Schema Therapy (Behary & Dieckmann, 2011), Cognitive-Behavioral Therapy for Personality Disorders (Leedy et al., 2007), Dialectical Behavior Therapy (Reed-Knight & Fischer, 2011), and Functional Analytic Psychotherapy (Callaghan et al., 2003).

At this time, there is no pharmacological treatment recommended for NPD. The use of pharmacological interventions with patients with NPD is limited to co-occurring symptomology and is driven by those symptoms (Caligor et al., 2015). Due to the frequent co-occurring presence of anxiety, depression, and emotional dysregulation, anxiolytics, anti-psychotics, antidepressants, and mood stabilizers may be prescribed as indicated (Rivas-Vazquez & Blais, 2002).

African American Cultural Perceptions of Diagnosis

Historically, African American Cultures perceive mental illness and diagnosis with skepticism and cynicism (Harris et al., 2020). These perceptions have been shaped and formed throughout decades regarding the authoritative issue of medicine and mental health (p. 5). Of note, the unethical practices of the Tuskegee Experiments are often cited as a main reason many African Americans are reluctant to seek health services, including mental health services (Peteet et al., 2022; Ward et al., 2009). Studies have shown that 30% of African American men report a mental health disorder, however, they are less likely to seek treatment (Holden et al., 2012). Of a sample of African American women with panic disorder only 13% sought treatment (Ward et al., 2009). Of the 70 participants within another study of individuals diagnosed with mental health conditions, only 37% of African American men and women have received some counseling or mental health therapy (Matthews et al., 2006).

Several studies have identified barriers to help-seeking behavior within the African American community, including cultural norms, stigma, financial constraints, lack of knowledge, and preference for alternative resources (Harris et al., 2020).

Growing up, individuals in this community did not observe their loved ones seeking professional help as it meant they were weak or unable to handle life stressors (p. 20). Furthermore, when experiencing emotional discomfort, they were often told to bury it, suck it up, pray about it, or put up a front (Matthews et al., 2006). In addition, African Americans choose not to discuss mental illness, let alone seek help, as they do not want to experience a higher level of discrimination or be labeled as "crazy" (White, 2017). This way of thinking is passed down from generation to generation (Matthews et al., 2006).

African Americans may lack mental health knowledge as they try not to ask for help in most situations (Matthew et al., 2006). Historically, members of the African American community have been "underserved, disenfranchised, marginalized, and still recovering from the generational residue of slavery" (Jones, 2020, p. 304). At the same time, the death rate among African Americans is high while the life expectancy is low compared to white individuals (p. 304). In addition, members of this community are killed by homicide more than any ethnic group in the United States (p. 304). Such experiences could cause extreme trauma and bring about many stressors that may develop into mental illness (Jones, 2020; Woods-Giscombe et al., 2016). Asking for help requires vulnerability, which many people, especially the African American community, are uncomfortable with (Harris et al., 2020). They may feel ashamed that they cannot handle something independently or may be shamed by others for wanting to utilize resources (p. 17). Therefore, they would rather suffer in silence than place themselves in a situation where they have to be vulnerable, experience shame within their community, or experience a greater level of discrimination (Ward et al., 2009).

While many African Americans choose not to utilize mental health services, some find seeking help daunting and costly (Harris et al., 2020). Compared to Hispanics ($40,766), whites ($55,096), and Asians ($66,935), African Americans have the lowest average annual household income, $34,001 (Kawaii-Bogue et al., 2017). Moreover, research has shown that lower socioeconomic groups face a more significant challenge of obtaining and maintaining quality health care (p. 15). Even if they have quality insurance, the copay may be too significant to pay when they have other financial obligations (Dempsey et al., 2016). They may, in turn, consider paying a cash rate or even locating a facility with a sliding scale fee; however, they still may not be able to afford it (p. 76). Therefore, the thought of utilizing mental health services would end before it could truly begin.

African American Cultural Perceptions of NPD

Across six studies, Maples et al. (2015) found that Americans and non-Americans, regardless of age or ethnicity, are substantially and problematically narcissistic.

According to recent studies, African Americans have reported high levels of self-esteem (Maples et al., 2015). More often than not, this community will have, or at least try to maintain, self-reliance (ex. strong black woman, masculinity, pride) and resilience due to the stigmatization of their group (Harris et al., 2020; Robinson et al., 2018). While strides have been made, there is still a significant amount of stigma surrounding mental health within the African American community due to racism and discrimination within healthcare, misdiagnoses, and mistrust (Harris et al., 2020; Holden et al., 2012; Matthews et al., 2006).

Black and minority ethnic groups tend to be over-represented in mental health diagnoses. Acknowledging and understanding local norms before diagnosing personality disorder is critical (McGillowary et al., 2010). Studies have shown that the diagnoses of personality disorders are often criticized as culturally biased (p. 1). In many ways, African Americans view themselves as strong, resilient individuals as a means to protect themselves from the uncertainties of being Black in America (Burt et al., 2017; Ziegler-Hill & Wallace, 2011). In some instances, their strength, resilience, and highly positive self-views may be perceived as Narcissistic behavior (Ziegler-Hill & Wallace, 2011). However, they may reject the diagnosis as it is considered a sign of weakness, something they do not acknowledge, nor feel they need treatment or medical intervention (Robinson et al., 2018; Ward et al., 2009). Furthermore, if a diagnosis is acknowledged, it is common for those in the African American community to compartmentalize or rely on themselves, God, or their family to help them cope (Harris et al., 2020).

Alternative Perceptions of Mental Health

Studies suggest that African Americans experience mental health concerns at the same rate as other Americans (e.g., Buser, 2009; Constantine et al., 2004). However, this population tends to underutilize available counseling services (Buser, 2009). Several studies have examined treatment utilization patterns and the causes for poor treatment adherence among this population (Jackson et al., 2007; Sussman, 2004). Authors have identified a number of potential barriers to successful treatment, including cultural mistrust (Whaley, 2001), stigma regarding mental illness, racism within the therapeutic exchange (Parham, 2002), and treatment modalities failing to address the cultural values and worldview of the client (Constantine et al., 2005; Duran et al., 2008). In part, because of the aforementioned barriers, African Americans often rely on informal networks of support in lieu of seeking counseling (Harley & Dillard, 2005; Parhain, 2002).

These networks typically include family and community resources, religious leaders, and indigenous healers (Yeh et al., 2004). In fact, African Americans are more likely to seek religious or spiritual experiences rather than admit to mental health concerns (Harley & Dillard, 2005). More than 85% of African Americans have a relationship with God and feel more comfortable speaking with a church leader than a mental health professional (Dempsey et al., 2016; Peteet et al., 2022). Spiritual and mental health concerns are often viewed as interconnected; therefore, religious institutions have an extensive history of providing both spiritual guidance and counseling services (Harley & Dillard, 2005).

In fact, many churches offer individual and group counseling through their counseling ministry, where the person providing the services is often a church member, the pastor's wife, or the pastor himself (Dempsey et al., 2016). Following the connection with their church leaders, African Americans result to prayer as a means of treatment (Robinson et al., 2018). It is an important coping mechanism and is used to decrease or alleviate stress (p. 1097). Studies have shown that individuals within this community will choose prayer first before they will ever consider counseling (Dempsey et al., 2016; Matthews et al., 2006).

In addition to church systems in the African American community, indigenous African spiritual systems also have a long history of providing mental health services (Clarke & Heidrich, 2009). In fact, African Americans may rely on indigenous African spirituality as an alternative to Western forms of counseling (Boyd-Franklin, 2003). Although the scholarly literature has explored the therapeutic use of religion, little attention has been given to African-based spiritual systems used by African Americans as a mental health intervention (Boyd-Franklin, 2003; Constantine et al., 2005).

DISCUSSION

It is difficult to identify NPD as many individuals with the condition do not see themselves as disordered and do not seek treatment due to the nature of the condition. When this difficulty is compounded with mistrust in the medical establishment it further complicates the identification and treatment of NPD in African Americans. This poses a significant problem as NPD has drastic impacts on not only the individual with the condition but on those close to them. Adding to this difficulty, sources of therapy are often limited by financial barriers that are more likely present for African Americans.

To meet these needs, mental health providers must make changes to the typical ways of doing things. As there is justified critique of assessment and diagnosis of African Americans, common personality assessments for NPD will need to be replaced with more appropriate options for the population. Specifically, test instruments need to undergo more elaborate development so as to not show racial bias.

Furthermore, treatment must not only be made financially and logistically accessible, but also needs to be culturally accessible. To be culturally accessible, it must meet people where they are and work with the systems already present in their lives. This will likely mean the development of partnerships between African American churches and mental health providers. To do that, there will have to be trust built within African American communities as well as with potential funding sources to help facilitate a manner of providing care that does not fit into the standard mold of siloed care.

Implications

African Americans are diagnosed with mental illness, including NPD Disorder, at the same rate as other individuals from different ethnic communities (Constantine et al., 2004). However, they are still less likely to seek treatment than any other community (Ward et al., 2009). Unfortunately, utilization of services will continue to decline if measures are not implemented to assist the African American community. African Americans view NPD as they would any other diagnosis, something they can handle by themselves, with the help of the church elders, or something they choose not to acknowledge (Dempsey et al., 2016). Several studies have shown that individuals within this community have difficulty trusting those within the healthcare system (Holden et al., 2012; Peteet et al., 2022). They fear adverse treatment, misdiagnosis, and involuntary hospitalization. This fear stops them from seeking help, furthering the gap of lack of awareness. Even if they were ready, African Americans do not know where to go or how to research mental health resources (Matthews et al., 2006). Therefore, many mental health concerns go undiagnosed or untreated.

It is essential to note that many individuals within this community prefer to address mental health through alternative methods. Alternative methods consist of working through life stressors with their immediate family members or friends, speaking with church elders/churchgoers, and praying. Family, church, and prayer are meaningful to this community. Therefore, such should be considered when developing ways to help them utilize mental health services. For example, it would be beneficial to establish a relationship with the church pastor (Dempsey et al., 2016). Developing a partnership with the pastor will allow the congregation and community to feel more comfortable trusting someone in the mental health field if their pastor trusts them (p. 82). Furthermore, if they feel more comfortable with mental health professionals, African Americans can build awareness and, in turn, address their mental health (p. 82).

LIMITATIONS

Research on African American and NPD is very limited. Therefore, it is difficult to assess and analyze the perceptions of NPD among African Americans. In addition, there are limited peer-reviewed studies on the effects of African Americans and any personality disorders as many individuals within this community do not recognize NPD or personality disorders as an issue. In order to gain more research in this area, it is crucial to address the disparities in the African American community regarding health care and mental health.

Furthermore, when examining NPD in correlation with the African American community, it is essential to separate and define identity vs. NPD. Due to racial bias, some professionals may assume an African American's identity is so grandiose that it fits the description of NPD. However, it may be how they identify as Black or African American.

Lastly, research and case studies on implementing different strategies to assist the African American community are scarce. Community members will not participate in research if they believe it will cause them more harm. More importantly, they will not consider mental health resources if the healthcare system and mental health professionals do not consider and consciously try to learn more about culture and identity before working with this community. It is imperative to change the narrative and work to alleviate or decrease the stigma highly attached to mental health in the African American community.

Future Research

Partnerships with African American churches could help close the mental health gap within the African American community. For future research, it may be necessary to consider dialog-based interventions through community-academic partnerships (CAP) "involving community stakeholders as partners in research" (Dempsey et al., p. 4, 2016; Peteet et al., 2022). When working with this community and possibly partnering with church leaders, it would be beneficial to have members of the research team who are culturally competent and understand their values and morals as black people (Dempsey et al., 2016). This type of research is often referred to as participatory action research (PAR, Baum et al., 2006), a form of research that includes those most affected by the research in the entire research process and that is recommended for use with minority populations. The purpose of this kind of research is to ensure to the greatest extent possible that the research is meaningful and helpful to the populations it affects.

In partnering with the church, it would be beneficial to connect with church members who are mental health professionals. There are more than 65,000 churches with predominantly African American members (Plunkett, 2014). Among the thousands of members that attend the church, some may include licensed professional counselors, licensed masters' and clinical social workers, psychologists, and even school counselors. A level of trust may already be established with these church members. Therefore, church members and the African American community may feel more comfortable speaking with those individuals, learning about resources, and possibly working with community mental health agencies.

Researchers may also benefit from examining the effects of church members partnering with mental health agencies and professionals to establish counseling ministries. For example, many African American churches provide various services/ministries, including health resources, education, food services, financial assistance, and youth programs (Campbell & Littleton, 2018). If they have not already, churches could implement a counseling ministry where African American community members can receive services from licensed professionals within the church.

Equally important, further research could determine the effectiveness of a sliding fee scale and if it will encourage individuals to utilize mental health services. A sliding fee allows individuals to pay a rate based on their income and not necessarily use their insurance (Kawaii-Bogue et al., 2017). Therefore, if African American community members are empowered and can address their mental health status without placing themselves in financial hardship, they may feel more inclined to seek services.

Through community partnership, research needs to be completed to meet the previously stated needs. First, research needs to address questions of racial bias in diagnosis and assessment (Males, 2018). Second, research needs to address solutions to overcoming the well-earned mistrust of the medical and mental health professions experienced by many African Americans (Dempsey et al., 2016; Peteet et al., 2022). Finally, there is little research in effective treatment for NPD and to the authors knowledge none that directly addresses effectiveness for treatment of NPD in the African American cultural context.

REFERENCES

American Psychiatric Association. (2022). Personality disorders. In Diagnostic and statistical manual of mental disorders (5th ed., text rev.). APA.

Baum, F., MacDougall, C., & Smith, D. (2006). Participatory action research. *Journal of Epidemiology and Community Health*, *60*(10), 854–857. doi:10.1136/jech.2004.028662 PMID:16973531

Behary, W. T., & Dieckmann, E. (2011). The art of empathetic confrontation, limit-setting, and leverage. In W. K. Campbell & J. D. Miller (Eds.), *The handbook of narcissism and narcissistic personality disorder: Theoretical approaches, empirical findings, and treatments* (pp. 445–456).

Boyd-Franklin, N. (2003). Black families in therapy: Understanding the African American experience. New York: Guilford.

Burt, C. H., Lei, M. K., & Simons, R. L. (2017). Racial discrimination, racial socialization, and crime: Understanding mechanisms of resilience. *Social Problems, 64*(3), 414–438. doi:10.1093ocpropw036

Callaghan, G. M., Summers, C. J., & Weidman, M. (2003). The treatment of histrionic and narcissistic personality disorder behaviors: A single-subject demonstration of clinical improvement using functional analytic psychotherapy. *Journal of Contemporary Psychotherapy, 33*(4), 321–339. doi:10.1023/B:JOCP.0000004502.55597.81

Campbell, K. W., & Miller, J. D. (2011). *The handbook of narcissism and narcissistic personality disorder: Theoretical approaches, empirical findings, and treatments.* John Wiley & Sons. doi:10.1002/9781118093108

Campbell, R. D., & Littleton, T. (2018). Mental health counseling in the Black American church: Reflections and recommendations from counselors serving in a counseling ministry. *Mental Health, Religion & Culture, 21*(4), 336–352. doi:10.1080/13674676.2018.1494704

Constantine, M. G., Myers, L. J., Kindaichi, M., & Moore, J. L. III. (2004). Exploring indigenous mental health practices: The roles of healers and helpers in promoting well-being in people of color. *Counseling and Values, 48*(2), 110–125. doi:10.1002/j.2161-007X.2004.tb00238.x

Day, N. J., Bourke, M. E., Townsend, M. L., & Grenyer, B. F. (2020). Pathological narcissism: A study of burden on partners and family. *Journal of Personality Disorders, 34*(6), 799–813. doi:10.1521/pedi_2019_33_413 PMID:30730784

Dempsey, K., Butler, S. K., & Gaither, L. (2016). Black churches and mental health professionals: Can this collaboration work? *Journal of Black Studies, 47*(1), 73–87. doi:10.1177/0021934715613588

Diamond, D., & Hersh, R. G. (2020). Transference-focused psychotherapy for narcissistic personality disorder: An object relations approach. *Journal of Personality Disorders, 34*(Supplement), 159–176. doi:10.1521/pedi.2020.34.supp.159 PMID:32186988

Drozek, R. P., & Unruh, B. T. (2020). Mentalization-based treatment for pathological narcissism. *Journal of Personality Disorders, 34*(Supplement), 177–203. doi:10.1521/pedi.2020.34.supp.177 PMID:32186985

Duran, E., Firehammer, J., & Gonzalez, J. (2008). Liberation psychology as the path toward healing cultural soul wounds. *Journal of Counseling and Development, 86*(3), 288–295. doi:10.1002/j.1556-6678.2008.tb00511.x

Harley, D. A., & Dillard, J. M. (Eds.). (2005). *Contemporary mental health issues among African Americans*. Amer Counseling Assn.

Harris, J. R., Crowe, A., & McKinney, J. G. (2020). African Americans' perceptions of mental illness and preferences for treatment. *Journal of Counselor Practice, 11*(1), 1–33. doi:10.22229/afa1112020

Holden, K. B., McGregor, B. S., Blanks, S. H., & Mahaffey, C. (2012). Psychosocial, socio-cultural, and environmental influences on mental health help-seeking among African-American men. *The Journal of Men's Health, 9*(2), 63–69. doi:10.1016/j.jomh.2012.03.002 PMID:22905076

Jackson, J. S., Neighbors, H. W., Torres, M., Martin, L. A., Williams, D. R., & Baser, R. (2007). Use of mental health services and subjective satisfaction with treatment among Black Caribbean immigrants: Results from the National Survey of American Life. *American Journal of Public Health, 97*(1), 60–67. doi:10.2105/AJPH.2006.088500 PMID:17138907

Jauk, E., Ulbrich, L., Jorschick, P., Höfler, M., Kaufman, S. B., & Kanske, P. (2022). The nonlinear association between grandiose and vulnerable narcissism: An individual data meta-analysis. *Journal of Personality, 90*(5), 703–726. doi:10.1111/jopy.12692 PMID:34860434

Jones, W. (2020). The lives of Douglass, Du Bois, and Washington: Self-actualization among African American males. *Journal of Humanistic Psychology, 60*(3), 303–329. https://doi-org.proxy.tamuc.edu/10.1177/0022167817739761. doi:10.1177/0022167817739761

Kawaii-Bogue, B., Williams, N. J., & MacNear, K. (2017). Mental health care access and treatment utilization in African American communities: An integrative care framework. *Best Practices in Mental Health, 13*(2), 11–29.

King, R. M., Grenyer, B. F., Gurtman, C. G., & Younan, R. (2020). A clinician's quick guide to evidence-based approaches: Narcissistic personality disorder. *Clinical Psychologist, 24*(1), 91–95. doi:10.1111/cp.12214

Leedy, M. J., Jackson, M., & Callahan, J. L. (2007). Treating depression and compensatory narcissistic personality style in a man with chronic Lyme disease. *Clinical Case Studies*, *6*(5), 430–442. doi:10.1177/1534650106295847

Males, M. (2018). Racial implications of the narcissistic personality inventory reinterpreting popular depictions of narcissism trends. *Journal of Psychology and Psychiatry*, *2*(1), 1–4. doi:10.15761/JPP.1000106

Matthews, A., Corrigan, P., Smith, B., & Aranda, F. (2006). A qualitative exploration of African-Americans' attitudes toward mental illness and mental illness treatment seeking. *Rehabilitation Education*, *20*(4), 253–268. doi:10.1891/088970106805065331

McGilloway, A., Hall, R. E., Lee, T., & Bhui, K. S. (2010). A systematic review of personality disorder, race and ethnicity: Prevalence, aetiology, and treatment. *BMC Psychiatry*, *10*(1), 1–14. doi:10.1186/1471-244X-10-33 PMID:20459788

Miller, J. D., Back, M. D., Lynam, D. R., & Wright, A. G. (2021). Narcissism today: What we know and what we need to learn. *Current Directions in Psychological Science*, *30*(6), 519–525. doi:10.1177/09637214211044109

Miller, J. D., Maples, J. L., Cai, H., Kisbu-Sakarya, Y., LoPilato, A., Sedikides, C., Buffardi, L., Gentile, B., Kwan, V. S., Pendry, L. F., Siedor, L., & Campbell, W. K. (2015). Narcissism and United States' culture: The view from home and around the world. *Journal of Personality and Social Psychology*, *109*(6), 1068–1089. doi:10.1037/a0039543 PMID:26389797

Nelson, S. M., Griffin, C. A., Hein, T. C., Bowersox, N., & McCarthy, J. F. (2022). Personality disorder and suicide risk among patients in the veterans affairs health system. *Personality Disorders*, *13*(6), 563–571. doi:10.1037/per0000521 PMID:34726449

Pederson, A., Tsai, A. C., Hawkins, D., Moskowitz, J., & Dixon, L. (2023). Understanding the association between mental health knowledge and mental health service utilization among black adults. *Community Mental Health Journal*, *59*(1), 57–67. doi:10.100710597-022-00988-w PMID:35794413

Peteet, B., Watts, V., Tucker, E., Brown, P., Hanna, M., Saddlemire, A., Rizk, M., Belliard, J. C., Abdul-Mutakabbir, J. C., Casey, S., & Simmons, K. (2022). Faith, fear, and facts: A covid-19 vaccination hesitancy intervention for black church congregations. *Vaccines*, *10*(7), 1–11. doi:10.3390/vaccines10071039 PMID:35891203

Plunkett, D. (2014). The black church, values, and secular counseling: Implications for counselor education and practice. *Counseling and Values, 59*(2), 208–221. doi:10.1002/j.2161-007X.2014.00052.x

Reed-Knight, B., & Fischer, S. (2011). Treatment of narcissistic personality disorder symptoms in a dialectical behavior therapy framework: A discussion and case example. In W. K. Campbell & J. D. Miller (Eds.), *The handbook of narcissism and narcissistic personality disorder: Theoretical approaches, empirical findings, and treatments* (pp. 466–475). doi:10.1002/9781118093108.ch42

Rivas-Vazquez, R. A., & Blais, M. A. (2002). Pharmacologic treatment of personality disorders. *Professional Psychology, Research and Practice, 33*(1), 104–107. doi:10.1037/0735-7028.33.1.104

Robinson, M. A., Jones-Eversley, S., Moore, S. E., Ravenell, J., & Adedoyin, A. C. (2018). Black male mental health and the black church: Advancing a collaborative partnership and research agenda. *Journal of Religion and Health, 57*(3), 1095–1107. doi:10.100710943-018-0570-x PMID:29417396

Stinson, F. S., Dawson, D. A., Goldstein, R. B., Chou, S. P., Huang, B., Smith, S. M., Ruan, W. J., Pulay, A. J., Saha, T. D., Pickering, R. P., & Grant, B. F. (2008). Prevalence, correlates, disability, and comorbidity of DSM-IV narcissistic personality disorder: Results from the wave 2 national epidemiologic survey on alcohol and related conditions. *The Journal of Clinical Psychiatry, 69*(7), 1033–1045. doi:10.4088/JCP.v69n0701 PMID:18557663

Sussman, L. K. (2004). The role of culture in definitions, interpretations, and management of illness. In U. P. Gielen, J. M. Fish, & J. G. Draguns (Eds.), *Handbook of culture, therapy, and healing* (pp. 37–65). Lawrence Erlbaum Associates Publishers.

Tolin, D. F., McKay, D., Forman, E. M., Klonsky, E. D., & Thombs, B. D. (2015). Empirically supported treatment: Recommendations for a new model. *Clinical Psychology: Science and Practice, 22*(4), 317–338. doi:10.1037/h0101729

Ward, E., Clark, L. O., & Heidrich, S. (2009). African American women's beliefs, coping behaviors, and barriers to seeking mental health services. *Qualitative Health Research, 19*(11), 1589–1601. doi:10.1177/1049732309350686 PMID:19843967

Whaley, A. (2001). Cultural mistrust and mental health services for African Americans: A review and meta-analysis. *The Counseling Psychologist, 29*(4), 513–531. doi:10.1177/0011000001294003

White, T. (2017). *Semi-structured interviews: African American clergy perceptions regarding mental health.* Sage Publications. doi:10.4135/9781526424136

Woods-Giscombe, C., Robinson, M., Carthon, D., Devane-Johnson, S., & Corbie-Smith, G. (2016). Superwoman schema, stigma, spirituality, and culturally sensitive providers: Factors influencing African American women's use of mental health services. *Journal of Best Practices in Health Professions Diversity : Research, Education and Policy*, *9*(1), 1124–1144. PMID:33043323

Yeh, C. J., Hunter, C. D., Madan-Bahel, A., Chiang, L., & Arora, A. K. (2004). Indigenous and interdependent perspectives of healing: Implications for counseling and research. *Journal of Counseling and Development*, *82*(4), 410–419. doi:10.1002/j.1556-6678.2004.tb00328.x

Zeigler-Hill, V., & Wallace, M. (2011). Racial differences in narcissistic tendencies. *Journal of Research in Personality*, *45*(5), 456–467. doi:10.1016/j.jrp.2011.06.001

Chapter 9
Major Depressive Disorder Among African-Americans

Elizabeth Wachira
https://orcid.org/0000-0003-4219-7545
Texas A&M University, Commerce, USA

Priscilla W. Wachira
Texas Woman's University, USA

Rahmatu Kassimu
Dr. K.'s Health Minute, USA

ABSTRACT

Major depressive depression is a common but serious mood disorder, and the leading cause of disability globally. It is associated with poorer physical health and higher rates of disability, as traumatic experiences can trigger a depressive episode. This chapter presents an overview of major depressive disorder, and highlights the pathways that lead to African Americans being disproportionately affected. It discusses the social determinants of health among African Americans that lead to depression being underreported and undertreated in this demographic group. This discussion extends to reinforce once again how systemic racism "a pandemic in a pandemic" shape the availability, quality, and use of mental healthcare access. The chapter concludes with a discussion on lessons learned and recommendations on how to aid in equitable and targeted interventions that are culturally relevant and attentive to the unique needs of this population.

DOI: 10.4018/978-1-6684-8918-5.ch009

INTRODUCTION

This chapter presents an overview of major depressive disorder and highlights the pathways that lead to African Americans being disproportionately affected. It discusses the social determinants of health among African Americans that lead to depression being underreported and undertreated in this demographic group. This discussion extends to reinforce once again how systemic racism “a pandemic in a pandemic” shapes the availability, quality, and use of mental healthcare access. The chapter concludes with a discussion of lessons learned and recommendations on how to aid in equitable and targeted interventions that are culturally relevant and attentive to the unique needs of this population.

Major depressive depression (MDD), frequently referred to as major depression, is a common but serious mood disorder, and the leading cause of disability globally (National Institute of Mental Health [NIMH], 2022; Yelton et al., 2022). It causes severe symptoms that affect “how you feel, think, and manage daily activities, such as sleeping, eating, or working that typically interrupts the ability to sleep, work, or perform additional daily tasks (Mayo Clinic, 2023; NIMH, 2022). In the United States, approximately twenty-one million adults, or 8.4% of the U.S. population have had at least one major depressive episode (NIMH, 2022). Although data on the exact burden of MDD remains ambiguous, those with the highest prevalence rates are women (10.5%), those aged 18-25 (17%), and who report having multiple (two or more) races (15.9%) (NIMH, 2022).

Accurate diagnosis of depression is crucial for also knowing disease burden and ensuring proper response and treatment. For clinicians to properly diagnose an individual with depression, symptoms must be present for at least two weeks. Symptoms include having persistently low or depressed mood, decreased interest in pleasurable activities (anhedonia), feelings of guilt or worthlessness, lack of energy, poor concentration, appetite changes, psychomotor retardation or agitation, sleep disturbances, or suicidal thoughts (Bains & Abdijadid, 2022). MDD is a clinical diagnosis and clinicians determine this through specific inquiries; they conduct a physical exam, draw lab tests (blood count, thyroid tests), do a psychiatric evaluation to assess thoughts, feelings, and behavior patterns in greater detail, and lastly, use the criteria listed in the Diagnostic and Statistical Manual of Mental Disorders (DSM-5) to identify depressive disorders (Mayo Clinic, 2023). To ensure accurate diagnosis, the DSM-5 guidelines published by the American Psychiatric Association (APA) stipulate that an individual must have five of the symptoms, one being a depressed mood or anhedonia causing social or occupational impairment (Bains & Abdijadid, 2022). These are important checkpoints to note as depressive symptoms can be secondary to other physical and mental disorders such as Parkinson’s, thyroid disorders, diabetes, schizophrenia or even taking medications that alter mood or behavior (Bains & Abdijadid, 2022).

The main cause of depression is not fully known, but causes are considered multifactorial and include a combination of biological, environmental, genetic, and or even psychological factors. For example, those who have lived through traumatic or stressful events, such as the death of a relative, physical, emotional, and or sexual abuse have an increased risk of depression. Likewise, experiencing a major life change such as financial loss (losing a job), a medical diagnosis or illness, taking certain medications, or using alcohol or drugs can all increase one's risk for depression (Centers for Disease Control and Prevention [CDC], 2022).

MDD is associated with poorer physical health and higher rates of disability as traumatic experiences such as the ones mentioned above can trigger a depressive episode (CDC, 2023; Gutiérrez-Rojas et al., 2020). Studies have found commonalities between stressful life events (SLEs) and depression. SLEs are more prominent amongst racial minorities from low single-family socioeconomic backgrounds, who are often victims of racism, communal violence, and with histories of substance abuse. It is therefore not surprising that African Americans, given the constant traumatic experiences they live through, often tend to have more serious, chronic, and severely debilitating diseases when diagnosed with MDD (Bailey, Mokonogho, & Kumar, 2019).

DETERMINANTS OF MDD AMONG AFRICAN AMERICANS

Social determinants of health are the conditions that a person is born into, lives, learns, worships, works, plays, and age that affects their quality of life as well as overall health and functioning (Yelton et al., 2022). These span five domains: social and community context, economic stability, health care access and quality, education access and quality, and neighborhood and built environment. These domains offer several facets that increase the risk of mental illness among African Americans, a risk exacerbated by the effects of systematic racism across these domains (Hudson et al., 2016; 2023; Yelton et al., 2022). For example, access to healthcare, neighborhood safety, and quality of education and shaped by institutionally sanctioned redlining which then leads to insufficient community resources and limited social and economic capital. This "resource deficiency" is present across the various domains as a stressor that produces adverse health outcomes and increases psychological distress for African Americans; an effect that they experience for longer time periods compared to their white counterparts.

Sustained and situational instances of collective trauma over time can have harmful effects on one's mental health. For example, the COVID-19 pandemic and the subsequent policies associated with attempts to manage the virus had profound effects across the globe. The pandemic exacerbated mental health issues and studies show that depression rates globally increased exponentially between 2017 and 2022 from 3.4% to 25% respectively (Bueno et al., 2021). African Americans however were disproportionately impacted due to their socioeconomic status and already disadvantaged life experiences. The interplay of socioeconomic factors increased their vulnerability to exposure risks given they are more likely to be employed in "public facing" essential industries that require them to work in close proximity with the public and occupy positions where working from home was not an option and public transportation the main mode of travel (Burstrom et al., 2020; Webb et al., 2020). Furthermore, the additional stress and trauma associated with attempts to follow regulations, hospitalizations and deaths of loved ones, and discontinuation of community programs exacerbated their mental health status (Okoro et al., 2022).

AFRICAN AMERICAN PERSPECTIVES ON MENTAL HEALTH

On average, and overall, across all mental health illnesses, African Americans experience these conditions at or about the same frequency as white Americans (Mental Health America [MHA], n.d.). However, these issues are exacerbated by the unique confluence of trauma and violence they continuously experience at higher rates than their white American counterparts. Current systems rife with systematic racism affect access to and trust in these systems resulting in trauma when engaging with service providers. This daily trauma is often compounded by occurrences such as the COVID-19 pandemic and highly televised and debated instances of police brutality. The impact of these occurrences provides a rationale for why Black adults in the U.S. are more likely to report persistent emotional distress compared to white Americans (Office of Minority Health [OMH], 2023). Lastly, African Americans have complex perspectives on mental health which are influenced by individual and social aspects. These perspectives are not limited to one aspect of life, but a multitude of experiences. This unfortunately results in fear of social stigma and being vulnerable resulting in poor coping strategies and low help-seeking behavior (Ward et al., 2013).

MENTAL HEALTH TREATMENT AMONG AFRICAN AMERICANS

There are numerous issues that arise that negatively impact access to services or quality treatment outcomes. For one, African Americans are usually misdiagnosed and undertreated for schizophrenia and mood disorders compared to other demographic groups (MHA, n.d.). Additionally, fear of social reprisal prevents many of them from seeking treatment as they fear being considered "crazy" by their social networks (Ward et al., 2013). Despite a demonstrated need, only one in three African American adults with mental illness receives treatment (National Alliance on Mental Illness [NAMI], n.d.). They are also less likely to receive care consistent with guidelines or be included in research leaving their invaluable input missing to policies and care reformations (APA, 2017). Interestingly, they are more likely to utilize emergency care for psychiatric issues as opposed to mental health professionals. It is therefore important to explore why African Americans avoid treatment despite having the need for psychiatric and depression-related issues.

Insight into the poor help-seeking behavior must be considered historically as Black and African American people have undergone violence, oppression, and systematic disenfranchisement, which was the bedrock of several American systems and drivers of systematic racism (MHA, n.d.). Racism has infiltrated every system, from law enforcement to the healthcare system, increasing the number of socioeconomic disparities that African Americans experience and synergistically affecting the education, health, social, and economic domains (NAMI, n.d.). Within the healthcare system, racism has led to health inequities plaguing African Americans at higher rates leading to more death and disability compared to white Americans. These inequities, coupled with perceptions of provider racism and biases, increase distrust of medical professionals and the field overall, reducing the likelihood that they will seek services when they need help.

Access to healthcare is also another issue that impacts help-seeking behavior largely due to affordability and insurance coverage. African Americans have higher uninsured or underinsured rates (10.4%) compared with their white counterparts (7.5%) (CDC, 2019). For example, 58.2% of African Americans ages 18 to 25 and 50.1% of adults ages 26 to 49 with serious mental illness did not receive treatment (CDC, 2019). Furthermore, these respondents had already been diagnosed with a mental health condition but received no mental health services in the year prior to the study. Therefore, help-seeking behavior among African Americans extends beyond individual choice or knowledge to social and economic factors inclusive of financial constraints and medical distrust reducing the likelihood that African Americans will seek treatment.

Stigma and Social Norms

Another factor that shapes help-seeking behavior is societal norms and resulting stigma. Negative attitudes about those with mental illnesses are pervasive in the U.S. but are likely to be more prevalent or debilitating among African American communities (NAMI, n.d.). The fear of appearing "less than" discourages many from seeking care, particularly African American men. Studies looking at the treatment-seeking behavior find that a potential barrier to seeking help is the perception that psychotherapy is associated with diminished weakness and pride (Bailey, Mokonogho & Kumar, 2019). While attitudes can vary by population demographics, older African Americans are more likely to view mental illness as a "personal weakness." These views negatively impact social norms and lead to a feeling of shame and worry that anyone experiencing a mental illness will be shunned, misunderstood, or experience discrimination in their social circles (Stare & Fernando, 2019). Moreover, they may also believe that discussions about mental health may not be appropriate in their social circles, leading them to suffer in silence as they fear that a diagnosis can lead to social isolation (Abdullah & Brown, 2020).

In the African American community, the notion that concerns such as mental illness should be resolved within the family or religious organization leads some to utilize faith-based support for mental health instead of a mental healthcare provider (Bailey, Mokonogho & Kumar, 2019; NAMI, 2023). Research well supports that familial or congregational social support provides tangible, emotional, and informational benefits that impact psychological well-being, treatment-seeking, adherence,and recovery (Yelton et al., 2022). The reliance or preference on "in-house" help among African Americans has created a divide between faith and medicine, instead of working in tandem. Churches are uniquely positioned and often represent trusted sources in communities for healing, community, and camaraderie. Studies show that faith-based interventions can help reduce feelings of isolation, help reduce stigma and provide easily accessible, culturally competent community-based mental health services and interventions (Campbell & Winchester, 2020). Therefore, while older generations of African Americans may have viewed the church in opposition to seeking mental health services, a collaborative, integrative model could significantly reduce not only risk factors and social stigma but also the prevalence and length of mental health issues.

DISPARITIES OF MDD AMONG AFRICAN AMERICANS

Historically, African Americans experience worse health outcomes due to social and cultural factors shaping availability and access to quality care. These differences in outcomes are termed "health disparities" and affect groups who have systematically experienced greater identity –based obstacles. The consequence of these experience includes having differential health outcomes associated with, and contributing to further social, environmental, or economic disadvantage (HP2030; Maura & de Mamani, 2017). For example, compared to white adults, African Americans are more likely to report persistent symptoms of emotional distress such as sadness or feeling hopeless at 2.6% compared to 4.2% respectively (NAMI, n.d.). The prevalence of MDD among African Americans can be misleading in that it shows that African Americans have a lower prevalence compared to whites at 12.9% compared to 18.7% (National Institute of Mental Health (NIMH, 2022).

This discrepancy is attributed to other key factors that shape access to quality mental health care based on interrelated factors discussed previously such as discrimination, mistrust of healthcare providers to inaccuracies of diagnostic methods utilized (Assari & Caldwell, 2018; Bailey et al., 2009; 2011; Bor et al., 2019; Hudson et al., 2016, 2023; Laurencin & Walker, 2020; Yelton et al., 2022). As discussed earlier, an important driver of these disparities, which cuts across these social-cultural domains are the continued experience and presence of racism in society. For example, when prevalence rates are compared based on gender, African American women present with more depressive symptoms and experiences with racism, sexism, and poverty increase this risk with symptoms expressed through hopelessness, suicide, and alcohol addiction (Bailey et al., 2009, 2011; Yelton et al., 2022). When prevalence is compared based on socioeconomic status (SES), African American men with higher SES have increased depressive risk and symptoms, an occurrence that is not seen among African American women or white men and women (Assari & Caldwell, 2018; Hudson et al., 2016, 2023). This is surprising considering the opportunities and resources that an increase in education or income has. However, due to increased exposure to racial discrimination, an increase in SES for African American men is associated with increased mental costs (Hudson et al., 2016, 2023).

Discrimination is a potent stressor related to both an increase in levels of depression symptoms and increased odds of depression (Hudson et al., 2016, 2023; Yelton et al., 2022). The "high effort coping" used to overcome stressful situations comes at a "mental health cost" for African Americans, particularly men, due to discrimination's overt and covert occurrences. Upward social mobility changes the composition of social networks such that African American men experience increased exposure to racism due to being in socially segregated work or living settings. Furthermore, this coupled with the decreased availability of social support, creates these differential outcomes based on both race and gender (Assari & Caldwell, 2018; Hudson et al., 2016, 2023; Yelton et al., 2022).

As mentioned before, discrimination cuts across the various determinants that shape health experiences and outcomes for African Americans. An expression of discrimination in society is the increase in hate crimes, particularly during the COVID-19 pandemic, hence termed a "pandemic on a pandemic" (Bor et al., 2019; Laurencin & Walker, 2020; Yelton et al., 2022). A study conducted by Bor et al. (2019) found that police killings had a spillover effect on mental health for African Americans in the general population as racism can also be experienced vicariously (Bor et al., 2019; Yelton et al., 2022). Specifically, they compared the effects of exposure to police killings of unarmed African American men and found that poor mental health days increased for African Americans, but no changes in days were noted among white Americans (Bor et al., 2019). The killings of African American men such as George Floyd and Ahmaud Arbery, to name a few, are examples of the pervasiveness of racism, since African Americans are more likely to experience police brutality than whites. This calls attention to the occurrence and continued disadvantage in the physical and mental health impact of this "pandemic on a pandemic" (Bor et al., 2019; Laurencin & Walker, 2020; Yelton et al., 2022). Therefore, police brutality is considered a social determinant of health that results in a heightened perception of systematic racism, lack of fairness, increased fear of victimization, increased vigilance and "high effort coping" among African Americans. (Bor et al., 2019). The spillover effects of this are diminished trust in social institutions such as law enforcement and medical institutions which ultimately leads to the perpetuation of health disparities among African Americans (Laurencin & Walker, 2020).

Disparities in Diagnosis and Management of MDD

MDD is a common disorder in the United States, and is associated with poorer physical health, high comorbidity, and higher rates of disability, making it the leading cause of disability globally (Yelton et al., 2022). Although it affects people of all races and ethnicities, African Americans are disproportionately affected despite having lower MDD prevalence rates due to differential diagnosis, treatment, and management received. Studies show that African Americans experience different symptoms and challenges in getting quality care for mental health disorders (Bailey et al., 2011; Martin et al., 2013). For example, African Americans with depression are frequently underdiagnosed and inadequately managed due to numerous individuals, service provider, and treatment setting factors (Bailey et al., 2009, 2011; Yelton et al., 2022). They are more likely to be poor, uninsured, and have a service provider from a different cultural background which contributes to the occurrences of inaccurate diagnosis and bias in a low access setting (Bailey et al., 2009, 2011; Yelton et al., 2022). The outcome of this is that African Americans are less likely to receive a proper diagnosis, and treatment and more likely to have depression for a long time and suffer greater disability (Bailey et al., 2009, 2011).

The disparities associated with mis or under-diagnosis of MDD among African Americans are attributed to differences in symptoms reported. Studies show that African Americans are more likely to report somatic symptoms that impact the recognition and diagnosis of MDD resulting in improper treatment. African American women present with more severe and psychosocial stressors and distress due to economic, educational, and discriminating factors (Bailey et al., 2009; 2011; Yelton et al., 2022). These include sleep disturbances, appetite or weight loss, versus more emotional sadness making it difficult to detect MDD. For men, due to both racism and gendered expectations of masculinity, diagnosis may be even lower as they are more hesitant to seek treatment or present with different symptoms that differ from traditional diagnostic symptoms (Martin et al., 2013). It is important to note that the traditional signs and symptoms of depression based on the DSM-5 diagnostic guidelines are "socially unacceptable habits" for men based on gendered norms (Bains & Abdijadid, 2022; Martin et al., 2013; Mayo Clinic, 2023; Yelton et al., 2022). Therefore, it is not surprising that they may present with alternate symptoms including anger, irritability, self-destruction, numbing pain, or distraction through substance abuse, gambling, or workaholic (Martin et al., 2013). Symptoms of depression in men and women using alternative diagnostic symptoms found that men reported higher rates of anger attacks, aggression, substance abuse,and risk-taking compared to women (Martin et al., 2013). Interestingly, when alternative scales were used, depression was more prevalent among men than women; this finding helps further explain why depression rates among African Americans, specifically men, are lower despite the expectation they should be higher given the numerous risk factors they have and experience (Bailey, Mokonogho, & Kumar, 2019; Martin et al., 2013).

Effective management and treatment of MDD depend on early and accurate diagnosis. Given the misdiagnosis and underdiagnosis among African Americans, it is not surprising that they are less likely to receive adequate and quality care. Alegría et al. (2008) looked at access to mental health care among adults with depression and found that African Americans had lower access utilization rates with 58.8% not accessing care compared to 42% among whites (Alegría et al., 2008). Of these, 85-90% had recent contact with the healthcare system further highlighting the inadequacies in diagnosis and MDD detection by providers. Studies show that African Americans are less likely to receive mental health services, and when they do, it is through emergency or crisis services resulting in fragmented care compared to whites treated in the outpatient setting by their primary care doctors ensuring continuity of care (Henry et al., 2020; Maura & de Mamani, 2017; Olfson et al., 2023). As such, treatment outcomes are poor, with African Americans having higher dropout rates from these services due to poor satisfaction and engagement with providers (Maura & de Mamani, 2017; Olfson et al., 2023). Reasons for poor engagement include mistrust of providers, different cultural or religious views on treatment, low preference for medication management,and associated mental health stigma (Alegría et al., 2008; Bailey et al., 2011; Maura & de Mamani, 2017; Olfson et al., 2023).

Aside from differential diagnosis and treatment outcomes, there are notable differences in the treatment and management of MDD among African Americans. They are less likely to receive psychotropic medications and more likely to receive psychotherapy (Henry et al., 2020; Maura & de Mamani, 2017; Olfson et al.,

2023). The preference for psychotherapy over medication treatment may be due to concerns about etiology of depression, the safety and effectiveness of antidepressants, and the role of religious/spiritual coping or interventions (Bailey, Mokonogho & Kumar, 2019). Despite the preference for psychotherapy, there are still notable pharmacological differences such that African Americans are more likely to be prescribed more antipsychotics (Maura & de Mamani, 2017; Olfson et al., 2023). The metabolic risk of these along with the small to modest effects as adjunctive treatments coupled with the higher rates of obesity and diabetes compound safety concerns for blacks and prompt concern for why these variations and overuse exist (Olfson et al., 2023).

LESSONS LEARNED AND RECOMMENDATIONS FOR FUTURE PRACTICE

MDD is associated with high comorbidity of physical and mental health diseases. For example, chronic diseases such as diabetes, stroke, obesity, and hypertension increase the risk of MDD by 50% as they can trigger a traumatic experience that leads to a depressive episode and vice versa (Gutiérrez-Rojas et al., 2020). More recently, the COVID-19 pandemic resulted in an increase in depression globally coupled with service disruptions and access that negatively affected high-risk groups such as African Americans. Factors that contribute to higher rates of MDD among this group include exposure to traumatic events tied to racism and poverty resulting in poor access to quality mental health care, having higher rates of chronic diseases, and lastly, stigma and cultural beliefs that shape treatment-seeking behavior. Therefore, improving mental health among African Americans requires multifaceted approaches that addresses the unique challenges and cultural factors affecting this population. Doing so can ultimately reduce stigma and increase access to mental health care.

Approaches to improving mental health outcomes solutions can be broadly grouped into three major focus areas that include: addressing the social determinants of mental health, reducing mental health-related stigma by addressing cultural beliefs and values, and lastly, increasing the representation of African American mental health practitioners. It is important to note that these solutions should be implemented in collaboration with African American communities to ensure that they are culturally sensitive and effective.

Addressing social determinants of health can help increase access to quality and effective mental health care. Some approaches for this include addressing the key interrelated drivers to mental health disparities among African Americans including poverty and racism. Systemic racism shapes the quality of one's built environment, educational access, and quality. Therefore, increasing access to education and job opportunities in low-income neighborhoods can improve poverty outcomes and requires tackling occurrences of discrimination that shape access to resources and upward mobility for African Americans. Another way to address access barriers among African Americans is to integrate mental health services into primary care settings (Olfson et al., 2023). Another way is to provide a voucher program for providers to be able to practice and accept clients in disenfranchised neighborhoods to increase access to mental health resources.

Culturally appropriate health education information on mental health can reduce stigma and provide resources to encourage African Americans seek help. Educational efforts should be aimed at the individual and group level. For example, educational efforts targeting community gatekeepers such as clergy, community health workers, and youth can ensure that continuous awareness and education is ongoing in the places where people live, work, and worship. This can be through health education programs targeting different demographic groups such as youth, parents, or clergy and integrating these into various community initiatives and locations such as community centers, places of worship, recreational centers, and libraries. Another way is to develop social media campaigns that use material and actors that represent this demographic and provide avenues for African American mental health providers to do the education and awareness.

African Americans face unique and nuanced interactions between social determinants of health that make them at higher risk of developing poor mental health. These same interactions also make African Americans more likely to suffer from these conditions leading to longer and more persistent episodes of negative mental health outcomes. This requires addressing cultural beliefs and values by developing culturally tailored interventions that are respectful of traditional beliefs and values. Therefore, promoting culturally sensitive education and care can help improve engagement and increase treatment-seeking behavior. For example, integrating traditional health practices such as spiritual and community support enables service providers to work in tandem with trusted gatekeepers such as community leaders, faith-based organizations, and traditional healer. This should also extend to community-driven approaches to mental health research to help increase the visibility of MDD, decrease stigma, and increase literacy (Algeria et al, 2008; World Health Organization [WHO], 2022; Yelton et al. 2022).

African Americans vary in their openness to seeking treatment due to fear of social reprisal, stigma, and a lack of access to quality, culturally competent mental health services. Aside from informing treatment and care, cultural values can also cause help-seeking barriers as among African Americans, as depression is seen as a personal failure or weakness. Therefore, strategies to reduce stigma-related barriers are also needed. This is especially true for men given the gendered social norms that limit help-seeking and even shape the symptoms they report resulting in occurrences of MDD misdiagnosis and under-diagnosis. Therefore, culturally appropriate education that tackles myths associated with MDD, and highlights the importance of emotional health and well-being is needed. This also extends to understanding the cultural and gendered differences in MDD expression that can lead to inaccurate diagnosis. As such, screening tools must be diversified to include culturally appropriate education on MDD “expression” particularly among men (Gutiérrez-Rojas et al., 2020)

Another major barrier to seeking care is the lack of understanding among mental health providers. As discussed previously, African Americans have historically experienced discrimination and prejudice in the healthcare system, and these experiences persist (NAMI, n.d.). Sadly, these experiences are often related to societal or provider implicit and explicit biases and inadequate poor cultural competency training that leads to higher misdiagnosis rates. Therefore, in line with promoting culturally sensitive care, it is also important to improve cultural understanding among current mental health providers who are not African American. Cultural competency training are many and should be extended to educate providers on anti-racist, anti-biases techniques to ensure effective communication and engagement when working with African Americans and highlight the importance of rapport building. Doing so can help increase trust and reduce fear of discrimination by ensuring they validate feelings of mistrust and invest time in building trust (Henry et al., 2020). Education should also extend to raising awareness among service providers that clinical representation of MDD may differ by culture and gender and alternative screening tools may be needed to accurately diagnose clients (Gutiérrez-Rojas et al., 2020; Martin et al., 2013). Furthermore, raises awareness that African Americans are more likely to experience persistent mental health conditions as opposed to periodic or sporadic episodes.

When polled, a study found that African Americans who screened positive for depression reported that they would seek help at higher rates than others in the general population (MHA, n.d.). Furthermore, it is known that African American people have better mental health outcomes when they are serviced by African American mental health. However, African Americans comprise a small percentage of mental health care providers. Therefore, increasing the representation of African American mental health providers can help reduce access barriers. Some strategies entail developing effective recruitment programs and plans that reduce discrimination and access-related barriers to program entry. In addition, work to facilitate programs that encourage peer-led educational programs that normalizes mental health treatment through mentorship programs and peer support groups (Alegría et al., 2008). Implemented in tandem, increasing representation and ensuring education efforts are community-led can help reduce stigma and increase access to care and support.

CONCLUSION

When an individual experiences numerous traumatic and painful events throughout the course of their life, the adverse experiences and emotions attached to them are normally pushed past or forgotten as a form of resilience. According to Socioemotional Selectivity Theory, as people age, they become more motivated to reserve positive experiences while separating themselves from negative ones (Carstensen et al, 1999; Grossmann et al., 2014). As a result, these individuals lack the mental and emotional space necessary to address these experiences accurately, due to the consistent denial or avoidance, also known as suppression. APA (n.d.) defines suppression as "the conscious intentional exclusion from the consciousness of a thought or feeling" and something that can negatively impact both physical and mental well-being.

African Americans are more likely to express their mental health issues through physical ailments such as chest and stomach pain. A mental health care provider who is not culturally competent would miss these signs of depression and misdiagnosis or not diagnose altogether. Additionally, physicians who service African Americans are 33% less likely to utilize patient-centered communication, opting for authoritarian styles and making patients feel devalued in interactions (APA, 2017). This confluence of factors often leads to higher risks of inadequate care, meaning that if African Americans seek care, they will not continue as they feel their needs are not being met. This suggests the need for integrated models of care that are evidence-based, culturally appropriate, and delivered by professionals that whom patients can be comfortable with and experience kinship (Henry et al., 2020). As such, improving mental health among African Americans requires ongoing and multifaceted approaches that attend to the unique challenges and needs of this community.

REFERENCES

Abdullah, T., & Brown, T. L. (2020). Diagnostic labeling and mental illness stigma among Black Americans: An experimental vignette study. *Stigma and Health*, *5*(1), 11–21. doi:10.1037ah0000162

Algeria, M., Chatterji, P., Wells, K., Cao, Z., Chen, C. N., Takeuchi, D., & Meng, X. L. (2008). Disparity in depression treatment among racial and ethnic minority populations in the United States. *Psychiatric Services (Washington, D.C.)*, *59*(11), 1264–1272. doi:10.1176/ps.2008.59.11.1264 PMID:18971402

American Psychological Association. (2017). *Mental health disparities: African Americans*. APA. *https://www.psychiatry.org/File%20Library/Psychiatrists/Cultural-Competency/Mental-Health-Disparities/Mental-Health-Facts-for-African-Americans.pdf*

American Psychological Association. (n.d). *APA Dictionary of Psychology*. APA. https://dictionary.apa.org/

Assari, S., & Caldwell, C. H. (2018). High risk of depression in high-income African American boys. *Journal of Racial and Ethnic Health Disparities*, *5*(4), 808–819. doi:10.100740615-017-0426-1 PMID:28842841

Bailey, R. K., Blackmon, H. L., & Stevens, F. L. (2009). Major depressive disorder in the African American population: Meeting the challenges of stigma, misdiagnosis, and treatment disparities. *Journal of the National Medical Association*, *101*(11), 1084–1089. doi:10.1016/S0027-9684(15)31102-0 PMID:19998635

Bailey, R. K., Mokonogho, J., & Kumar, A. (2019). Racial and ethnic differences in depression: Current perspectives. *Neuropsychiatric Disease and Treatment*, *15*, 603–609. doi:10.2147/NDT.S128584 PMID:30863081

Bailey, R. K., Patel, M., Barker, N. C., Ali, S., & Jabeen, S. (2011). Major depressive disorder in the African American population. *Journal of the National Medical Association*, *103*(7), 548–559. doi:10.1016/S0027-9684(15)30380-1 PMID:21999029

Bains, N., & Abdijadid, S. (2022, June 1). Major Depressive Disorder In *StatPearls [Internet]*. StatPearls. https://www.ncbi.nlm.nih.gov/books/NBK559078/

Bor, J., Venkataramani, A. S., Williams, D. R., & Tsai, A. C. (2018). Police killings and their spillover effects on the mental health of black Americans: A population-based, quasi-experimental study. *Lancet*, *392*(10144), 302–310. doi:10.1016/S0140-6736(18)31130-9 PMID:29937193

Bueno-Notivol, J., Gracia-García, P., Olaya, B., Lasheras, I., López-Antón, R., & Santabárbara, J. (2021). Prevalence of depression during the COVID-19 outbreak: A meta-analysis of community-based studies. *International Journal of Clinical and Health Psychology*, *21*(1), 100196. doi:10.1016/j.ijchp.2020.07.007 PMID:32904715

Burström, B., & Tao, W. (2020). Social determinants of health and inequalities in COVID-19. *European Journal of Public Health*, *30*(4), 617–618. doi:10.1093/eurpub/ckaa095 PMID:32638998

Campbell, R. D., & Winchester, M. R. (2020). Let the Church say...: One congregation's views on how the Black church can address mental health with Black Americans. *Social Work & Christianity*, *47*(2), 105–122. doi:10.34043wc.v47i2.63

Carstensen, L. L. IsAfrican Americancowitz, D. M., & Charles, S. T. (1999). Taking time seriously: A theory of socioemotional selectivity. *American Psychologist, 54*(3), 165–181. https://doi-org.ezp.twu.edu/10.1037/0003-066X.54.3.165

Centers for Disease Control and Prevention. (2019, November 5). Table A-8. *National Health Interview Survey.* CDC. https://www.cdc.gov/nchs/nhis/shs/tables.htm

Centers for Disease Control and Prevention. (2022, September 14). *Mental Health Conditions: Depression and Anxiety.* CDC. https://www.cdc.gov/tobacco/campaign/tips/diseases/depression-anxiety.html

Grossmann, I., Karasawa, M., Kan, C., & Kitayama, S. (2014). A cultural perspective on emotional experiences across the life span. *Emotion (Washington, D.C.)*, *14*(4), 679–692. https://doi-org.ezp.twu.edu/10.1037/a0036041. doi:10.1037/a0036041 PMID:24749641

Gutiérrez-Rojas, L., Porras-Segovia, A., Dunne, H., Andrade-González, N., & Cervilla, J. A. (2020). Prevalence and correlates of major depressive disorder: A systematic review. *The British Journal of Psychiatry*, *42*(6), 657–672. doi:10.1590/1516-4446-2020-0650 PMID:32756809

Henry, T. L., Jetty, A., Petterson, S., Jaffree, H., Ramsay, A., Heiman, E., & Bazemore, A. (2020). Taking a closer look at mental health treatment differences: Effectiveness of mental health treatment by provider type in racial and ethnic minorities. *Journal of Primary Care & Community Health*, *11*, 2150132720966403. doi:10.1177/2150132720966403 PMID:33089752

Hudson, D., Collins-Anderson, A., & Hutson, W. (2023). Understanding the Impact of Contemporary Racism on the Mental Health of Middle Class Black Americans. *International Journal of Environmental Research and Public Health*, *20*(3), 1660. doi:10.3390/ijerph20031660 PMID:36767028

Hudson, D. L., Neighbors, H. W., Geronimus, A. T., & Jackson, J. S. (2016). Racial discrimination, john henryism, and depression among African Americans. *The Journal of Black Psychology*, *42*(3), 221–243. doi:10.1177/0095798414567757 PMID:27529626

Laurencin, C. T., & Walker, J. M. (2020). A pandemic on a pandemic: Racism and COVID-19 in Blacks. *Cell Systems*, *11*(1), 9–10. doi:10.1016/j.cels.2020.07.002 PMID:32702320

Martin, L. A., Neighbors, H. W., & Griffith, D. M. (2013). The experience of symptoms of depression in men vs women: Analysis of the National Comorbidity Survey Replication. *JAMA Psychiatry*, *70*(10), 1100–1106. doi:10.1001/jamapsychiatry.2013.1985 PMID:23986338

Maura, J., & Weisman de Mamani, A. (2017). Mental health disparities, treatment engagement, and attrition among racial/ethnic minorities with severe mental illness: A review. *Journal of Clinical Psychology in Medical Settings*, *24*(3-4), 187–210. doi:10.100710880-017-9510-2 PMID:28900779

Mayo Clinic. (2022, October 14) *Depression (major depressive disorder)*. Mayo Clinic. https://www.mayoclinic.org/diseases-conditions/depression/diagnosis-treatment/drc-20356013

Mental Health America. (n.d.). *Black and African American Communities and Mental Health.* MHA. https://www.mhanational.org/issues/black-and-african-american-communities-and-mental-health

National Alliance on Mental Illness. (n.d). Black/African American. *National Alliance on Mental Illness.* NAMI. https://www.nami.org/Your-Journey/Identity-and-Cultural-Dimensions/Black-African-American

National Institute of Mental Health. (2022, January). *Mental Health Information.* NAMI. https://www.nimh.nih.gov/health/statistics/major-depression

Office of Minority Health. (2023, February 17). *Mental and behavioral health-African Americans.* Office of Minority Health. https://www.minorityhealth.hhs.gov/omh/browse.aspx?lvl=4&lvlid=24

Okoro, O., Vosen, E. C., Allen, K., Kennedy, J., Roberts, R., & Aremu, T. (2022). COVID-19 impact on mental health, healthcare access and social wellbeing–a Black community needs assessment. *International Journal for Equity in Health*, *21*(1), 1–11. doi:10.118612939-022-01743-z PMID:36138403

Olfson, M., Zuvekas, S. H., McClellan, C., Wall, M. M., Hankerson, S. H., & Blanco, C. (2023). Racial-ethnic disparities in outpatient mental health care in the United States. *Psychiatric services.*

Stare, B. G., & Fernando, D. M. (2019). Black American men's treatment experiences in mental health court: A phenomenological analysis. *Journal of Addictions & Offender Counseling*, *40*(1), 17–35. doi:10.1002/jaoc.12054

Ward, E., Wiltshire, J. C., Detry, M. A., & Brown, R. L. (2013). African American men and women's attitude toward mental illness, perceptions of stigma, and preferred coping behaviors. *Nursing Research*, *62*(3), 185–194. doi:10.1097/NNR.0b013e31827bf533 PMID:23328705

Webb Hooper, M., Nápoles, A. M., & Pérez-Stable, E. J. (2020). COVID-19 and racial/ethnic disparities. *Journal of the American Medical Association*, *323*(24), 2466. doi:10.1001/jama.2020.8598 PMID:32391864

World Health Organization. (2022, March 2). *Mental health and COVID-19: early evidence of the pandemic's impact: scientific brief.* WHO. https://apps.who.int/iris/handle/10665/352189

Yelton, B., Friedman, D. B., Noblet, S., Lohman, M. C., Arent, M. A., Macauda, M. M., Sakhuja, M., & Leith, K. H. (2022). Social determinants of health and depression among African American adults: A scoping review of current research. *International Journal of Environmental Research and Public Health*, *19*(3), 1498. doi:10.3390/ijerph19031498 PMID:35162519

APPENDIX

CHAPTER DISCUSSION QUESTIONS

1. Why do African Americans have lower rates of depression despite experiencing numerous risk factors?

2. How do cultural beliefs and norms contribute to the mis and under-diagnosis of MDD among African Americans?

3. How does systemic racism contribute to worse mental health outcomes for African Americans?

4. What are effective ways to reduce the stigma surrounding mental health in African Americans?

5. What are some ways we can engage community gatekeepers in faith-based leaders to promote mental health awareness in their community?

6. How can we encourage cultural competency among current mental health providers?

7. How can service providers build and maintain trust in the African American population?

8. What incentives can we provide to encourage more African American college students to pursue careers in mental health?

9. Read the two case studies below, and for each one:

a. Identify the problem and explain why it may exist.

b. Identify at least three distinct solutions for each scenario presented.

c. Discuss what you would do differently if you were the service provider.

Case Study One

Star, a 22-year-old African American female university student is referred to the campus counseling center. Upon arrival, she is met with an intake form, and shortly after, given brochures on stress management and told to return when she experiences an increase physically in her stress levels. Already stressed, she tells the intake counselor that she is in dire need of counseling services and would like assistance. The intake counselor makes it clear that her intake form's symptoms do not appear evident or serious enough to place on the counselor's list, so she is again encouraged to refer to the educational material she has been given and incorporate more sleep into her lifestyle. Immediately, she sees one of her classmates Laura who is of European descent enter the center for the same reasons, and not long is advised to wait in the seating area for the next counselor. As they exchange their hellos & goodbyes, it becomes evident to Star that her mental health needs are not of importance in comparison to students who may look like her friend Laura. At a crossroads, Star decides to follow through with her concerns and presents them to the University's Student Health director.

Case Study Two

Corey, a 14-year-old African American boy is known amongst his teachers as bright, talkative, curious, and funny. He is always willing to help and is always prepared in class. Lately, though, Corey has been late to multiple classes. He is unprepared and often falls asleep in class. When questioned, he becomes angry or requests to go to the nurse stating that his head hurts. He no longer socializes with friends and teachers have started to notice that he now sits alone during lunch. Additionally, his grades are starting to fall. Worried, his biology teacher pulls him aside to try to figure out what is going on. Corey lashes out, with tears in his eyes, stating that she wouldn't understand and runs away. Recognizing that something is seriously wrong, the teacher immediately emails the counselor to refer Corey for services.

Section 2

Addressing Mental Health in the African-American Community

Chapter 10
Promoting Black or African-American Men's Mental Health Through Empowering Masculinity

Daniel Bates
https://orcid.org/0000-0003-0964-4892
Truman State University, USA

ABSTRACT

There is a critical need for community advocates to understand the mental health needs of Black or African American (BA) men and the hesitancy in regard to accessing mental health services. Traditional, western masculinity powerfully influences how BA men perceive mental health struggles and vice versa, how reaching out for help and support affects an individual is perceived as being a man. Racial discrimination, marginalization and institutional oppression need to be taken into account when exploring mental health among BA men, especially in how these experiences interact with the enactment of masculinity. There is a great need for those who work with BA men to be aware of the mental health trends of this population, and the sociopolitical dynamics in the United States that contribute to them, equipped to effectively employ gender-adapted strategies with BA men, and familiar with evidenced-based approaches for promoting BA men's health and wellbeing in a way that is culturally responsive.

DOI: 10.4018/978-1-6684-8918-5.ch010

INTRODUCTION

There is a critical need for counselors, researchers, educators, community leaders and advocates, and policymakers to understand the mental health needs of Black or African American (BA) men and the hesitancy in regard to accessing mental health services. Traditional, Western masculinity powerfully influences how BA men perceive mental health struggles and vice versa, how reaching out for help and support affects an individual is perceived as being a man. As if these issues weren't complex enough, racial discrimination, marginalization and institutional oppression need to be considered when exploring mental health among BA men, especially in how these experiences interact with the enactment of masculinity. The intersection of adherence to traditional masculine norms and exposure to racial injustice has contributed to several alarming health disparities among BA men. There is a great need for those who work with BA men to be aware of the mental health trends of this population, and the sociopolitical dynamics in the United States that contribute to them, equipped to effectively employ gender-adapted strategies with BA men, and familiar with evidenced-based approaches for promoting BA men's health and wellbeing in a way that is culturally responsive.

In this chapter, evidence covering trends in men's physical and mental health, and specifically BA men's physical and mental health in the United States will be explored. Contributors to those concerning physical and mental health trends that are unique to BA men will be discussed not exhaustively, but with enough information so that the reader is aware of the sociopolitical and economic realities that affect BA men's stress, presentation of mental illness, opportunities for treatment, and overall perception of thriving in a system that has historically disadvantaged them. The chapter will conclude with a case study and in-depth discussion of how a culturally responsive and gender adapted approach may be successfully applied.

MEN'S MENTAL AND PHYSICAL HEALTH IN THE UNITED STATES

Mental Health Trends Among Men in the United States

Compared to women, men are far less likely to access psychological and medical services (NSDUH, 2021), which affects the course, longevity, and severity of treatable psychological conditions and subsequently contributes to their worsening over time. Men seemingly put off addressing problems and reaching out for help until the very last minute when issues are at their worst. Seeking out counseling services is usually in response to family and friends' requests usually accompanied by a crisis (Seidler et al., 2016; Seidler et al., 2017). Crisis are typically more fraught to treat and have a lower likelihood of sustained positive outcomes. This is evidenced by men using more emergency services, and to a far greater extent, BA men (Snowden et al., 2009). It provides an insight into why the suicide rate is so high among men: men comprise 78% of those who die by suicide in the United States (NSDUH, 2020); men's suicide rate is three to seven times higher than women (Nock, 2008); and suicide is listed as one of the top three causes of mortality among men in Canada (British Columbia Vital Statistics Agency, 2002; Bilsker and White, 2011). The rate of suicide is even worse for vulnerable groups within the male population, such as young men, men of color, sexually minoritized men, and men in a lower SES bracket (Blumberg et al., 2015; Chandra et al., 2009; Cummings, 2014; National Institute of Mental Health, 2019; Parent et al., 2018). Men are 1.5 times as likely as women to use illicit drugs and twice as likely to engage in heavy alcohol consumption (CDC, 2021). Men are more likely to die due to drug overdose, as well as the death rate associated with chronic liver disease and cirrhosis (NCHS, 2018). Men who have higher rates of hypertension (aged 45-64) are twice as likely to be unaware of their hypertension as compared to women (aged 20-44) (NCHS, 2018). Men, compared to women, have higher rates of being overweight and obese (NCHS, 2018).

If men do seek out help, they often encounter systemic gender bias toward adult men in the mental health field (Mahalik et al., 2012). For example, therapeutic services are designed to appeal more so to potential female clients (Morison et al., 2014), and less so to men's treatment preferences (Liddon et al., 2017). Face-to-face, talk therapy runs into conflict with traditional male socialization, values (Levant, 2006), and masculine norms (Mahalik et al., 2003; McCarthy & Holliday, 2004; Wong & Rochlen, 2005).

Gender stereotyping by clinicians pose a barrier to men getting the services they need (Ali et al., 2010; Yourstone et al., 2009). Treatment effectiveness could be at risk if mental health providers possess biases towards men and masculinity (Kiselica & Englar-Carlson, 2013), or racial biases (citation). A lack of representation of men in counselor roles, especially BA men, may also play a role since only 17% of the American Counseling Association membership is composed of men, and 19.6% of counselors in the United States are BA (Baggerly et al., 2017). According to the 2013 U.S. Census Bureau report, 83.6% of active psychologists identify as White (U.S. Census Bureau, 2005–2013), which is consonant with the American Psychological Association's (APA) 2015 demographic data showing 81% of their members identify as White and only 2-3% identify as BA (APA, 2015) with that number increasing up to 4% as of 2018 (APA, 2022).

Physical Health Trends Among Men in the United States

Reluctance to access medical and psychological services contributes to a variety of physical and mental health gender disparities that disproportionately affect men's quality of life. The primary cause of death for men in the United States is cardiovascular disease killing 382,776 men in 2020, which is roughly 1 out of every 4 male deaths (CDCP, 2022). Skin, lung, and prostate cancer are the most common forms of cancer among men in the United States (ACS, 2021). Regarding prostate cancer, the American Cancer Society (ACS) expects roughly 288,300 new cases in the United States by 2023 resulting in 34,700 deaths (ACS, 2021). Over a man's lifetime, 1 in 8 will be diagnosed with prostate cancer and has a higher likelihood of developing among older men and non-Hispanic BA men, with the average age of men when first diagnosed at 66 (ACS, 2021). Other health issues that significantly impact men are testicular cancer, lung cancer, erectile dysfunction, sexually transmitted infections, and diabetes among others (Neukrug et al., 2013). Compared to females, men have higher mortality and lower life expectancy (Murphy et al., 2020). Males are more likely to engage in risky behavior, such as substance use (Abuse, 2019), and less likely to take preventive health measures, such as wearing seatbelts (SAMHSA, 2013).

BA MEN'S MENTAL AND PHYSICAL HEALTH IN THE UNITED STATES

Mental Health Trends Among BA Men in the United States

Over 2021, roughly 16% of the U.S. population that identifies as BA adults indicated experiencing a mental illness (Reinhart et al., 2021). For BA and Hispanic men ages 18-44 who regularly experienced symptoms of depression and anxiety, a mere 26.4% were likely to access mental health services as opposed to 45.4% of White men (NCHS Data Brief No. 206, 2015). BA men are hesitant to out mental health services and treatment when needed (Blumberg et al., 2015; Cummings, 2014; NIMH, 2019; Parent et al., 2018), which is concerning for a number of reasons, namely the symptomology of depression among BA has a powerfully negative impact in terms of severity and persistence, and is more treatment-resistant when compared to White people (Bailey et al., 2019). This higher risk of struggling with depressive symptoms yet have a lower likelihood of accessing mental health services (Plowden et al., 2016) is a dangerous combination. However, BA adults had the highest rate of mental health-related ED visits (96.8 visits per 1,000 adults), which also extended to specific mental health-related disorders such as substance use disorders, anxiety disorders, and mood disorders (Peters et al., 2023). This suggests, similarly to what was discussed above regarding the general population of men delaying accessing services until issues reach a crisis point, is even more evident among BA men.

Physical Health Trends Among BA Men in the United States

Cardiovascular disease is the primary cause of death for BA men in the United States (citation). BA men, in comparison to White men, face greater morbidity and premature mortality from preventable medical issues, while engaging with preventative health services significantly less (National Healthcare Disparities Report, 2006; Arias, 2004; Wong et al., 2006; Hertz et al., 2005; Nelson et al., 2002). Globally, BA men possess the highest rates of hypertension (Douglas, 2005), which, in the age range of 30-39, makes BA men, as compared to White men, susceptible to other medical conditions such as kidney failure (USRDS, 2005). BA men compared to White men are 60% more likely to die of a stroke, 30% more likely to die of heart disease, and more likely to die of diabetes (The Office of Minority Health, 2008). Death by homicide rate is significantly higher for BA men relative to White men (National Urban League, 2007). BA men have a higher likelihood of developing lung cancer relative to White men (Zerhouni, 2002) and oral cancer compared to any racial/ethnic group in the United States (NIDCR, 2009). And BA men are nine times more likely to die from HIV/AIDS relative to White men (The Office of Minority Health, 2008).

Barriers to Accessing Mental Health Services

BA men are one of the most underserved groups in the United States regarding access to medical and mental health services, contributing to negative health outcomes (Smedley et al., 2003). BA adults, 18 years and older, received less than half the mental health services compared to White adults (SAMHSA, 2019), yet BA adults reported experiencing greater levels of sadness (CDC, 2019), and greater levels of suicide ideation (CDC, 2019). BA men are 4 times more likely to die by suicide than BA women (CDC, 2019), with suicide being the second leading cause of death for BA adults between the ages of 15-24 in 2017 (CDC, 2017). There are several barriers that contribute to the reluctance to access mental health services such as socioeconomic status, traditional masculine norms, racial discrimination, unawareness regarding the necessity for preventative medical care, religious doctrines, and peer influences (Cheatham et al., 2008). There is also a great deal of stigma attached to mental illness and mental health services within the BA community, especially among men. Several studies highlight key sex differences between BA women and men regarding health attitudes and practices, revealing that BA men are far less likely to engage in medical health services (Watson, 2014), mental health services

(Courtenay et al., 2002), more likely to engage in unhealthy coping behaviors (Courtenay, 2000), and hold negative beliefs about mental health services (Ward et al., 2013). Researchers believe that BA men's notions about masculinity play a large role in men's overall physical and mental health (Courtenay, 2000; Cheatham et al., 2008; Vogel et al., 2011). Hammond (2011) found in a sample of 216 BA men that perceived racism in healthcare organizations was significantly associated with medical mistrust even after all other variables in the model were controlled for. Furthermore, masculine role identity played a strong role in the trust-building process between patient and physician.

In terms of health-promoting practices, BA and mixed heritage men reported less medical compliance, increased risky behaviors involving substance abuse, and increased risky health-related beliefs regarding masculinity compared to European American men (Courtenay et al., 2002). These findings reveal the presence of a complex set of relationships between stigma associated with mental illness in the BA community, mistrust in medical and mental health services and service providers based on past experiences such as the Tuskegee Syphilis Trial (Gamble, 1997), the intersection of cultural beliefs around masculinity that prevent men from accessing services until a crisis has unfolded, and specific barriers related to membership in the BA community related to racial discrimination and marginalization. In the following two sections, health-promoting attitudes and adherence to traditional masculine norms will be examined more closely in so far as their contribution to racial health disparities leading to a discussion on specific ways those active in the BA community can specifically target the beliefs and attitudes of BA men towards their own physical health and wellbeing, accessing services, and the interplay of masculinity.

HEALTH ATTITUDES AND PRACTICES OF BA MEN

As discussed previously, BA men are less likely to seek mental health services and receive treatment when needed compared to White men (Blumberg et al., 2015; Cummings, 2014; NIMH, 2019; Parent et al., 2018). The racial disparity in accessing mental health services is only a small part of a larger trend related to health attitudes, behaviors, and practices that significantly vary by race and ethnicity (Thorpe et al., 2015). For example, Courtenay et al. (2002) used an exploratory factor analysis to examine risky behaviors and risky health-related beliefs among a diverse sample of 1816 undergraduate students. They found several gender and ethnicity differences among respondents such as men engaging in less preventive behaviors, less medical compliance, riskier substance abuse behaviors, and riskier health-related beliefs than women. BA and mixed heritage men reported less medical compliance, riskier substance abuse behaviors, and riskier health-related beliefs regarding masculinity than European American men. These health-related beliefs and behavior differences play a significant role in health outcomes.

More recent research has uncovered similar findings to that of Courtenay et al. (2002). Ward et al., (2013) conducted a study on 272 BA men and women ages 25-72. A third of the sample, not parsed by gender, reported experiencing mental illness or receiving treatment for mental illness. They also found that men felt that having a mental illness could lead to negative consequences. BA women held similar attitudes, but, unlike the men, felt that professional services could treat mental illness. Young BA men were the least likely to be open and or seek out psychological help. Both men and women expressed a significant level of concern regarding the stigma associated with mental health and an interest in religious coping.

Health Attitudes and Behaviors, and the Rest of the Story

Xanthos et al. (2010) noted in their study investigating the social determinants that affect BA men's health, "Health behavior determines health to some extent, it is important to recognize that social and environmental factors place minorities such as African–American men at a significant disadvantage with regard to health and disease" (pg. 11). In a study on race-related stressors, Williams (2018) said "We do not currently have a clear sense of either the levels of mental health status for the major racial/ethnic groups in the U.S. or the patterning of the various indicators of mental health status for all these minority populations" (pg. 4). However, Williams went on to explain there is a consensus among many researchers that social contextual factors like stressors related to stigmatized racial and ethnic minority communities play a role in the health disparities observed across racial groups. Racial discrimination bears a negative relationship to racial identity development, which is important for a number of key health-related psychological variables (Cross, 1991; Cross & Fhagen-Smith, 2001) and is associated with depressive symptoms among BA youth (Wong et al., 2003). Traditional masculine ideals such as stoicism, self-reliance, risk-taking, toughness, and being a problem-solver often isolate men from seeking out help and worsen the psychological impact of exposure to marginalization, racial discrimination, poverty, aggressive policing, and incarceration, a topic that will be explored in more detail in the following section.

TRADITIONAL MASCULINITY AND BA MEN

Traditional masculinity has been defined as the "endorsement and internalization of cultural belief systems about masculinity and the male gender" (Pleck et al.

1993, p. 88). Yet, the construct of masculinity extends beyond the endorsement and internalization of cultural beliefs associated with masculinity to how those norms are enacted. Scholars have developed the term *hegemonic masculinity*, which is the normative cultural expectations of men as defined by the dominant group (Connell & Messerschmidt, 2005), to capture the specific way in which Western cultural understandings of masculinity are strongly swayed by the social groups that hold the most sociopolitical influence. And, how those notions of masculinity have harmed BA men. BA masculinity has been historically viewed through the lens of White dominant culture masculine norms (Connell, 1995). BA men are simultaneously judged and excluded by hegemonic norms. Lorber (1997) in discussing multiple systems of oppression that converge on subordinate groups, points out that "Black men are punished for their masculinity" (pg. 26).

Masculinity-related concepts need to be considered from an intersectional perspective in order to fully understand how BA men construct masculinity. To conceptualize masculinity (and construct it impacts such as help-seeking beliefs, health-related attitudes and practices, and coping skills) without accounting for race/ethnicity would be wholly insufficient. As of the last 20 years, researchers have used qualitative research designs to understand self-defined BA masculinity, which has opened up new lines of research into positive masculinity among BA men. The development of constructs like positive masculinity conceptualized from a multicultural and intersectional lens bears the promise of better understanding and reaching BA men and the potential to mitigate the physical and mental health disparities between BA men and White men.

Among men in general, conformity to traditional masculine norms has been linked with negative mental health outcomes (Addis & Mahalik, 2003; Englar-Carlson, 2006), whereas positive masculinity has been associated with psychological strengths (Hammer & Good, 2010) and greater mental health service utilization (Sileo & Kershaw, 2020). It is not yet clear if these findings extend to BA men, and no study has explored positive masculinity themes in this population. Until this gap can be addressed through research, approaches targeting BA men's health behavior, help-seeking attitudes, and treatment programs designed for BA men will continue to be hindered by a scarcity of information about elements of masculinity associated with positive health outcomes. There is a critical need for research to develop the positive masculinity construct among BA men to inform the development of culturally sensitive masculinity measures and interventions. For effective engagement and treatment to be successfully achieved, advocates in the BA community need to be aware of the intersection of masculinity and racial/ethnic identity in health promotion.

Mental Health Stigma and Masculinity

Vogel et al. (2011) found that conceptualizations of masculinity significantly affected BA men's health behaviors and health outcomes. Lease et al. (2019) examined whether endorsement of traditional masculinity ideology differed between White men and BA men and if those differences affected health-promoting behaviors like physical activity, stress management, and health responsibility. No direct effects were found which runs contrary to past research linking the endorsement of masculine norms being linked with few health-promoting behaviors. If anything, the results revealed a more complex picture than has been previously imagined. Self-efficacy and outcome expectations mediated the effects of endorsement of traditional masculine norms on intent and health-promoting behaviors. Using a Multigroup analysis, Lease and colleagues compared model fit for White (n = 194) and BA (n = 158) men and found that the stronger a male study participant endorsed traditional masculine ideology was associated with lower self-efficacy and more negative outcome expectations. Lease and colleagues did not find differences between White and BA men's enactment of traditional masculine ideology relative to the performance of health-promoting behaviors. Both groups were similar. However, researchers did find a significant indirect effect "between endorsement of traditional masculinity and physical activity behaviors via outcome expectations (perceived barriers and benefits) for BA men, but not for White men" (pg. 128).

The association between the endorsement of traditional masculine norms and lower self-efficacy is a result of these behaviors being considered feminine (Leaper & Van, 2008). Masculinity threat deters men from engaging in health-promoting behaviors. As it relates to outcome expectations, previous research has also demonstrated an association between a fatalistic outcome expectations and endorsement of traditional masculine norms (Mahalik et al., 2007; Sloan et al., 2015). Most notably, results revealed a significant indirect effect: increased endorsement of traditional masculinity ideology corresponded with a decrease in positive outcome expectations, intentions to act, and health-promoting behaviors.

Men engage in health behaviors associated with negative physical outcomes (Courtenay, 2000a) and underutilize, delay and engage less in medical and preventative care (Addis & Mahalik, 2003; Courtenay et al., 2002; Galdas et al., 2005; Levant et al., 2009). It is important to note that a person may be limited in pursuing health-promoting behavior like annual doctor's visits due to the economic cost of taking time off of work and decreased ability to support one's family (Wexler et al., 2009). Outside of an emergency situation, the threat of being perceived as less masculine dissuaded men from engaging in health-related behaviors (Noone & Stephens, 2008; Tyler & Williams, 2014).

Additionally, engagement in health behaviors varies by race and ethnicity (Thorpe et al., 2015). As mentioned earlier, Courtenay et al. (2002) found a gender and ethnicity difference among a diverse sample of 1816 undergraduate students. Self-management and health-related protective behaviors are perceived as non-masculine resulting in the avoidance of help-seeking and poor physical and mental health outcomes (Bjordahl et al., 2015; Boon, 2005; Capraro, 2000; Johnson et al., 2015; Mahalik et al., 2003). Mount et al. (2012) found that BA men held fatalistic attitudes towards health conditions, feeling that death was inevitable regardless of how they responded to preventable diseases.

Racial Discrimination and Masculinity

BA men experience a number of disadvantages when compared to other, more advantaged groups (Gehlert et al., 2008), which include, but is not limited to race-related stress, aggressive policing, poverty, over-representation of the prison population, and racial discrimination and marginalization. Social contextual factors like race-related stress among stigmatized racial and ethnic minority communities play a role in the health disparities observed across racial groups (Williams, 2018). Research also highlights the impact of aggressive policing tactics (e.g., frequent stops, intrusive, disrespectful encounters, and perceived injustice) were positively correlated with PTSD symptomology and anxiety (Geller et al., 2014). According to Chetty et al. (2018) BA U.S. citizens, compared to White citizens, have considerably higher rates of downward mobility and lower rates of downward mobility, leading to substantial economic disparities continuing from generation to generation. As of 2019, BA comprises 14% of the total population in the United States yet represent 33% of individuals incarcerated (the majority of which are men), a number that increases to 46% when looking specifically at individuals who have already served at least 10 years (Nellis, 2021). Also, exposure to racial discrimination instills a sense of disempowerment and reinforces feelings of powerlessness among BA men and other individuals who share membership in a minoritized racial/ethnic group (Foster & Matheson, 1998; Operario & Fiske, 2008), and increases a sense of marginalization and instability among BA men (Hammond & Mattis, 2005; Matthews et al., 2013). Research demonstrated not only a negative psychological impact but also a strong link between racial discrimination and negative health outcomes for BA men (Branscombe et al., 1999; Hammond, 2012; Mays et al., 2007).

The experience of racial discrimination contributed to a heightened vigilance to masculinity threats and a subsequent greater endorsement of male gender norms relative to a control group that was not exposed to racial discrimination. The perceived threat to masculinity increased BA men's masculine-typed behaviors (e.g., doing push-ups). Osa et al. (2021) found evidence in support of the hypothesis that racial discrimination functioned as a threat to masculinity, resulting in BA men having higher levels of DFM. Drive for muscularity (DFM) has been linked with a number of negative physical and psychological health symptoms among non-Hispanic White men. Correspondingly, recent studies have found comparable levels of negative physical and psychological symptoms among men of marginalized ethnic groups (McCreary, 2012; Swami, 2016). DFM is a way men *do* or perform masculinity (Hunt et al., 2013). Threats to masculinity increase DFM. Racial discrimination bears a negative relationship to racial identity development (Cross, 1991; Cross & Fhagen-Smith, 2001) and is associated with depressive symptoms among BA youth (Wong et al., 2003).

Marginalization and Structural Oppression Influence Masculinity

Marginalization and structural oppression limit the ways in which BA men are able to enact culturally bound, hegemonic, Western, Traditional masculine norms. As a result, BA men have found adaptive ways to enact masculine norms within the limits imposed by marginalization and structural oppression. This is in keeping with previous research showing that racial minorities construct masculinity differently than dominant White culture (Levant, 2011). The performance of masculinity for BA men serves multiple purposes: a means of racial and ethnic identification which signifies social capital and sustains group solidarity and differentiation (Bashi & Mcdaniel, 2016; Connell & Messerschmidt, 2005; Swami, 2016). And, it demonstrates social capital to other ethnic groups who possess more power and status (Griffith, 2015). Structural marginalization and oppression put limits on how BA men can endorse and enact hegemonic masculine norms (Connell & Messerschmidt, 2005; Griffith, 2015). As a result, BA men have developed unique strategies for navigating masculinity that are distinctive from the hegemonic norms (Hammond & Mattis, 2005; Harris, 1995; Levant et al., 2010), by emphasizing alternative hegemonic norms like muscularity (e.g., autonomy, leadership, and toughness), or hypermasculinity (Brennan et al., 2015; Ward, 2005).

Health-Related Behaviors and Masculinity Threat

Lease et al. (2019) examined whether endorsement of traditional masculinity ideology differed between White men and BA men and if those differences affected health promoting behaviors like physical activity, stress management, and health responsibility. No direct effects were found which runs contrary to past research linking the endorsement of masculine norms being linked with few health-promoting behaviors. If anything, the results revealed a more complex picture than has been previously imagined. Self-efficacy and outcome expectations mediated the effects of endorsement of traditional masculine norms on intent and health-promoting behaviors. Using a Multigroup analysis, Lease and colleagues compared model fit for White (n = 194) and BA (n = 158) men and found that the stronger a male study participant endorsed traditional masculine ideology was associated with lower self-efficacy and more negative outcome expectations. Lease and colleagues did not find differences between White and BA men's enactment of traditional masculine ideology relative to the performance of health promoting behaviors. Both groups were similar. However, researchers did find a significant indirect effect "between endorsement of traditional masculinity and physical activity behaviors via outcome expectations (perceived barriers and benefits) for Black/African American men, but not for White men" (pg. 128).

The association between the endorsement of traditional masculine norms and lower self-efficacy is a result of these behaviors being considered feminine (Leaper & Van, 2008). Masculinity threat deters men from engaging in health promoting behaviors. As it relates to outcome expectations, previous research has also demonstrated an association between fatalistic outcome expectations and endorsement of traditional masculine norms (Mahalik et al., 2007; Sloan et al., 2015). Most notably, results revealed a significant indirect effect: increased endorsement of traditional masculinity ideology corresponded with a decrease in positive outcome expectations, intentions to act, and health-promoting behaviors.

Men engage in health behaviors associated with negative physical outcomes (Courtenay, 2000a) and underutilize, delay and engage less in medical and preventative care (Addis & Mahalik, 2003; Courtenay et al., 2002; Galdas et al., 2005; Levant et al., 2009). It is important to note that a person may be limited in pursuing health promoting behavior like annual doctor's visits due to the economic cost of taking time off of work and decreased ability to support one's family (Wexler et al., 2009). Outside of an emergency situation, the threat of being perceived as less masculine dissuaded men from engaging in health-related behaviors (Noone & Stephens, 2008; Tyler & Williams, 2014). Mount et al. (2012) found that BA men held fatalistic attitudes towards health conditions, feeling that death was inevitable regardless of how they responded to preventable diseases.

A CULTURALLY RESPONSIVE AND GENDER-ADAPTED APPROACH THAT EMPOWERS BA MASCULINITY

The research conducted on BA men has historically been dominated by a deficit focus. Research up until the 1970's viewed BA men as "irresponsible and even deviant" (Rogers, et al., 2015, pg. 416) and not even considered men (Franklin, 1986). Rogers et al. (2015) study of masculinity among BA men from an intersectional feminist theory describes the history of research on BA men. He describes the efforts early researchers made to explain the shortcomings of BA men. Frazier (1939) theorized that due to a history of slavery and oppression, the patriarchal family system was eroded and, in its place, a matriarchal system emerged. This female-dominated familial system resulted in an impaired male role performance (Moynihan, 1965). Staples (1978) countered the deficit model by pointing out its many issues and argued for a more positive and unbiased perspective of BA men. Cazenave (1979, 1984) empirically investigated Staples' challenge to the deficit model and discovered that BA men constructed masculinity differently than White, Western masculine norms, most notably, BA men expanded the role of provider to include financial as well as emotional needs. Franklin (1986) and later Majors and Bilson (1992) developed the concept of Black male role expectations, a set of expectations developed in response to oppression that is meant to communicate "pride, strength and control" (Majors & Bilson, 1992, pg. 4).

New lines of research have emerged that focus on the ways in which BA men define masculinity for themselves. Hunter and Davis (1992, 1994) found that BA men when asked what they thought about masculinity, elicited four key domains: self-determination and accountability, family, pride and spirituality, and humanism. Hammond and Mattis (2005) surveyed BA men and discovered similar findings. BA men endorse masculine norms of responsibility-accountability, self-determination, autonomy, providing-waymarking, spirituality-religiosity, moral rectitude/virtues, and family centeredness. Chaney (2009) studied a group of BA men's perceptions of masculinity from varying levels of socioeconomic status. Several themes emerged from the data, such as maturity, autonomy (and taking responsibility for oneself), providing for one's family financially, emotionally, and spiritually, and awareness of oneself. Chaney (2009) drew out the subtle point that traditional, Western masculinity, even the aspects of it that are positive, are insufficient to capture the way marginalization plays into BA men's conceptualization and enactment of masculinity. Duck (2009) found that BA men strongly endorse, adhere, and conform to traditional masculine norms, although are simultaneously excluded from full participation in masculine practice. Duck (2009) suggests that, although excluded and marginalized, BA men still enact traditional masculinity so as to receive the gendered social benefits of not being subordinate to women, whilst still experiencing disparate social, economic, educational, and political outcomes compared to White men.

Roberts-Douglas and Curtis-Boles (2013) using an open-ended interview questionnaire, investigated what factors from adolescence predicted healthy and adaptive masculine identities among young BA men. Nine key themes emerged; most notably, 86% of the respondents indicated a family member as a role model was a key factor in their masculinity development, and of that majority, 73% indicated their father as the role model. Roberts-Douglas and Curtis-Boles (2013) stated that "African American males in this study, while frequently exposed to traditional masculinity norms, can and do form definitions of masculinity and self-perception with intentional inclusion of positive schemas (provider, education) and resilience against negative schemas (violence, misogyny)" (pg. 10).

Rogers et al. (2015) used a qualitative research design with a sample of 17 BA men to understand the intersection of race and gender. Several key themes emerged from the data analysis: leadership, structural oppression, African American values, traditional masculinity, familial relationships, and self-definition. Mincey et al. (2014) used a qualitative study design to investigate how BA men understood masculinity in general, masculinity relative to their race/ethnicity, and the influences on masculinity development. The sample consisted of BA male college students: one group of students attended a historically Black college and university (HBCU), and another group attended a predominantly White university. Five themes emerged from this examination of 'what it means to be a Black man': something to prove, responsibility to uphold one's history, strength, attitude (personal sense of honor and power), and overcoming stereotypes.

The masculine-related ideals, values, and traits revealed by the aforementioned research evince a critical distinction in how BA men understand themselves to be men, lying in direct contrast to traditional, Western notions of masculinity. What is considered to be adaptive and maladaptive is context-dependent and culturally bound. In the view of Connell (1995), Lorber (1997), and Wade & Rochlen (2013), the sociopolitical milieu in the United States invalidates BA manhood. BA men do not have the power and privilege to enact traditional masculine norms successfully (Harris, 1995), as a result, are left with maladaptive alternatives (Majors, 1989), which inflict harm on men and communities of color (Majors & Bilson, 1992). As the evidence shows, attempting to fulfill those masculine expectations comes at the cost of BA men's physical and mental health. Conversely, when asked directly, BA men conceptualize masculinity differently from the dominant cultural group in important and meaningful ways. Ways that, in fact, strengthen mental health and racial identity development. Yet, there is a complexity to navigate as demonstrated by Coleman-Kirumba et al.'s (2023) research. Among a sample of 160 BA men located in the United States, BA masculinity predicted the public stigma of help-seeking. Public stigma has been shown to predict self-stigma of help-seeking among BA men (Cadaret & Speight, 2018). Public stigma predicts self-stigma of help-seeking and indirectly less psychological help-seeking, whereas traditional masculinity was negatively associated with publicstigma, and indirectly increases psychological help-seeking. Given these complex results, Coleman-Kirumba and colleagues (2023) suggest a nuanced and targeted approach to effectively engage BA men.

Engaging and encouraging BA men's development of positive masculinity entails the deconstruction of traditional masculinity as defined by the dominant culture, and, as Coleman-Kirumba et al.'s (2023) research shows, the deconstruction of BA masculinity as well. The aim is to reconstruct masculinity that empowers BA men to enact masculinity in ways that are adaptive to their social location and produce well-being for themselves, their families and their communities. Initial evidence discussed in the following section suggests positive masculinity is linked with positive physical and mental health outcomes. There is, therefore, an empirical basis to assume positive masculinity if increased among BA men will produce positive physical and mental health results and thus reduce the health disparity gap.

MENTAL HEALTH BENEFITS OF EMPOWERING MASCULINITY

White (2008) explored how a diverse sample of 20 BA men exercised their creative agency to define for themselves the assumptions and practices of manhood, enact social change, and create egalitarian relationships with women, children, and other men. Sileo and Kershaw (2020) sought to understand the relationship between specific dimensions of masculine norms (status, toughness, and anti-femininity) with better or worse mental health outcomes among a diverse sample of 119 emerging adult men (ages 18–25 years) over a 6-month period who have been historically underrepresented in research of this kind (i.e., younger, lower SES, and racial minority). 63.2% of the study participants identified as BA, and 18.8% identified as multiracial (all of which identified one of their racial/ethnic identifiers as BA). Results demonstrated an association between status with less depressive symptoms, toughness was associated with greater substance abuse, and anti-femininity was associated with greater hostility. The former masculine trait was associated with greater mental health service utilization, whereas the latter two masculine traits were associated with less mental health service utilization. The sample included a greater level of racial diversity than has been present in previous studies, however, there was a lack of diversity regarding sexual identity since the sample was made up of heterosexual young men.

These findings are consistent with research conducted on samples of men of other racial/ethnic identities. Among a sample of predominantly White men, Hammer and Good (2010) investigated the positive, strength-based aspects of masculinity. They found that endorsement of some traditional Western masculine norms (e.g., risk-taking, dominance, the primacy of work, and pursuit of status) was associated with positive psychology constructs including personal courage, autonomy, endurance, and resilience. That is, results revealed men's endorsement of traditional Western masculine norms was associated with higher levels of psychological strengths.

Specifically, they found that the pursuit of status was associated with both positive strengths (e.g., courage) and negative outcomes (e.g., lack of grit, defined as perseverance for long-term goals). Iwamoto and colleagues (2010) found complex correlation patterns between Asian American men's endorsement of masculine norms with harmful and protective mental health outcomes.

Researchers have discovered an association between *machismo*, exhibited by Mexican American men, and negative characteristics of sexism, chauvinism, and hypermasculinity (Anders, 1993; Ingoldsby, 1991; Mosher & Tompkins, 1988), and negative outcomes such as greater levels of alexithymia. Yet, some scholars have criticized the research on machismo as negative and restrictive (e.g., Casas et al., 1994; Felix-Ortiz et al., 2001), and for failing to recognize positive features such as being nurturing, defending the physical safety and honor of one's family, valuing dignity, being wise, hardworking, accountability, being spiritual, and connected emotionally (Casas et al., 1994; Mirande´, 1988, 1997). Scholars have used the term *caballerismo* to describe the positive aspects of machismo. The term has a rich socio-historical meaning. And as a construct, caballero bears a positive association with affiliation, racial/ethnic identity, and coping through problem-solving (Arciniega et al., 2008). Research investigating other masculinity measures, not designed to capture positive masculine traits, has uncovered complex correlational patterns, where subscales are largely correlated with negative health outcomes, yet many subscales are uncorrelated with health-related outcomes or bear a positive relationship to health-related outcomes (Gerdes & Levant, 2018).

Consider appealing to men's strengths and a desire for personal improvement to recruit male participants in wellness programs like mindfulness training. A mechanism surrounding self-regulation and stress reduction, mindfulness is a complex and adaptive process that requires paying attention to the present moment in a receptive and non-judgmental attitude. It encourages an emotion-regulation strategy that disarms the pathways of stressor reactivity such that exposure to a stressor is no longer hazardous to one's health (de Frias & Whyne, 2014). In studies that have explored mindfulness among BA adults, it has been shown that mindfulness is inversely associated with suicide ideation and elevated suicide risk with clinical implications of mindfulness' potential utility as a psychological buffer and tool for reducing anxious arousal and distress (Brooks et al., 2021).

Yet, getting BA men, or any man in general, interested and motivated to engage in mental health services is challenging provided all the reasons already discussed. Therefore, it is necessary to present mental health services and programs from a strengths-based perspective that appeals to masculine norms. The way counseling services are advertised, described, and explained may serve to attract or detract men from accessing services. Scholars have argued that the current structure and design of counseling services are "feminized" (Morison et al., 2014) and incommensurate with traditional, masculine values (Levant, 2006). Yet, appealing to masculine values and male interests may pique the curiosity of men by describing counseling as "health discussions" and building a sense of "brotherhood" with other men (Gross et al., 2016). Some programs have used creative titles to advertise services such as the "DUDES Club" (Gross et al., 2016), "Bromatters" (Wang et al., 2016), and "HeadsUpGuys" (HeadsUpGuys, 2017). These are just some examples from experts launching innovative programs; there is room for creativity and innovation in how to present services to potential male clients.

It is also extremely critical when exploring how BA men construct and enact masculinity is to recognize the importance of culture, social status, religion/spirituality, and class. These intersecting forces of identity significantly impact how men come to see manhood, and how they embody or violate those standards. For example, researchers have identified among Mexican and Mexican-American men, masculinity constructs such as *Machismo* and *Caballerismo* that represent detrimental and positive dimensions of masculinity that are deeply rooted in Hispanic culture and history (Arciniega et al., 2008). Yet, whatever change is being encouraged in a BA male, the desired change needs to make sense in the individuals social context. Drawing from Uri Bronfenbrenner's ecological model is the notion of *ecological validity* (Cook, 2015), which forces us to think in terms of what makes sense to the individual and their context.

Importantly, scholars have suggested that community advocates should think of masculinity and the men who strongly adhere to traditional notions of masculinity as a kind of cultural group. If advocates adopt this view from a culturally responsive perspective (Calloway & Creed, 2021), it allows for curiosity and openness to the impact of masculinity on a BA male life. It creates space for a safe and supportive relationship to be developed, where real questions about masculinity can be discussed. Being curious and *culturally humble* (Hook et al., 2013) allows advocates to make discoveries and connections that would not be possible if they were closed and culturally insulated. And, as discussed previously, it is critical to examine the intersection of overlapping identities such as gender, culture, race, and class, and discuss the physical and psychological impact on their mental health (Cho et al., 2013; Sanchez-Peña et al., 2016). Effective engagement cannot be successfully achieved without taking into account the intersection of masculinity and racial/ethnic identity in health promotion.

CONCLUSION

In order to effectively work with BA men, it is necessary to have a general understanding of BA male socialization, masculine norms and values, and trends in BA men's mental and physical health (Englar-Carlson & Kiselica, 2013). Being able to appreciate how masculinity plays a role in a BA man's physical and mental health, for better or worse, is critical. From a position of respect and understanding, advocates can help BA men identify their own gendered history, discussing key people and influences that shaped their conceptions of what it means to be a man (Wilson et al., 2022). Uncovering this rich material can help BA men see what aspects of masculinity they may want to challenge, adjust, or reinforce, that are consistent with their own self-image, goals, and values. Borrowing from Martín-Baró's (1994) liberation psychology theory, community advocates have the opportunity to support BA men and their communities to transform their own oppression and world. Advocates can assist BA men in recognizing the harmful impact traditional masculinity on their mental health (see Alaniz, 1996; Neff, Prihoda, & Hoppe, 1991; Beaver, Gold, & Prisco, 1992; Mosher & Sirkin, 1984; Mayo & Resnick, 1996; Fragoso & Kashubeck, 2000; Liang, Salcedo, Miller, 2011; Glass & Owen, 2010), and offer guidance in how to reconstruct positive masculinity in an ecologically valid manner (Cook, 2015).

Recent findings show a clear link between positive masculinity and positive mental health benefits for men. These results have serious implications for reducing the physical and mental health gaps among BA men. Worldwide, men are three to seven times more likely to die by suicide than women (Nock, 2008). The situation is even more dire among BA men who are less likely to seek mental health services and receive treatment when needed (Blumberg et al., 2015; Chandra et al., 2009; Cummings, 2014; NIMH, 2019; Parent et al., 2018). BA men, in comparison to White men, face greater morbidity and premature mortality from preventable medical issues, while engaging with preventative health services significantly less (AHRQ, 2006; Arias, 2004; Thom et al., 2006; Wong et al., 2006; Hertz et al., 2005; Nelson et al., 2002). BA men experience a number of disadvantages when compared to other, more advantaged groups (Gehlert et al., 2008). Masculinity plays a significant role in health-promoting behaviors and patterns of BA men (Courtenay et al., 2002). Therefore, it is critically important to effectively engage BA men and encourage, not diminish, their sense of masculinity in a more expanded, health-promoting perspective that is ecologically valid.

REFERENCES

Abuse, S. (2019). *Mental Health Services Administration. (2019). Key substance use and mental health indicators in the United States: Results from the 2018 National Survey on Drug Use and Health (HHS Publication No. PEP19-5068, NSDUH Series H-54).* Rockville, MD: Center for Behavioral Health Statistics and Quality. Substance Abuse and Mental Health Services Administration. https://www. samhsa. gov/data

Addis, M. E., & Mahalik, J. R. (2003). Men, masculinity, and the contexts of help seeking. *The American Psychologist*, *58*(1), 5–14. doi:10.1037/0003-066X.58.1.5 PMID:12674814

Affleck, W., Carmichael, V., & Whitley, R. (2018). Men's mental health: Social determinants and implications for services. *Canadian Journal of Psychiatry*, *63*(9), 581–589. doi:10.1177/0706743718762388 PMID:29673270

Ali, A., Caplan, P. J., & Fagnant, R. (2010). Gender stereotypes in diagnostic criteria. In *Handbook of gender research in psychology* (pp. 91–109). Springer., doi:10.1007/978-1-4419-1467-5_5

American Psychological Association. (2015). *Demographic characteristics of division 12 members by membership status, 2015*. APA. http://www.apa.org/about/division/officers/services/div-12-2015.pdf

American Psychological Association. (2022). *Demographics of U.S. Psychology Workforce [Interactive data tool]*. APA. https://www.apa.org/workforce/data-tools/demographics

Anders, G. (1993). Machismo: Dead or alive? *Hispanic*, *3*, 14–20.

Arciniega, G. M., Anderson, T. C., Tovar-Blank, Z. G., & Tracey, T. J. (2008). Toward a fuller conception of Machismo: Development of a traditional Machismo and Caballerismo scale. *Journal of Counseling Psychology*, *55*(1), 19–33. doi:10.1037/0022-0167.55.1.19

Arias, I. (2004). Report from the CDC. The legacy of child maltreatment: Long-term health consequences for women. *Journal of Women's Health*, *13*(5), 468–473. doi:10.1089/1540999041280990 PMID:15257839

Baggerly, J., Tan, T. X., Pichotta, D., & Warner, A. (2017). Race, ethnicity, and gender of faculty members in APA-and CACREP-accredited programs: Changes over five decades. *Journal of Multicultural Counseling and Development*, *45*(4), 292–303. doi:10.1002/jmcd.12079

Bailey, R. K., Mokonogho, J., & Kumar, A. (2019). Racial and ethnic differences in depression: Current perspectives. *Neuropsychiatric Disease and Treatment*, *15*, 603–609. doi:10.2147/NDT.S128584 PMID:30863081

Bashi, V., & Mcdaniel, A. (2016). A theory of immigration and racial stratification. *Journal of Black Studies*, *27*(5), 668–682. doi:10.1177/002193479702700505

Beel, N., Jeffries, C., Brownlow, C., Winterbotham, S., & Du Preez, J. (2018). Recommendations for male-friendly individual counseling with men: A qualitative systematic literature review for the period 1995–2016. *Psychology of Men & Masculinity*, *19*(4), 600–611. doi:10.1037/men0000137

Benjamin, E. J., Virani, S. S., Callaway, C. W., Chamberlain, A. M., Chang, A. R., Cheng, S., Chiuve, S. E., Cushman, M., Delling, F. N., Deo, R., de Ferranti, S. D., Ferguson, J. F., Fornage, M., Gillespie, C., Isasi, C. R., Jiménez, M. C., Jordan, L. C., Judd, S. E., Lackland, D, & Muntner, P. (2018). Heart disease and stroke statistics—2018 update: A report from the American Heart Association. *Circulation*, *137*(12), e67–e492. doi:10.1161/CIR.0000000000000558 PMID:29386200

Bilsker, D., & White, J. (2011). The silent epidemic of male suicide. *British Columbia Medical Journal*, *53*(10).

Bjordahl, K. K., Salgado, D. S., & Johnson, B. (2015, May). *Associations between men's concern for heterosexual self-presentation and attitudes towards psychological help seeking*. Poster session presented at the 95th Annual Convention of the Western Psychological Association, Las Vegas, NV.

Blumberg, S. J., Clarke, T. C., & Blackwell, D. L. (2015). Racial and ethnic disparities in men's use of mental health treatments. *National Center for Health Statistics Data Brief No.*, (206), 1–8. PMID:26079520

Boon, K. A. (2005). Heroes, metanarrative, and the paradox of masculinity in contemporary western culture. *Journal of Men's Studies*, *13*(3), 301–312. doi:10.3149/jms.1303.301

Branscombe, N. R., Schmitt, M. T., & Harvey, R. D. (1999). Perceiving pervasive discrimination among African Americans: Implications for group identification and well-being. *Journal of Personality and Social Psychology*, *77*(1), 135–149. doi:10.1037/0022-3514.77.1.135

Brennan, D. J., Souleymanov, R., George, C., Newman, P. A., Hart, T. A., Asakura, K., & Betancourt, G. (2015). Masculinity, muscularity, and HIV sexual risk among gay and bisexual men of color. *Psychology of Men & Masculinity*, *16*(4), 393–403. doi:10.1037/a0038725

British Columbia Vital Statistics Agency. (2011). *Selected vital statistics and health status indicators: Annual Report 2002*. VS Agency. www.vs.gov.bc.ca/ stats/annual/2002/

Brooks, J. R., Lebeaut, A., Zegel, M., Walker, R. L., & Vujanovic, A. A. (2021). Anxiety sensitivity and suicide risk: Mindfulness as a psychological buffer for Black adults. *Journal of Affective Disorders*, *289*, 74–80. doi:10.1016/j.jad.2021.04.012 PMID:33945917

Calloway, A., & Creed, T. A. (2022). Enhancing CBT consultation with multicultural counseling principles. *Cognitive and Behavioral Practice*, *29*(4), 787–795. doi:10.1016/j.cbpra.2021.05.007

Capraro, R. L. (2000). Why college men drink: Alcohol, adventure, and the paradox of masculinity. *Journal of American College Health*, *48*(6), 307–315. doi:10.1080/07448480009596272 PMID:10863874

Casas, J. M., Wagenheim, B. R., Banchero, R., & Mendoza-Romero, J. (1994). Hispanic masculinity: Myth or psychological schema meriting clinical consideration. *Hispanic Journal of Behavioral Sciences*, *16*(3), 315–331. doi:10.1177/07399863940163009

Cazenave, N. A. (1979). Middle-income Black fathers: An analysis of the provider role. *The Family Coordinator*, *28*(4), 583–593. doi:10.2307/583522

Cazenave, N. A. (1984). Race, socioeconomic status, and age: The social context of American masculinity. *Sex Roles*, *11*(7-8), 639–656. doi:10.1007/BF00288117

Centers for Disease and Prevention. (2017). *National Center for Injury Prevention and Control. Web-based Injury Statistics Query and Reporting System*. WISQARS.

Centers for Disease and Prevention. (2019). Summary Health Statistics: National Health Interview Survey: 2017. *Table A-7*. [Data set]. CDC. https://www.cdc.gov/nchs/nhis/shs/tables.htm

Centers for Disease and Prevention. (2019). National Vital Statistics Report, Table 10. [Data set]. CDC. https://www.cdc.gov/nchs/data/nvsr/nvsr68/nvsr68_09.pdf

Centers for Disease Control and Prevention, National Center for Health Statistics. (2022). About Multiple Cause of Death, 1999–2020. CDC WONDER Online Database website. Centers for Disease Control and Prevention., Retrieved February 21, 2022, from.

Chan, J. W. (2018). School-based karate-do: Supporting the well-being of gay male youth. *Canadian Journal for New Scholars in Education/Revue canadienne des jeunes chercheures et chercheurs en éducation, 9*(1).

Chandra, A., Scott, M. M., Jaycox, L. H., Meredith, L. S., Tanielian, T., & Burnam, A. (2009). Racial/ethnic differences in teen and parent perspectives toward depression treatment. *The Journal of Adolescent Health*, *44*(6), 546–553. doi:10.1016/j.jadohealth.2008.10.137 PMID:19465318

Chaney, C. (2009). Boys to men: How perceptions of manhood influence the romantic partnerships of black men. *The Western Journal of Black Studies*, *33*, 110–112.

Cheatham, C. T., Barksdale, D. J., & Rodgers, S. G. (2008). Barriers to health care and health-seeking behaviors faced by Black men. *Journal of the American Academy of Nurse Practitioners*, *20*(11), 555–562. doi:10.1111/j.1745-7599.2008.00359.x PMID:19128339

Chetty, R., Friedman, J. N., Hendren, N., Jones, M. R., & Porter, S. R. (2018). *The opportunity atlas: Mapping the childhood roots of social mobility* (No. w25147). National Bureau of Economic Research. doi:10.3386/w25147

Coleman-Kirumba, L. M., Cornish, M. A., Horton, A. J., & Alvarez, J. C. (2023). Experiences of Black men: Forms of masculinity and effects on psychological help-seeking variables. *The Journal of Black Psychology*, *49*(1), 32–57. doi:10.1177/00957984221098122

Connell, R. W. (1995). *Masculinities*. Routledge.

Connell, R. W., & Messerschmidt, J. W. (2005). Hegemonic masculinity rethinking the concept. *Gender & Society*, *19*(6), 829–859. doi:10.1177/0891243205278639

Cook, E. P. (2015). *Understanding people in context: The ecological perspective in counseling*. John Wiley & Sons., doi:10.1002/9781119222743

Courtenay, W. H. (2000). Constructions of masculinity and their influence on men's well-being: A theory of gender and health. *Social Science & Medicine*, *50*(10), 1385–1401. doi:10.1016/S0277-9536(99)00390-1 PMID:10741575

Courtenay, W. H., McCreary, D. R., & Merighi, J. R. (2002). Gender and ethnic differences in health beliefs and behaviors. *Journal of Health Psychology*, *7*(3), 219–231. doi:10.1177/1359105302007003216 PMID:22114246

Cross, W. E. Jr. (1991). *Shades of Black: Diversity in African-American identity*. Temple University Press.

Cross Jr, W. E., & Fhagen-Smith, P. (2001). Patterns of African American identity development: A life span perspective. *New perspectives on racial identity development: A theoretical and practical anthology*, 243-270.

Cummings, J. R. (2014). Contextual socioeconomic status and mental health counseling use among US adolescents with depression. *Journal of Youth and Adolescence, 43*(7), 1151–1162. doi:10.100710964-013-0021-7 PMID:24114588

de Frias, C. M., & Whyne, E. (2014). Stress on health-related quality of life in older adults: The protective nature of mindfulness. *Aging & Mental Health, 19*(3), 201–206. doi:10.1080/13607863.2014.924090 PMID:24940847

DeAngelis, T. (2021, September 1). Black men's mental health matters. Monitor on Psychology. APA. https://www.apa.org/monitor/2021/09/ce-black-mental-health

Douglas, J. G. (2005). Clinical guidelines for the treatment of hypertension in African Americans. *American Journal of Cardiovascular Drugs, 5*(1), 1–6. doi:10.2165/00129784-200505010-00001 PMID:15631532

Duck, W. (2009). Black male sexual politics: Avoidance of HIV/AIDS testing as a masculine health practice. *Journal of African American Studies, 13*(3), 283–306. doi:10.100712111-009-9097-2

Englar-Carlson, M. (2006). Masculine norms and the therapy process. In M. Englar-Carlson & M. A. Stevens (Eds.), *In the room with men: A casebook of therapeutic change* (pp. 13–47). American Psychological Association., doi:10.1037/11411-002

Englar-Carlson, M., & Kiselica, M. S. (2013). Affirming the strengths in men: A positive masculinity approach to assisting male clients. *Journal of Counseling and Development, 91*(4), 399–409. doi:10.1002/j.1556-6676.2013.00111.x

Felix-Ortiz, M., Abreu, J. M., Briano, M., & Bowen, D. (2001). A critique of machismo measures in psychological research. In F. Columbus (Ed.), *Advances in psychology research* (Vol. III, pp. 63–90). NOVA Science Publishers.

Fleming, P. J., Lee, J. G., & Dworkin, S. L. (2014). "Real men don't": Constructions of masculinity and inadvertent harm in public health interventions. *American Journal of Public Health, 104*(6), 1029–1035. doi:10.2105/AJPH.2013.301820 PMID:24825202

Foster, M. D., & Matheson, K. (1998). Perceiving and feeling personal discrimination: Motivation or inhibition for collective action? *Group Processes & Intergroup Relations, 1*(2), 165–174. doi:10.1177/1368430298012004

Franklin, C. W. (1986). Conceptual and logical issues in theory and research related to Black masculinity. *The Western Journal of Black Studies, 10*, 161–166.

Frazier, E. F. (1939). *The Negro Family in the United States*. University of Chicago Press., doi:10.2307/2292637

Galdas, P. M., Cheater, F., & Marshall, P. (2005). Men and health help-seeking behaviour: Literature review. *Journal of Advanced Nursing*, *49*(6), 616–623. doi:10.1111/j.1365-2648.2004.03331.x PMID:15737222

Gamble, V. N. (1997). The Tuskegee Syphilis Study and women's health. *Journal of the American Medical Women's Association (1972)*, *52*(4), 195-196.

Gehlert, S., Sohmer, D., Sacks, T., Mininger, C., McClintock, M., & Olopade, O. (2008). Targeting health disparities: A model linking upstream determinants to downstream interventions. *Health Affairs*, *27*(2), 339–349. doi:10.1377/hlthaff.27.2.339 PMID:18332488

Geller, A., Fagan, J., Tyler, T., & Link, B. G. (2014). Aggressive policing and the mental health of young urban men. *American Journal of Public Health*, *104*(12), 2321–2327. doi:10.2105/AJPH.2014.302046 PMID:25322310

Gerdes, Z. T., & Levant, R. F. (2018). Complex relationships among masculine norms and health/well-being outcomes: Correlation patterns of the conformity to masculine norms inventory subscales. *American Journal of Men's Health*, *12*(2), 229–240. doi:10.1177/1557988317745910 PMID:29219033

Goff, P. A., Di Leone, B. A. L., & Kahn, K. B. (2012). Racism leads to pushups: How racial discrimination threatens subordinate men's masculinity. *Journal of Experimental Social Psychology*, *48*(5), 1111–1116. doi:10.1016/j.jesp.2012.03.015

Griffith, D. M. (2015). "I AM a Man": Manhood, minority men's health, and health equity. *Ethnicity & Disease*, *25*(3), 287–293. doi:10.18865/ed.25.3.287 PMID:26672674

Gross, P. A., Efimoff, I., Patrick, L., Josewski, V., Hau, K., Lambert, S., & Smye, V. (2016). The DUDES Club: A brotherhood for men's health. *Canadian Family Physician Medecin de Famille Canadien*, *62*(6), e311–e318.

Hammer, J. H., & Good, G. E. (2010). Positive psychology: An empirical examination of beneficial aspects of endorsement of masculine norms. *Psychology of Men & Masculinity*, *11*(4), 303–318. doi:10.1037/a0019056

Hammond, W. P. (2010). Psychosocial correlates of medical mistrust among African American men. *American Journal of Community Psychology*, *45*(1-2), 87–106. doi:10.100710464-009-9280-6 PMID:20077134

Hammond, W. P., & Mattis, J. S. (2005). Being a Man About It: Manhood Meaning Among African American Men. *Psychology of Men & Masculinity*, *6*(2), 114–126. doi:10.1037/1524-9220.6.2.114

Harris, S. M. (1995). Psychosocial development and Black male masculinity: Implications for counseling economically disadvantaged African American male adolescents. *Journal of Counseling and Development, 73*(3), 279–287. doi:10.1002/j.1556-6676.1995.tb01749.x

HeadUpGuys. (n.d.). *Manage & Prevent Depression in Men. Vancouver (BC).* HeadsUpGuys. https://headsupguys.org

Heron M. (2018). Deaths: leading causes for 2016 [PDF-2.3M]. *National Vital Statistics Report, 67*(6), 1–77.

Hertz, R. P., Unger, A. N., Cornell, J. A., & Saunders, E. (2005). Racial disparities in hypertension prevalence, awareness, and management. *Archives of Internal Medicine, 165*(18), 2098–2104. doi:10.1001/archinte.165.18.2098 PMID:16216999

Hunter, A. G., & Davis, J. E. (1992). Constructing gender: An exploration of Afro-American men's conceptualization of manhood. *Gender & Society, 6*(3), 464–479. doi:10.1177/089124392006003007

Hunter, A. G., & Davis, J. E. (1994). Hidden voices of Black men: Meaning, structure, and complexity of manhood. *Journal of Black Studies, 25*(1), 20–40. doi:10.1177/002193479402500102

Ingoldsby, B. (1991). The Latin American family: Familism vs. machismo. *Journal of Comparative Family Studies, 1*(1), 57–64. doi:10.3138/jcfs.22.1.57

Iwamoto, D. K., Liao, L., & Liu, W. M. (2010). Masculine norms, avoidant coping, Asian values, and depression among Asian American men. *Psychology of Men & Masculinity, 11*(1), 15–24. doi:10.1037/a0017874 PMID:20657794

Johnson, B. L., McShane, T. O., & Salgado, D. M. (2015, May). *Effects of masculine norms on health behaviors in men.* Poster presented at the Western Psychological Association Convention, Las Vegas, NV.

Kiselica, M. S. (2011). Promoting positive masculinity while addressing gender role conflict: A balanced theoretical approach to clinical work with boys and men. In C. Blazina & D. S. Shen-Miller (Eds.), An international psychology of men: Theoretical advances, case studies, and clinical innovations (pp. 127–156). Routledge/Taylor & Francis Group.

Kiselica, M. S., & Englar-Carlson, M. (2010). Identifying, affirming, and building upon male strengths: The positive psychology/positive masculinity model of psychotherapy with boys and men. *Psychotherapy (Chicago, Ill.), 47*(3), 276–287. doi:10.1037/a0021159 PMID:22402085

Kiselica, M. S., Englar-Carlson, M., Horne, A. M., & Fisher, M. (2008). A positive psychology perspective on helping boys. *Counseling troubled boys: A guidebook for professionals*, 31-48.

Leaper, C., & Van, S. R. (2008). Masculinity ideology, covert sexism, and perceived gender typicality in relation to young men's academic motivation and choices in college. *Psychology of Men & Masculinity, 9*(3), 139–153. doi:10.1037/1524-9220.9.3.139

Lease, S. H., Shuman, W. A., & Gage, A. N. (2019). Incorporating traditional masculinity ideology into health promotion models: Differences for African American/Black and White men. *Psychology of Men & Masculinity, 20*(1), 128–141. doi:10.1037/men0000151

Levant, R. F. (2006). Forward. In M. Englar-Carlson & M. A. Stevens (Eds.), *In the room with men: A casebook of therapeutic change* (pp. xv–xx). American Psychological Association.

Levant, R. F. (2011). Research in the psychology of men and masculinity using the gender role strain paradigm as a framework. *The American Psychologist, 66*(8), 765–776. doi:10.1037/a0025034 PMID:22082409

Levant, R. F., Rankin, T. J., Williams, C. M., Hasan, N. T., & Smalley, K. B. (2010). Evaluation of the factor structure and construct validity of scores on the Male Role Norms Inventory—Revised (MRNI-R). *Psychology of Men & Masculinity, 11*(1), 25–37. doi:10.1037/a0017637

Levant, R. F., Wimer, D. J., Williams, C. M., Smalley, K. B., & Noronha, D. (2009). The relationships between masculinity variables, health risk behaviors and attitudes toward seeking psychological help. *International Journal of Men's Health, 8*(1), 3–21. Advance online publication. doi:10.3149/jmh.0801.3

Liddon, L., Kingerlee, R., & Barry, J. A. (2017). Gender differences in preferences for psychological treatment, coping strategies, and triggers to help-seeking. *British Journal of Clinical Psychology, 57*(1), 42–58. doi:10.1111/bjc.12147 PMID:28691375

Lorber, J. (1997). *The Variety of Feminisms and Their Contributions to Gender Equality*. Germany: Bis.

Mahalik, J. R., Burns, S. M., & Syzdek, M. (2007). Masculinity and perceived normative health behaviors as predictors of men's health behaviors. *Social Science & Medicine, 64*(11), 2201–2209. doi:10.1016/j.socscimed.2007.02.035 PMID:17383784

Mahalik, J. R., Good, G. E., Tager, D., Levant, R. F., & Mackowiak, C. (2012). Developing a taxonomy of helpful and harmful practices for clinical work with boys and men. *Journal of Counseling Psychology, 59*(4), 591–603. doi:10.1037/a0030130 PMID:23088685

Majors, R., & Billson, J. (1992). *Cool pose: The dilemmas of Black manhood in America*. Touchstone.

Mathis, J. E. (2018). *Comparing Treatment Outcomes of Young Adult Males and Females in Wilderness Therapy Programs through a Gender Schema Lens* [Doctoral dissertation, Northcentral University].

Matthews, L. R., Gerald, J., & Jessup, G. M. (2021). Exploring men's use of mental health support offered by an Australian Employee Assistance Program (EAP): Perspectives from a focus-group study with males working in blue-and white-collar industries. *International Journal of Mental Health Systems, 15*(1), 1–17. doi:10.118613033-021-00489-5 PMID:34348756

Mays, V. M., Cochran, S. D., & Barnes, N. W. (2007). Race, race-based discrimination, and health outcomes among African Americans. *Annual Review of Psychology, 58*(1), 201–225. doi:10.1146/annurev.psych.57.102904.190212 PMID:16953796

McCarthy, J., & Holliday, E. L. (2004). Help-seeking and counseling within a traditional male gender role: An examination from a multicultural perspective. *Journal of Counseling and Development, 82*(1), 25–30. doi:10.1002/j.1556-6678.2004.tb00282.x

McCreary, D. R. (2012). Muscularity and body image. Encyclopedia of Body Image and Human Appearance, 2, 561–567. doi:10.1016/B978-0-12-384925-0.00088-2

Mincey, K., Alfonso, M., Hackney, A., & Luque, J. (2014). Understanding masculinity in undergraduate African American men: A qualitative study. *American Journal of Men's Health, 8*(5), 387–398. doi:10.1177/1557988313515900 PMID:24356494

Mirande´, A. (1988). Chicano fathers: Traditional perceptions and current realities. In P. Bronstein & C. P. Cowan (Eds.), *Fatherhood today: Men's changing role in the family* (pp. 93–106). Wiley.

Mirande´, A. (1997). *Hombres y machos: Masculinity and Latino culture*. Westview Press.

Morison, L., Trigeorgis, C., & John, M. (2014). Are mental health services inherently feminised? *The Psychologist, 27*(6), 414–416.

Mosher, D., & Tompkins, S. (1988). Scripting the macho man: Hypermasculine socialization and enculturation. *Journal of Sex Research*, *25*(1), 60–84. doi:10.1080/00224498809551445

Mount, D. L., Johnson, D. M., Rego, M. I., Schofield, K., Amponsah, A., & Graham, L. F. (2012). Preliminary findings exploring the social determinants of Black males' lay health perspectives. *American Journal of Men's Health*, *6*(1), 71–79. doi:10.1177/1557988311420993 PMID:22105065

Moynihan, D. P. (1965). *The Negro family: The case for national action*. Washington, DC: U. S. Government Printing Office.

Murphy, S. L., Kochanek, K. D., Xu, J. Q., & Arias, E. (2021). *Mortality in the United States, 2020. NCHS Data Brief, no 427*. National Center for Health Statistics., doi:10.15620/cdc:112079

National Center for Health Statistics (US). (2018). *Health, United States, 2017: With Special Feature on Mortality*. National Center for Health Statistics.

National Institute of Mental Health. (2019). *Mental health information, statistics. Major Depression*. NIH. https://www.nimh.nih.gov/health/statistics/major-depression.shtml

National Urban League. (2007). *State of Black America: Portrait of the Black Male*. Beckham Publications Group.

Nellis, A. 2021. *The Color of Justice: Racial and Ethnic Disparity in State Prisons*, The Sentencing Project. https://policycommons.net/artifacts/3351700/the-color-of-justice-racial-and-ethnic-disparity-in-state-prisons/.

Nelson, K., Norris, K., & Mangione, C. M. (2002). Disparities in the diagnosis and pharmacologic treatment of high serum cholesterol by race and ethnicity: Data from the Third National Health and Nutrition Examination Survey. *Archives of Internal Medicine*, *162*(8), 929–935. doi:10.1001/archinte.162.8.929 PMID:11966345

Neukrug, E., Britton, B. S., & Crews, R. C. (2013). Common health-related concerns of men: Implications for counselors. *Journal of Counseling and Development*, *91*(4), 390–397. doi:10.1002/j.1556-6676.2013.00109.x

NIDCR. (2009). *Oral Cancer: What African American Men Need to Know*. Bethesda, MD: National Institute of Dental and Craniofacial Research. http://www.nidcr.nih.gov/Oral Health/Topics/OralCancer/AfricanAmericanMen.htm

Nock, M. K., Borges, G., Bromet, E. J., Alonso, J., Angermeyer, M., Beautrais, A., Bruffaerts, R., Chiu, W. T., de Girolamo, G., Gluzman, S., de Graaf, R., Gureje, O., Haro, J. M., Huang, Y., Karam, E., Kessler, R. C., Lepine, J. P., Levinson, D., Medina-Mora, M. E., & Williams, D. (2008). Cross-national prevalence and risk factors for suicidal ideation, plans and attempts. *The British Journal of Psychiatry*, *192*(2), 98–105. doi:10.1192/bjp.bp.107.040113 PMID:18245022

Noone, J. H., & Stephens, C. (2008). Men, masculine identities, and health care utilisation. *Sociology of Health & Illness*, *30*(5), 711–725. doi:10.1111/j.1467-9566.2008.01095.x PMID:18564976

Operario, D., & Fiske, S. (2008). Stereotypes: Content, structures, processes, and context. In Social Cognition (pp. 22–44). doi:10.1002/9780470693421.ch2

Osa, M. L., & Kelly, N. R. (2021, March 4). Experiences of Discrimination Are Associated With Drive for Muscularity Among African American Men. *Psychology of Men & Masculinity*, *22*(2), 365–374. doi:10.1037/men0000287

Parent, M. C., Hammer, J. H., Bradstreet, T. C., Schwartz, E. N., & Jobe, T. (2018). Men's mental health help-seeking behaviors: An intersectional analysis. *American Journal of Men's Health*, *12*(1), 64–73. doi:10.1177/1557988315625776 PMID:29226771

Peters, Z. J., Santo, L., Davis, D., & DeFrances, C. J. (2023). *Emergency department visits related to mental health disorders among adults, by race and Hispanic ethnicity: United States, 2018–2020. National Health Statistics Reports; no 181*. National Center for Health Statistics. doi:10.15620/cdc:123507

Pleck, J. H., Sonenstein, F. L., & Ku, L. C. (1993). Masculinity ideology: Its impact on adolescent males' heterosexual relationships. *The Journal of Social Issues*, *49*(3), 11–29. doi:10.1111/j.1540-4560.1993.tb01166.x

Plowden, K. O., Thompson Adams, L., & Wiley, D. (2016). Black and blue: Depression and African American men. *Archives of Psychiatric Nursing*, *30*(5), 630–635. doi:10.1016/j.apnu.2016.04.007 PMID:27654249

Reinert, M., Fritze, D., & Nguyen, T. (2021). *The State of Mental Health in America 2022*. Mental Health America, Alexandria VA.

Rice, S. M., Fallon, B. J., Aucote, H. M., & Möller-Leimkühler, A. M. (2013). Development and preliminary validation of the male depression risk scale: Furthering the assessment of depression in men. *Journal of Affective Disorders*, *151*(3), 950–958. doi:10.1016/j.jad.2013.08.013 PMID:24051100

Roberts-Douglass, K., & Curtis-Boles, H. (2013). Exploring positive masculinity development in African American men: A retrospective study. *Psychology of Men & Masculinity*, *14*(1), 7–15. doi:10.1037/a0029662

Rogers, B. K., Sperry, H. A., & Levant, R. F. (2015). Masculinities among African American men: An intersectional perspective. *Psychology of Men & Masculinity*, *16*(4), 416–425. doi:10.1037/a0039082

Seidler, Z. E., Dawes, A. J., Rice, S. M., Oliffe, J. L., & Dhillon, H. M. (2016). The role of masculinity in men's help-seeking for depression: A systematic review. *Clinical Psychology Review*, *49*, 106–118. doi:10.1016/j.cpr.2016.09.002 PMID:27664823

Seidler, Z. E., Rice, S. M., River, J., Oliffe, J. L., & Dhillon, H. M. (2017). Men's mental health: The case for a masculinities model. *Journal of Men's Studies*, *26*(1), 92–104. doi:10.1177/1060826517729406

Sileo, K. M., & Kershaw, T. S. (2020). Dimensions of masculine norms, depression, and mental health service utilization: Results from a prospective cohort study among emerging adult men in the United States. *American Journal of Men's Health*, *14*(1), 1557988320906980. doi:10.1177/1557988320906980 PMID:32079448

Sloan, C., Conner, M., & Gough, B. (2015). How does masculinity impact on health? A quantitative study of masculinity and health behavior in a sample of U.K. men and women. *Psychology of Men & Masculinity*, *16*(2), 206–217. doi:10.1037/a0037261

Smedley, B. D., Stith, A. Y., & Nelson, A. R. (2003). Racial and ethnic disparities in diagnosis and treatment: a review of the evidence and a consideration of causes. *Unequal treatment: Confronting racial and ethnic disparities in health care.*

Snowden, L. R., Catalano, R., & Shumway, M. (2009). Disproportionate use of psychiatric emergency services by African Americans. *Psychiatric Services (Washington, D.C.)*, *60*(12), 1664–1671. doi:10.1176/ps.2009.60.12.1664 PMID:19952158

Staples, R. F. (1978). Masculinity and race: The dual dilemma of Black men. *The Journal of Social Issues*, *34*(1), 169–183. doi:10.1111/j.1540-4560.1978.tb02547.x

Substance Abuse and Mental Health Services Administration. (2013). Addressing the Specific Behavioral Health Needs of Men. Treatment Improvement Protocol (TIP) Series 56. HHS Publication No. (SMA) 13-4736. Rockville, MD: Substance Abuse and Mental Health Services Administration.

Substance Abuse and Mental Health Services Administration. (2019). Results from the 2018 National Survey on Drug Use and Health: Mental Health Detailed Tables. *Table 8.17B*. [Data set]. SAMHSA. https://www.samhsa.gov/data/report/2018-nsduh-detailed-tables

Swami, V. (2016). Masculinities and ethnicities: Ethnic differences in drive for muscularity in British men and the negotiation of masculinity hierarchies. *British Journal of Psychology*, *107*(3), 577–592. doi:10.1111/bjop.12162 PMID:26592864

The Office of Minority Health. (2008). *Stroke and African Americans. Rockville, MD: U.S. Department of Health & Human Services.* Office of Minority Health. http://www.omhrc.gov/templates/content.aspx?lvl=2&lvlID=51&ID=3022

The Office of Minority Health. (2008). *African American Profile*. U.S. Department of Health & Human Services. http:// www.omhrc.gov/templates/browse.aspx?lvl=2&lvlID=51

Thorpe, R. J. Jr, Kennedy-Hendricks, A., Griffith, D. M., Bruce, M. A., Coa, K., Bell, C. N., Young, J., Bowie, J. V., & LaVeist, T. A. (2015). Race, social and environmental conditions, and health behaviors in men. *Family & Community Health*, *38*(4), 297–306. doi:10.1097/FCH.0000000000000078 PMID:26291190

Tyler, R. E., & Williams, S. (2014). Masculinity in young men's health: Exploring health, help-seeking and health service use in an online environment. *Journal of Health Psychology*, *19*(4), 457–470. doi:10.1177/1359105312473784 PMID:23493865

United States Renal Data System. (2005). *Home*. National Institute of Diabetes and Digestive and Kidney Diseases. Available at: http://www.usrds.org/

U.S. Census Bureau. (2005-2013). *American Community Survey 1-Year PUMS file*. US Census Bureau. http://www.census. gov/programs-surveys/acs/data/ pums.html

Vogel, D. L., Heimerdinger-Edwards, S. R., Hammer, J. H., & Hubbard, A. (2011). "Boys don't cry": Examination of the links between endorsement of masculine norms, self-stigma, and help-seeking attitudes for men from diverse backgrounds. *Journal of Counseling Psychology*, *58*(3), 368–382. doi:10.1037/a0023688 PMID:21639615

Wade, J. C., & Rochlen, A. B. (2013). Introduction: Masculinity, identity, and the health and well-being of African American men. *Psychology of Men & Masculinity*, *14*(1), 1–6. doi:10.1037/a0029612

Wang, J., Patten, S. B., Lam, R. W., Attridge, M., Ho, K., Schmitz, N., Marchand, A., & Lashewicz, B. M. (2016). The effects of an e-mental health program and job coaching on the risk of major depression and productivity in Canadian male workers: Protocol for a randomized controlled trial. *JMIR Research Protocols*, *5*(4), e6350. doi:10.2196/resprot.6350 PMID:27847352

Ward, E., Wiltshire, J. C., Detry, M. A., & Brown, R. L. (2013). African American men and women's attitude toward mental illness, perceptions of stigma, and preferred coping behaviors. *Nursing Research*, *62*(3), 185–194. doi:10.1097/NNR.0b013e31827bf533 PMID:23328705

Ward, E. G. (2005). Homophobia, hypermasculinity and the US black church. *Culture, Health & Sexuality*, *7*(5), 493–504. doi:10.1080/13691050500151248 PMID:16864218

Watkins, D. C., Green, B. L., Rivers, B. M., & Rowell, K. L. (2006). Depression and black men: Implications for future research. *Journal of Men's Health & Gender*, *3*(3), 227–235. doi:10.1016/j.jmhg.2006.02.005

Watson, J. (2014). Young African American males: Barriers to access to health care. *Journal of Human Behavior in the Social Environment*, *24*(8), 1004–1009. doi:10.1080/10911359.2014.953416

Wexler, R., Elton, T., Pleister, A., & Feldman, D. (2009). Barriers to blood pressure control as reported by African American patients. *Journal of the National Medical Association*, *101*(6), 597–603. doi:10.1016/S0027-9684(15)30947-0 PMID:19585931

White, A. (2008). *Ain't I a feminist? African American men speak out on fatherhood, friendship, forgiveness, and freedom*. State University of New York Press.

Williams, D. R. (2018). Stress and the Mental Health of Populations of Color: Advancing Our Understanding of Race-related Stressors. *Journal of Health and Social Behavior*, *59*(4), 466–485. doi:10.1177/0022146518814251 PMID:30484715

Wilson, M., Gwyther, K., Swann, R., Casey, K., Featherston, R., Oliffe, J. L., Englar-Carlson, M., & Rice, S. M. (2022). Operationalizing positive masculinity: A theoretical synthesis and school-based framework to engage boys and young men. *Health Promotion International*, *37*(1), daab031. doi:10.1093/heapro/daab031 PMID:33842967

Wong, C. A., Eccles, J. S., & Sameroff, A. (2003). The influence of ethnic discrimination and ethnic identification on African American adolescents' school and socioemotional adjustment. *Journal of Personality*, *71*(6), 1197–1232. doi:10.1111/1467-6494.7106012 PMID:14633063

Wong, M. D., Chung, A. K., Boscardin, J. W., Li, M., Hsieh, H.-J., Ettner, S. L., & Shapiro, M. F. (2006). The contribution of specific causes of death to sex differences in mortality. *Public Health Reports (Washington, D.C.)*, *121*(6), 746–754. doi:10.1177/003335490612100615 PMID:17278410

Wong, Y. J., & Rochlen, A. B. (2005). Demystifying Men's Emotional Behavior: New Directions and Implications for Counseling and Research. *Psychology of Men & Masculinity*, *6*(1), 62–72. doi:10.1037/1524-9220.6.1.62

Xanthos, C., Treadwell, H. M., & Holden, K. B. (2010). Social determinants of health among African–American men. *The Journal of Men's Health*, *7*(1), 11–19. doi:10.1016/j.jomh.2009.12.002

Yourstone, J. Y., Lindholm, T., Grann, M., & Fazel, S. (2009). Gender differences in diagnoses of mentally disordered offenders. *International Journal of Forensic Mental Health*, *8*(3), 172–177. doi:10.1080/14999010903199316

Zerhouni, E. (2002). Prostate Cancer Research Plan FY 2003-FY 2008. NIH., Available at http://planning.cancer.gov/ pdfprgreports/prostateplan.pdf, Retrieved January 4, 2010, from.

Chapter 11
Schizophrenia:
Impact and Disparities in the Black Community

Avril W. Knox
Texas A&M University, Commerce, USA

ABSTRACT

Schizophrenia is a chronic psychotic illness that compromises a patient's ability to think clearly and maintain emotional stability. A patient's disease frequently makes interacting with others and forming enduring relationships challenging. It impacts a person's thoughts, feelings, and behavior as a severe mental disease. The diagnosis of schizophrenia among African Americans seeking mental health treatment is thus one of the most prominent and prevalent inequities. Environmental risk factors may be a part of the incidence rise. Black people's schizophrenia diagnoses may be biased, which can significantly impact the treatment provided. Determining and reducing diagnostic bias has been a critical strategy for reducing disparities in Black People's mental health outcomes.

INTRODUCTION

The history of schizophrenia and mental health generally are intertwined and have unique contextual repercussions. The English equivalent of the Greek term for schizophrenia is 'split mind.' This term, which in Latin translates to 'premature dementia' was created in 1908 by Swiss psychiatrist Paul Eugen Bleuler (1857-1939) to describe a range of mental diseases that German psychiatrist Emil Kraepelin (1856-1926) had named "dementia praecox" (Fraguas & Breathnach, 2009). A

DOI: 10.4018/978-1-6684-8918-5.ch011

leading cause of disability globally and a severe psychotic condition is schizophrenia (Bennett & Rosenheck, 2021). The disease often appears in late adolescence or early adulthood. It frequently results in years of incapacity, significant psychological suffering, social isolation, suicidality, drug misuse, unemployment, dependency on government aid, and homelessness.

Schizophrenia is a severe mental condition that impacts a person's thoughts, feelings, and actions. People living with schizophrenia may appear to have lost all sense of reality, which may upset them and their loved ones. Participating in everyday activities may be challenging for someone with schizophrenia, but effective therapies are available. Many people undergoing therapy can participate in school or the workforce, become independent, and value their connections with others (National Institute of Mental Health (NIMH), 2021). The condition is complex, protracted, and marked by various symptoms, including hallucinations, delusions, abnormal speech or behavior, and cognitive decline. The disease's early onset and persistence make it a devastating disorder for many individuals and their families. Disability is typically caused by the interaction of negative symptoms (characterized by loss or deficits) with cognitive symptoms, such as impairments in attention, working memory, or executive function. Positive signs, including suspicion, delusions, and hallucinations, may also cause relapse. Due to the disorder's inherent heterogeneity, its diagnostic criteria, etiology, and pathophysiology have not been established (Pate, 2014).

The most common type of functional psychosis is schizophrenia. Those with the illness may display various symptoms. Schizophrenia does not cause a *split personality*, despite how the disease is depicted in the media. Instead, it is a chronic psychotic disorder that affects the patient's ability to think clearly and feel emotionally stable. A patient's sickness often interferes with their ability to participate in social activities and form meaningful relationships. Although social withdrawal and other abnormal (schizoid) behaviors often precede a person's first psychotic episode, other persons may not exhibit any symptoms. Indicative of a psychotic episode are patient-specific signs and symptoms (psychotic features) that reflect the *false reality* the patient has created in their head. As noted, schizophrenia symptoms are divided into positive, negative, and cognitive categories. Therefore, the psychiatrist must carefully consider each sign to differentiate it from other psychotic disorders, such as schizoaffective disorder, a depressive disorder with psychotic symptoms, and bipolar disorder with psychotic characteristics. Positive signs, which may be called "psychotic acts not observed in healthy individuals," are the most obvious. These symptoms may include hallucinations, delusions, and abnormal motor behavior with varying degrees of severity. According to the NIMH (2021), each sign is defined. For example:

Hallucinations: When a person perceives sounds, tastes, smells, or sensations that are not truly present. People living with schizophrenia frequently hear voices. Before family or friends become aware of a problem, those who hear voices may continue to do so for some time.

Delusions: When someone holds firmly to false ideas that may appear unreasonable to others.

Abnormal Motor Behavior: When a person has strange or irrational thinking methods. Thought disorders can make it difficult for people to organize their words and ideas. For example, a speaker occasionally stops in the middle of a thought, switches topics abruptly, or uses meaningless phrases. Also, when a person displays strange body motions, people with movement disorders may repeatedly perform specific movements.

According to Pate (2014), positive symptoms are simpler to recognize but more likely to result in severe morbidity because they impact the patient's emotions and actions. McCutcheon (2020) wrote that the most common functional psychosis is schizophrenia, and those with the illness may display various symptoms. The most common detrimental effects are diminished emotional expressiveness and avolition (decreased initiation of goal-directed behavior). Anhedonia and analogy may also happen to patients. It is critical to understand that negative symptoms may be the primary reason for a diagnosis of schizophrenia or may be secondary to a concomitant psychotic disease, medication, or environmental factor. Cognitive symptoms are the most current grouping of schizophrenia symptoms. These symptoms are non-specific and must be severe enough for another to notice them. Cognitive symptoms, include impaired speech, cognition, attention, and gradually impaired communication abilities.

Further limitations and unpleasant settings for patients may result from schizophrenia symptoms. These individuals are more prone to substance misuse, which may include a variety of substances, including alcohol, cigarettes, and prescription medications. Anxiety, melancholy, panic attacks, and obsessive-compulsive disorder may exacerbate the symptoms of schizophrenia, in addition to being common in those with them. Also, they often do not know much about the illness. This thinking style has been linked to higher nonadherence and relapse rates, worse psychosocial functioning, uncleanliness, and worsened health outcomes (McCutcheon, 2020).

The fundamental signs of schizophrenia and its comorbid illnesses may lead to social and vocational impairment. The patient may find it challenging to locate and maintain a stable job due to inadequate or incomplete schooling. People with schizophrenia have few acquaintances and rely on others for daily assistance to manage relapses and recurring symptoms. Patients with schizophrenia often have an unclear outlook. Only 20% of patients say their therapies were effective. The remaining patients have chronic symptoms, a high frequency of psychotic episodes, and a poor response to antipsychotic drugs (Pate, 2014).

DIMENSION AND EFFECT

The World Health Organization (2023) estimated that over 24 million people (1 in 300, or 0.32%) worldwide have schizophrenia. For adults, the incidence is 1 in 222 (0.4%). It does not occur as frequently as other mental illnesses. The onset often occurs in late adolescence or the 20s and occurs sooner in men than women. Significant suffering and impairment in personal, familial, social, academic, occupational, and other critical aspects of life are typically linked to schizophrenia. These patients have a two-to-three times higher risk of dying young than the general population. Physical ailments, including viral, metabolic, and cardiovascular problems, are frequently the cause.

Theoretical Perspective: Etiology

Genetic Theory

It has been determined through epidemiological research (including those with twins, in adoption situations, and with siblings) that schizophrenia is heritable to 80% to 85%. In addition, genetic theories have explained the emergence of schizophrenia through molecular genetic investigations (Kim, 2016).

Neurobiological Theory

Kim (2016) also mentioned that the explanation for the origin of schizophrenia had been investigated with the advancement of neuroimaging. According to neurobiological theories, structural and functional abnormalities in the brain cause schizophrenia. This hypothesis to explain schizophrenia incorporates elements from several disciplines, including neuropathology, physiology, chemistry, and brain anatomy. The following are etiological findings: 1) Decreases in the white matter, 2) functional changes and poor functional connections in the prefrontal cortex, 3) decrease in neuronal and membrane integrity, and 4) abnormalities in the neurotransmitters.

Regarding adult neurogenesis, a key neuropathological finding of schizophrenia is decreased hippocampal volume. More advanced systematic methodologies are required to properly comprehend this hypothesis due to the complexity of the brain and neurobiological markers. The neurobiological explanation, however, is the most accepted due to its significance in explaining the pathways that lead to schizophrenia, identifying therapy targets, and predicting results (Kang et al., 2016).

The neurobiological theory aids in predicting the possible progression of schizophrenia. Every person with schizophrenia may proceed with their illness differently. There are typical illness progression patterns, however. Initially, classic psychotic symptoms like hallucinations or delusions appear due to improper neurotransmitter regulation. Those with schizophrenia will experience the following stage, known as the chronic stage, marked by less characteristic psychotic symptoms once this acute stage has been effectively controlled or treated with antipsychotics. However, a relapse might happen while the condition is chronic. One way to determine how well one's brain functions is to perform structural or functional brain imaging. Therefore, prefrontal structural and neurochemical abnormalities can be used to explain illness progression using various functional brain imaging techniques. Also, the progression of schizophrenia can be predicted by observing how antipsychotic medicines affect the body (Kim, 2016).

Several significant results that have increased our understanding of the disease's scientific foundation have come from recent research that used the neurobiological hypothesis to pinpoint the genesis of schizophrenia. Much research has concentrated on structural brain imaging, discovering the prefrontal lobe changes related to schizophrenia. Reduced neuronal and membrane integrity has also been demonstrated, and it has been postulated that the functional connection between the prefrontal areas may be compromised. Neurotransmitter dysregulation has also been noted. The research examined the correlation between schizophrenia's cortical and gray matter volumes and the severity of symptoms. According to the study, variations in cortical and grey matter volumes point to distinct neurobiological processes underpinning schizophrenia's two primary symptom categories, positive and negative. The right hemisphere's importance in the case of someone with decreased expressivity was emphasized. Neurodevelopmental epidemiological research cannot demonstrate the etiology of schizophrenia, but neurobiological investigations can explain the causal links. The scientific basis for schizophrenia has been well-established, despite certain discrepancies between study results that make it difficult to pinpoint pathophysiology (Roffman et al., 2005).

Neurodevelopmental Theory

According to Kim (2016), it has been proposed that neurodevelopmental theory is crucial to comprehending schizophrenia, in addition to the mounting evidence of genetic influences on schizophrenia. This hypothesis focuses on the relationship between genetics, environmental exposures, and pathogenic events. For example, pathological changes in the brain stem, cerebral cortex, cerebellar vermis, cerebral symmetry, and limbic system may result from adverse environmental exposures during the perinatal period, such as maternal virus infections, fetal starvation, or severe prematurity. Moreover, there is substantial evidence for a neurodevelopmental genesis for anatomical abnormalities such as lateral ventricular enlargement and third ventricle enlargement in the brains of schizophrenia patients.

DISPARITIES IN DIAGNOSING SCHIZOPHRENIA AMONG CULTURES

Although Schizophrenia has been found in persons from many different racial and ethnic origins worldwide, the disease's diagnosis has some peculiar traits in the United States. The 2010 U.S. Census counted 42,163,000 persons of African American ethnicity, of which 19,057,000 were men (U.S. Census, 2010). Unlike women, White men, and all other ethnic groups in the U.S., African American males—who make up 45% of the African American population—are disproportionately diagnosed with schizophrenia in inpatient settings (Barnes, 2008; Metzl, 2009; Snowden & Cheung, 1990). Schizophrenia affects men 1.4 times more frequently than women (Varcarolis & Halter, 2010). A higher percentage of Black American men are diagnosed with schizophrenia when seeking treatment, despite the distribution of the condition is only slightly more frequent in males than in the general community (Barnes, 2008; NIMH, 2008).

BLACK MEN AND SCHIZOPHRENIA

There are specific contextual differences affecting Black Americans, though their rates of mental illness are generally comparable to those of other Americans. For example, Black people are more than twice as likely to report having significant psychological distress if they live below the poverty line (American Psychological Association, 2023). Another example is that Black people's depressive symptoms are more incapacitating, persistent, and resistant to therapy than that of White (Bailey, 2019). Also, Black males are not getting the assistance they require for these issues. For instance, compared to 45.4% of non-Hispanic White males with the same symptoms, only 26.4% of Black and Hispanic men aged 18-44 reported using mental health services regularly (NCHS Data Brief, 2015). It can be challenging to locate Black psychologists when Black males seek therapy and prefer a same-race practitioner because they still comprise only about 4% of the doctoral-level psychology workforce (Conroy et al., 2023).

BLACKS AND SCHIZOPHRENIA

Eack et al. (2012) considered the more frequent diagnosis of schizophrenia among Black Americans seeking mental health treatment an example of glaring and persistent inequities not only in the mental healthcare system but as a reflection of the larger society. Although there is no specific genetic evidence to support a rise in frequency in this group, this phenomenon does exist. Some of the increase in prevalence may be due to environmental factors. Given that the approaches recommended for treating psychotic versus mood disorders differ significantly and receiving an unnecessary antipsychotic medication(s) may have serious side effects, bias in diagnosing schizophrenia among Black Americans significantly impacts care. Therefore, understanding and minimizing diagnostic bias has been a top concern in addressing inequities in mental health outcomes among African Americans.

Until recently, little information was available about the causes or processes of the overrepresentation of schizophrenia diagnoses in the African American community. Sociodemographic traits and clinical presentations of those seeking care have been the focus of efforts to identify the origins of diagnostic bias in this population. These studies have continued to show an increase in schizophrenia diagnoses among Blacks, even after adjusting for differences in socioeconomic status and symptoms (Eack et al., 2012).

Diagnosing psychotic disorders is widespread domestically and abroad. However, differences in such a diagnosis by race have been noted across time and in different mental health professions. Schwartz (2014) found an excessive prevalence of psychotic illness diagnoses among American Africans is one of the most reliable ways to relate race and diagnosis. For instance, studies reveal that Black Americans are around five times more likely than Euro-Americans to be admitted to state mental institutions with a diagnosis of schizophrenia. Surprisingly, the physicians' race does not appear to affect the diagnosis. The relationship between race and diagnostic patterns has been the subject of several investigations, but only a limited number of literature reviews have collected data for use in clinical settings. Nevertheless, the overwhelming body of research evidence, which first gained traction in the early 1980s, demonstrates how Black Americans are misdiagnosed more often than Euro-Americans.

Compared to White adults, Black Americans are more likely to exhibit symptoms of chronic emotional distress, including melancholy, despair, and a sense that everything is a struggle, according to the Office of Minority Health with the U.S. Department of Health and Human Services (2021). More than twice as many Black people who live below the poverty line report having substantial psychological distress compared to those who are financially secure. They are also between three and five times more likely to be given a diagnosis of schizophrenia than any other racial or ethnic group (Schwartz, 2014).

A study by Olbert et al. (2018) repeatedly noted that Blacks receive schizophrenia diagnoses at higher rates than Whites. The study illustrated the potential of data from meta-analytical literature reviews to analyze potential moderators, examine whether structured interview assessments help minimize racial diagnostic discrepancies in schizophrenia, and quantify the extent of these gaps. Studies that offered unique sample data and published data sufficient to compute ratios at the 0.05 confidence intervals for a schizophrenia diagnosis by race were included. A total of 14 studies Using structured-interview diagnostic evaluations and 41 studies Using unstructured assessments met the inclusion criteria. Even though there was many variety, there was not much evidence of publishing bias. Inverse heterogeneity models showed that Blacks were diagnosed with schizophrenia at higher rates than Whites with studies using unstructured and structured-instrument diagnostic evaluations.

Gara (2019) stated that Black Americans compared to other racial and ethnic groupings are more likely to receive a schizophrenia diagnosis in clinical settings in the United States. Previous studies repeatedly demonstrated that Blacks with mood disorders are substantially more likely than other ethnicities to receive a false-positive diagnosis of schizophrenia. "Racial diagnostic discrepancy in schizophrenia constitutes a persistent yet varied clinical phenomenon that has been stable for the past three decades." Gara also found that Black Americans showed a higher percentage (44%) of schizophrenia diagnoses compared to Euro-Americans (32%), with a statistically significant relationship between race and hospital admitting diagnosis. Comparing researchers' primary diagnosis and its relationship to race, Neighbors et al. (1989) found a statistically considerable clinician relationship that Blacks had a higher percentage (33%) of schizophrenia diagnoses compared to Whites (24%). These findings illustrate how clinicians perceive symptoms differently by race, particularly when assigning a diagnosis of schizophrenia.

Strawkowski et al. (1997) discovered that it is challenging to eliminate bias in clinical assessment. For individuals of color, receiving an evaluation or treatment from a racial majority group can have detrimental clinical effects such as depression. Biological and social-environmental factors may impact a specific racial or ethnic group and predispose it more than other groups to a specific condition such as schizophrenia. When a physician makes a differential diagnosis, non-medical aspects may also have an impact. Schizophrenia is, by definition, a diagnosis of exclusion. The difference between White and Black Americans being diagnosed with it is alarming, especially considering that a significant mood illness is an actual cause. Therefore, before this diagnosis is made, other possible causes, notably mood disorders, must be considered and ruled out. An alternative explanation is that severe depression is more frequently co-morbid in Blacks with schizophrenia, whether it occurred before, concurrent with, after, or unrelated to the diagnosis of schizophrenia (Gara, 2019).

VIEWS FROM THE COMMUNITY

The Centers for Disease Control and Prevention (2016) states that African Americans/Blacks experience more severe psychological discomfort than non-Hispanic Whites (3.4% of Blacks compared to 3.2% of Whites). Also, Blacks frequently experience melancholy, anxiety, and post-traumatic disorder (Hall, 2018; Office of Minority Health, 2016; SAMHSA, 2015). The difficulties Black communities face economically, socially, educationally, and physically may be contributing factors. Therefore, it is crucial to investigate African Americans' attitudes toward mental disease and treatment, given the differences in help-seeking and the propensity of Black Americans to develop mental illness. Schwartz and Blankenship (2014) suggested that race is another factor that impacts the diagnosis of psychotic diseases.

Implications for future research include examining hypotheses from the literature. It is plausible that clinician race affects clinical judgment and results in diagnostic prejudice. However, this has not been conclusively established. Instead, it was proposed in earlier work that the application of diagnostic criteria could vary based on the physician's race. When examining a Black patient, a doctor of another race may not consider certain cultural traits. Black individuals, for instance, often have lower levels of confidence in the healthcare system. Therefore, due to this mistrust, Black individuals may be less forthcoming about their symptoms and experiences. A physician of another race could interpret that hesitation as paranoia, a typical indication of schizophrenia.

Nagendra et al. (2022) wrote that racism has a role in the inequities of Blacks diagnosed with schizophrenia. These researchers reported that Black people suffer from poor mental and physical health due to marginalization and prejudice. Major instances of racial discrimination (e.g., being wrongfully dismissed from a job) and lesser ones (e.g., being followed around a store) are experienced by Blacks, and both have been linked to higher incidences of psychotic symptoms. In addition, many regularly used schizophrenia tests were created by and normed primarily based on Whites, whose daily encounters are very different from those of racially underrepresented cultures. It is unknown whether these metrics extend to other cultures. A higher level of suspicion among Blacks can be an adaptive reaction to discrimination rather than a sign of psychopathology. Therefore, assessing paranoia in this population is particularly difficult (Whaly, 2001).

Using a large, mixed sample of schizophrenia-spectrum diagnoses, those at high risk of developing psychosis, and non-psychiatric controls, Wolny et al. (2021) analyzed item-level racism for self-reported paranoia measured by the *Schizotypal Personality Questionnaire*. The results showed that even when they had the same latent levels of suspicion, Blacks scored higher than Whites on practically every question involving paranoia. These results indicated that rather than the classic psychopathology, Blacks might demonstrate ordinary and adaptive experiences that may mimic schizophrenia.

Some authors hypothesized that misinterpreting what is taken to be disruptive and socially deviant behaviors frequently associated with Black Americans was a contributing cause of misdiagnosis. Others have written that environmental factors were a cause for misdiagnosing schizophrenia. Structural racism, conditions in which individuals live, physical stress, lack of healthy foods, childcare, incarceration, homelessness, unemployment, and anxiety caused by discrimination have all been understood as stressors that increase the risk of schizophrenia. Other explanations for the long-term pattern mentioned above include unintended clinician biases and the underdiagnosis of major depressive disease and bipolar disorder among Black Americans in favor of a diagnosis of psychotic disorder. Hence, there may be different outcomes with treatment and resources from a mental health professional.

AVOIDING MENTAL HEALTH SERVICES

There are differing views about people who have mental health disorders. This is often the case in the Black community. According to the National Alliance on Mental Illness (2020), 63% of Blacks think having a mental health issue is a sign of personal weakness. People might feel ashamed of having a mental illness and concerned about being treated differently. Help-seeking among Black Americans is impacted by a lack of knowledge about the community's mental health resources, the high costs of mental health services, cultural beliefs about mental illness and treatment (including mistrust of medication), and the stigma associated with mental illness. As a result, they might turn to one another for help rather than risk having a poor experience with a professional of a different race (Avent Harris & Wong, 2018). Rather than seeking a diagnosis, many will turn to their church or another faith community they know for strength and to avoid isolation. However, the *Annual State of the Communities Report with Diverse Communities* (2020) reported that when asked about talking to loved ones, the faith community, family, and friends, only 12.5% of respondents who identified as African American/Black said they "strongly agree" or "agree," with that course of action. In contrast, 67% of those identified as White agreed with it.

The American Psychiatric Association (2017) stated that 13.3% of Americans identify as African American. The percentage of Black Americans in the United States is lower than non-Hispanic Whites, and the number of those seeking mental health services is still proportionately lower than that of their White counterparts (see Figures 1 and 2). Nonetheless, despite their need for mental health services, only one in three Blacks who need mental health treatment obtain it. In addition,

Mental Health Facts for Black Americans (American Psychiatric Association, 2017) lists the following:

- Less likely to get the treatment that complies with recommendations
- Are less likely to be in a research study
- They often use primary care providers or hospital emergency rooms and avoid using mental health professionals for treatment.

Figure 1. The distribution of Black Americans in the U.S.
(SAMHSA, 2012)

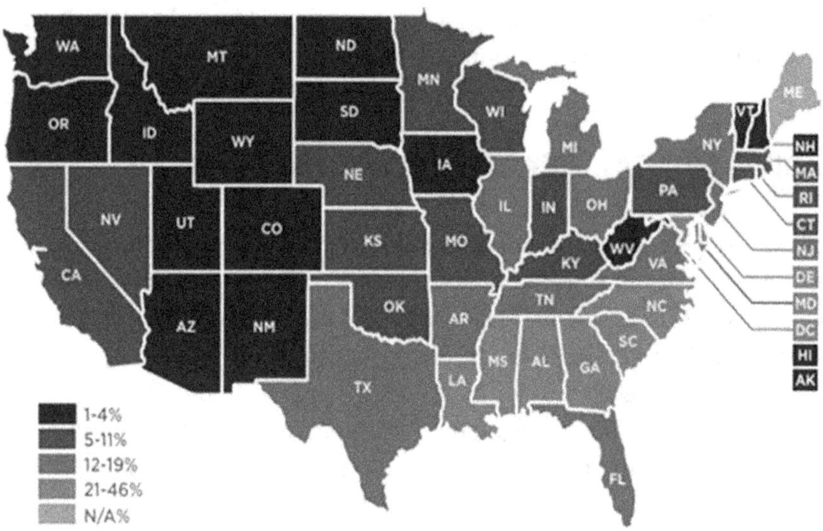

Figure 2. Mental health service use in the past year among adults, by race/ethnicity and gender
(SAMHSA, 2012)
Source: SAMHSA, Center for Behavioral Health Statistics and Quality (2012). https://www.samhsa.gov/data/sites/default/files/MHServicesUseAmongAdults/MHServicesUseAmongAdults.pdf

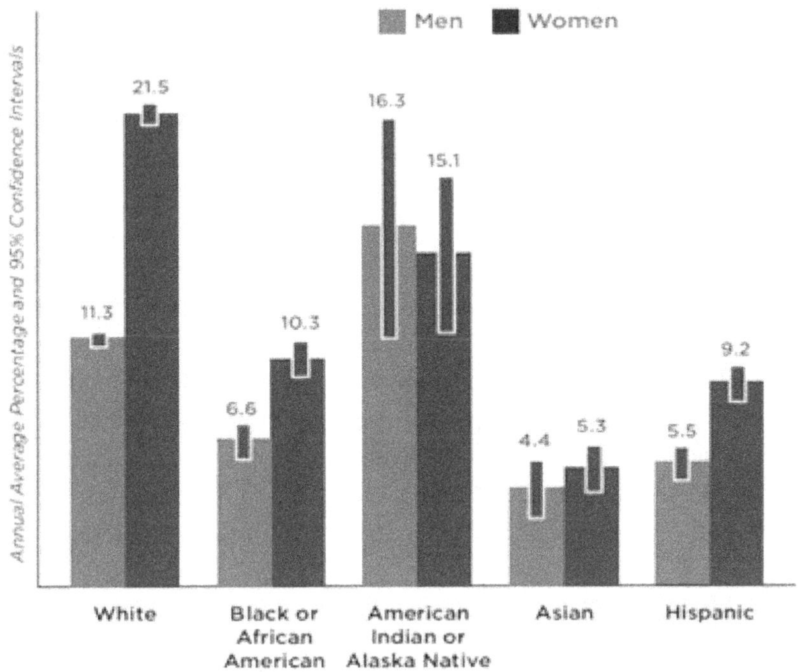

TREATMENT

A recent study conducted by Nagendra et al. (2022) concluded that psychosocial and clinical results for Blacks with schizophrenia are poorer than for Whites. While racism-related variables partially account for these discrepancies, another hypothesis might be that Blacks may respond less favorably to psychosocial therapies for psychotic illnesses. These researchers sought to determine how effective first-episode psychosis (FEP), evidenced-based treatment approaches are for Blacks and Whites. FEP allows the examination of treatment results by race without past therapy and a persistent condition as confounding variables. The treatment trajectories of Black and White Americans with FEP who received supportive individual or group therapy and medications have been examined in two studies (Nagendra et al., 2022). According to both studies, Blacks showed less improvement than White participants' symptoms and functioning over a year. Both groups received treatment from the same clinic.

Bennett and Rosenheck (2021) reported that recent investigations gave rise to optimism that early, intensive therapy can alter the course of this condition by easing symptoms and enhancing functioning. The RAISE-ETP study compared a coordinated specialty care intervention called NAVIGATE to ordinary community care for patients with first-episode psychosis. It was the most significant and longest test of this strategy in the U.S. The study revealed that NAVIGATE enhanced quality of life, decreased symptoms of psychosis, and was cost-effective.

A specialist care program was coordinated to evaluate long-term treatment in the same study conducted by Narendra et al. (2022). The *Recovery After an Initial Schizophrenia Episode Early Treatment Program* (RAISE-ETP), a two-year randomized controlled trial, was carried out at 34 locations around the U.S. (Narendra et al., 2022). Compared to standard community-based treatment, the coordinated specialist care program NAVIGATE was evaluated by RAISE-ETP for efficacy. Delivered by an integrated, multidisciplinary team, NAVIGATE is a multicomponent FEP treatment that includes medication management, family education, individual strengths, and resiliency-based therapy that supports employment and education. After two years, individuals in NAVIGATE care remained in care longer, had better medication management, and improved quality of life, overall symptoms, self-reported mental health, and psychosocial functioning more than those in community-based treatment.

Blacks in NAVIGATE encountered fewer instances of stigma than those receiving community-based therapy. This could be because of individual resiliency training, a NAVIGATE intervention in which clients are taught to identify and challenge their stigmatizing beliefs about psychosis, process the distress connected to psychotic experiences, develop strengths-based perspectives, and cultivate resilience. These activities, which reduce stigma, emphasize openly discussing and challenging stigma. Black participants may have related to the importance of resilience because Black culture highlights resilience as a strategy to deal with prevalent anti-Black racism. Through enhanced self-advocacy and a more positive outlook on interpersonal interactions, this strategy appears to have helped people suffer less stigma over time. The significance of coordinated specialized care for Blacks is indicated by the rise in stigma in coordinated specialty care, but a decline in NAVIGATE (Nagendra et al., 2022). The study's findings are conflicting, but it is plausible that NAVIGATE had more Black than White providers. By sharing a racial identity, Black providers were likely better able to relate to and address the difficulties associated with stigma experienced by Black clients. Although studies accounted for treatment attendance, no measure existed to assess treatment adherence or participation. Therefore, some patients may have gone to the clinic (perhaps due to requests from family or the court) but did not participate in therapeutic activities or take their prescribed medications as directed. Given that research suggests that Black and Latinx participants may have poorer treatment engagement and adherence rates, it is critical to better understand how participants interact with their care and how it affects outcomes (Bennett & Rosenheck, 2021).

There are several difficulties in treating schizophrenia. Though antipsychotic drugs have been the therapeutic foundation, first-generation antipsychotics often have side effects almost as unpleasant and crippling as the disorder. Second-generation antipsychotics have been a viable substitute since 1989. These newer formulations have fewer side effects and are at least as effective as earlier medications in treating psychotic illnesses. They may also be more successful in treating symptoms and cognitive deficits (Mallinger et al., 2006).

In a sample of veterans with schizophrenia receiving high-intensity community-based case management at a VA facility, Browne and Mohamed (2021) examined racialized disparities in service use and a variety of treatment outcomes (e.g., symptoms, suicidality, and justice system involvement). Compared to other outpatient treatment settings, the VA is better prepared to offer Black veterans fair access to care. The authors discovered that Black veterans had considerably higher recovery rates in anxiety/depression, thinking disorder, and withdrawal symptoms at clinically relevant thresholds. Moreover, no outcomes showed White veterans had superior treatment trajectories. Overall, service-use indicators for both groups were comparable. Therefore, when health systems remove obstacles to care and allow access to the best quality care, racial disparities in outcome trajectories can be reduced or even eliminated.

Schizophrenia: A Case Study

According to a study of phenomenology, Anderson (2014) discussed research that sought to advance knowledge of what it is like for African American guys to live with schizophrenia by applying interpretative phenomenology and a methodological framework developed by van Manen (1990, 1997). In this study, five men aged 21 to 57 recounted their lifestyles in the context of having a schizophrenia diagnosis. Four main themes emerged from the respondents' actual experiences. They actively try to test reality, express their autonomy, are aware that they have a mental illness, and perceive the fact that they perceive reality differently as a gift. It is critical to acknowledge the clients' capacity for asserting their autonomy and to value each man's perception of himself as distinctive and exceptional to give appropriate therapeutic assistance to African American males with schizophrenia diagnoses (Anderson, 2014).

Methods

The participants were men of African American descent who were aware they had been diagnosed with schizophrenia. Age of 18 years or older, independent living in the community, the capacity to consent to participate based on the assessment of the outpatient staff, and the ability to communicate his experience were the criteria for participation in the research. A primary dementia diagnosis served as a criterion for exclusion since this illness may interfere with abstract thought, which may already be impaired by schizophrenia. Three people were interviewed, and their descriptions of the occurrence were consistent. In the fourth interview, no novel or original concepts were revealed; the participant's comments were repeated and did not provide new details. The fifth participant reiterated the topics that had already been established. As a result, data saturation was reached (Fain, 2013).

Data Analysis

Anderson (2014), the researcher for the study, utilized flyers to solicit patients for the study through outpatient clinics and communications with mental health professionals. Through this recruitment, five men committed to the study. Informed consent was the strategy of the research process; then, face-to-face audio-taped interviews were conducted and transcribed. In in-person meetings with the other team members, the researcher provided the early readings of the narrative and his field notes. The team studied all of the interview narratives to gain comprehensive insight. The team then found the interview's linked themes. The transcripts were reviewed several times and then grouped into developing themes. All the participants' experiences influenced each piece. The following were the themes:

- They are aware of their mental illness.
- They go out of their way to test reality.
- They declare their independence.
- They view the fact that they perceive reality differently as a gift.

Findings

Anderson (2014) also mentioned that if participants had a concomitant diagnosis of cognitive impairment unrelated to schizophrenia, they were excluded from the study. Of the five participants, one had a bachelor's degree, while another had an associate degree. Four of these individuals had high school diplomas. The fifth subject had finished only the seventh grade. Each of the five participants was getting a disability benefit of some kind. All were unmarried or divorced at the time of the research; four had never married. They were now undergoing counseling or therapy as part of their psychiatric outpatient care. The five subjects were taking an atypical neuroleptic; two were each on an anti-Parkinsonian drug, one was being given an anti-anxiety medication, and another was taking an antidepressant. They followed their treatment plans exactly, including taking their antipsychotic prescriptions. The ages of the males varied from 13 to 33 years, with a mean of 21 years, at the time of their initial diagnosis of schizophrenia. For at least two years, each subject had a schizophrenia diagnosis. Three individuals reported many mental hospitalizations, and all participants said they received at least one inpatient therapy. In the twelve months prior, none had visited a hospital. One person said he had not seen the hospital in over 20 years. The participants were open about sharing their experiences, and their desire to candidly enriched the narrative. Notably, participants did not mention that their diagnosis of schizophrenia was made more difficult because they were male and African American, despite the literature's suggestion to the contrary.

The participants were able to express the effects that schizophrenia had on their lives while also articulating the symptoms with clarity. They paid close attention to the behaviors that led to hospitalizations and did their best to prevent them. In their assessment of longitudinal studies that looked at the long-term effects of poor insight for people with schizophrenia, Lincoln et al. (2007) discovered that most studies indicated a link between poor insight and low treatment adherence. The high degree of understanding shown by the study's subjects, therefore, lines up with their high levels of treatment adherence. Nevertheless, it is intriguing because while adhering to therapy, a few participants still reported experiencing some symptoms of schizophrenia. One participant said he still thought others could read his mind, while another said he occasionally had trouble telling what was true and what was false. To assist them in clarifying their thinking, two participants said that they occasionally talk about ideas and thoughts with other peer support group members. To avoid what may be a delusional evaluation from coloring outside information, research participants seemed to be hypervigilant and sensitive to using the traditional methods of thinking about others (Anderson, 2014).

Usher (2001) noticed the challenges that participants in her phenomenological research of drug adherence in people with schizophrenia reported having linked to side effects. Respondents described how side effects affected their bodies to "lose its transparency," making them distinct and stand out. All of these participants were taking newer, atypical psychotropic medications rather than the older, more traditional antipsychotic agents with more stigmatizing side effects like tardive dyskinesia may be one possible explanation for the lack of concerns expressed about medication side effects in these participants. These participants reported feeling good about themselves and expecting to be accepted "as is." The individuals identified as pleasant, sincere, modest, and caring. They did not feel a need to alter anything about themselves. This may have been influenced by the individuals' claimed support systems, which included family, friends, or therapists. These individuals were the Close Community (CC), which the participants rated as welcoming, devoted, and caring. The participants trusted the CC, and the males appeared to value the judgments and opinions of those in the CC.

Implications for Practice

The study is relevant and can be of practical use in the workplace. The client's capacity to discern who supports his autonomy and who does not support his sovereignty has important implications for therapy. Clients believe they can resist challenges to their autonomy and feelings of value because they have the information, skills, resources, and authority to do so. As a result, they have the authority to let employees in or not. The healing process requires collaboration between mental health professionals and their patients. These respondents also showed how important peer support is to their well-being. Ultimately, maintaining stability for people with schizophrenia depends on excellent outpatient treatment. Numerous access barriers have been identified by prior research, but these obstacles can only be removed with a deeper understanding of how non-recoverees encounter obstacles (Anderson, 2014).

This study's key conclusion is that individuals who reported successful symptoms participated in peer support groups, a low-cost intervention. Four of the five participants regularly attended peer support programs (at least monthly). Two of them worked as peer support organization counselors. The fifth man indicated engagement with his family but did not categorize it as positive or negative. Four of the men reported positive family support. It is advised to include peer group support that is therapeutically and philosophically sound when employing organizations that offer outpatient services to people with mental disorders. Ultimately, rather than functioning on an as-needed basis, these partnerships must be established in the provision of care (Anderson, 2014).

THE EXPRESSED EMOTIONS PERSPECTIVE

A family environment concept called "expressed emotion" (EE) measures how much negativity, antagonism, and emotional over-involvement a family member exhibits against a patient (Hooley, 2007, pp. 329–330). Poorer patient outcomes for schizophrenia and other diseases have typically been linked to high levels of EE in the family environment. Contrary to popular belief, high EE may be linked to a better symptom course in African American patients. EE, a psychosocial construct, gauges the emotional climate of the family setting by counting the number of times relatives criticize, become angry, or become too emotionally invested when discussing the patient (Hooley, 2007; Kopelowicz et al., 2002). High levels of EE in the family are known as a significant environmental risk for relapse and worsening symptoms (Cutting et al., 2006; Hooley et al., 1997). However, according to findings from research by Rosenfarb et al. (2006), African American patients responded better to more critical and invasive treatment practices. In particular, the authors discovered that over two years, lower levels of abnormal or unusual thinking (rated from the patient symptom profile) were associated with more critical remarks and intrusive behaviors from relatives (as coded from the *Family Problem Solving Task*, which the patient and their family member complete together).

It is also possible that patients' interpretations of 'criticism' may differ by ethnicity. Nonetheless, other studies contend that compared to White-American speech patterns, African-American speech tends to be livelier and more expressive (Davidson, 2001). Rogan and Hammer (1998) believed that Black Americans may value a more confrontational approach because they see it as a sign of authenticity and honesty. In African-American households, actions are often classified as high EE and may instead be seen by patients as indicating concern and care. Hence, high EE attitudes may alleviate symptoms in this population instead of aggravating them.

Having a family member considered high EE is often linked to more severe patient symptoms, according to the literature. However, research from Rosenfarb et al. (2006) found this may not be true for African-American patients. The current investigation aimed to look for comparable data to support that contradictory result. Our hypothesis was confirmed: African-American patients had greater symptom severity with caregivers who scored low on EE on the *Five-Minute Speech Sample*, which is an interview that assesses factors as a predictor of relapse in those with schizophrenia and major depressive illness (Mazza et al., 2022).

Gurak and Weisman De Mamani (2017) suggested that the content of such studies demonstrated how remarks made by high and low EE relatives may affect the intensity of the patient's symptoms. Among speech samples from family members, researchers identified three themes: Though low and high EE African-American relatives discussed the value of family collectivism and interdependence as valued constructs, it was surprisingly more common in high EE relatives; high EE family members appeared to be more direct and expressive in presenting their views; and low EE family members frequently expressed a passive attitude. African Americans may be culturally encouraged to take a vibrant, more directed, and interdependent caring style. As a result, African American patients from high EE families could experience empathy and genuine concern from their family members.

There is substantial evidence that African-American culture values family solidarity and reliance on family (Davidson, 2001; Kane, 2000; Kymalainen & Weisman de Mamani, 2008; Kymalainen et al., 2006). African-American families are known for having a strong network of relatives and for understanding that each family member is an essential part of the family (Davidson, 2001; Kane, 2000). Evidence from the current study suggests that in African American culture, patients may view some aspects of family members with a high EE more positively, as stated by Gurak and Weisman De Mamani (2017). While we do not advocate for raising EE in African-American families, attempts to lower high EE attitudes may harm this population. Conversely, mental health professionals may significantly influence symptoms by working with African-American families to boost dynamic demonstrations of care, concern, and commitment to their ill family members and help patients see their circumstances as an illness.

SEEKING CULTURALLY-COMPETENT CARE

The National Alliance on Mental Health (2023) reports that those struggling with mental health must receive the best care when symptoms are identified. It is also crucial that healthcare providers who treat them are knowledgeable about their culture. While we advise consulting a mental health expert, speaking with a primary care physician (PCP) is also an excellent place to begin. A primary care provider may provide an initial mental health examination and, if necessary, a referral to a mental health expert. There could be a list of local mental health professionals accessible from community and religious organizations given to patients as well. Asking questions to gauge a provider's cultural sensitivity level might be beneficial. Providers should anticipate and encourage questions from their patients or customers. Everyone should leave their meetings with the health care provider feeling heard and valued, whether seeking treatment from a PCP or a mental health expert. A crucial component of treatment is the interaction between the patient and their mental health professional. To obtain the best assistance and care, a person must believe that their caregiver understands who they are.

Consequently, schizophrenia is a persistent psychotic condition that impairs a patient's capacity for clear thought and emotional stability. A patient's illness frequently makes it difficult for them to engage in social interactions and build lasting connections. As a severe mental illness, it affects a person's ideas, feelings, and behavior. People with schizophrenia may appear to have lost all sense of reality, which can be unpleasant to them and those who care about them. For someone with schizophrenia, it could be challenging to engage in daily activities, but effective therapies are available. Many people who receive treatment can participate in their studies or careers, become independent, and cherish their relationships with others (NIMH, 2021). Some may not show symptoms, though social withdrawal and other odd behaviors frequently precede a person's first psychotic episode. To distinguish schizophrenia from other psychotic diseases, including schizoaffective disorder (a depressive condition with psychotic symptoms) and bipolar disorder with psychotic features, the psychiatrist must carefully evaluate each sign.

Psychiatrists have a role in helping Black patients live better lives by carefully considering the historical, social, and personal aspects that affect the treatment they get. Hence, one of the most prominent and pervasive inequalities is diagnosing schizophrenia among Black Americans seeking mental health care. Some of the growth in incidence may be related to environmental risk factors. Bias in the diagnosis of schizophrenia among Blacks can substantially influence the therapy given. The treatments advised for treating psychotic illness versus mood disorders differ significantly, and prescribing an inappropriate antipsychotic treatment can have harmful results. Hence, detecting and minimizing diagnostic bias has been one of the primary methods to reduce inequities in mental health outcomes for Black Americans (Eack et al., 2012).

Possible contributing variables to the inequities in mental health care for Blacks include the challenges Black communities experience in the economy, society, education, and physical health. Given the disparities in help-seeking and the tendency to disparage mental illness among Black Americans, examining how African Americans regard mental illness and treatment is imperative. Research has demonstrated that racism contributes to disparities in diagnosing and treating Black Americans with schizophrenia. According to these studies, racism and marginalization hurt Black people's physical and mental health. Blacks in the U.S. encounter overt and subtle forms of racial discrimination, and both types have been associated with higher rates of psychotic symptoms (Nagendra et al., 2022).

Mental illness is considered a sign of personal weakness by 63% of Black people, according to the National Alliance on Mental Illness (2020). As a result, it may make some people feel guilty and fear that they will receive unfavorable treatment, leading to debate on how Black Americans manage schizophrenia. In addition, various factors affect how often they seek assistance, including a lack of awareness about the community's mental health services, the high cost of mental health treatments, cultural beliefs about mental illness, its treatment, and the stigma associated with mental illness. These all influence how often Black Americans seek help (Avent Harris & Wong, 2018).

Physicians can significantly impact a patient's symptoms by working with African American families to promote dynamic demonstrations of care, concern, and dedication to their ill family members and assist them in identifying their conditions. In addition, communication between patients and their mental health providers is essential to treatment. For example, it is vital for schizophrenia-diagnosed individuals to feel their caregiver understands them to receive the best support and care.

REFERENCES

American Psychiatric Association. (2017). *Mental health disparities: African Americans.* APA. https://www.psychiatry.org/File%20Library/Psychiatrists/Cultural-Competency/Mental-Health-Disparities/Mental-Health-Facts-for-African-Americans.pdf

Anderson, L. B. (2014). African American males diagnosed with Schizophrenia: A phenomenological study. *Issues in Mental Health Nursing*, *35*(1), 580–587. doi:10.3109/01612840.2013.867464 PMID:25072210

Avent Harris, J. R., & Wong, C. D. (2018). African American college students, the Black church, and counseling. *Journal of College Counseling*, *21*(1), 15–28. doi:10.1002/jocc.12084

Bailey, R., Mokonogho, J., & Kumar, A. (2022). Racial and ethnic differences in depression: Current perspectives. *Neuropsychiatric Disease and Treatment*, *15*, 603–609. https://www.tandfonline.com/doi/full/10.2147/NDT.S128584. doi:10.2147/NDT.S128584 PMID:30863081

Barnes, A. (2008). Race and hospital diagnosis of schizophrenia and mood disorders. *Social Work*, *53*(1), 77–83. doi:10.1093w/53.1.77 PMID:18610823

Bennett, D., & Rosenheck, R. (2021). Socioeconomic status and the effectiveness of treatment for first-episode psychosis. *Health Services Research*, *56*(3), 409–417. doi:10.1111/1475-6773.13606 PMID:33231881

Blumberg, S., Clarke, T., & Blackwell, D. (2015). Racial and ethnic disparities in men's use of mental health treatments. *NCHS Data Brief*, *206*. https://files.eric.ed.gov/fulltext/ED578186.pdf PMID:26079520

Browne, J., & Mohamed, S. (2021). Evaluation of disparities in the impact of mental health intensive case management on 6-month symptoms, functioning, and quality of life between Black and White veterans diagnosed with schizophrenia. *Schizophrenia Research*. doi:10.1016/j.schres.2021.07.002 PMID:34247886

Centers for Disease Control and Prevention, U.S. Department of Health and Human Services. (2016). Health, United States, 2015: With special feature on racial and ethnic health disparities *DHHS Publication No. 2016-1232*. CDC. https://www.cdc.gov/nchs/data/hus/hus15.pdf

Conroy, J., Lin, L., & Stamm, K. (2023). *Center for workforce studies; graduate psychology studies opens doors*. American Psychiatric Association. https://www.apa.org/monitor/2021/09/datapoint-graduate

Cutting, L. P., Aakre, J. M., & Docherty, N. M. (2006). *Schizophrenic patients' perceptions of stress, expressed emotion, and sensitivity to criticism*. Schizophrenia Bulletin.

Davidson, M. N. (2001). *Know the adversary: The impact of race on styles of dealing with conflict*. Sex Roles.

Eack, S., Bahorik, A., Newhill, C., Neighbors, H., & Davis, L. (2012). *Interviewer-perceived honesty as a mediator of racial disparities in the diagnosis of schizophrenia*. Psychiatry Online., doi:10.1176/appi.ps.201100388

Fain, J. A. (2013). Reading, understanding, and applying nursing research (4th ed.). F. A. Davis.

Fraguas, D., & Breathnach, C. S. (2009). Problems with retrospective studies of the presence of schizophrenia. *History of Psychiatry*, *20*(1), 61–71. doi:10.1177/0957154X08089453 PMID:20617641

Gara, M., Minsky, S., Silverstein, S., Miskimen, T., & Strakowski, S. (2019). A naturalistic study of racial disparities in diagnoses at an outpatient behavioral health clinic. *Psychiatric Services (Washington, D.C.)*, *70*(2), 30–134. doi:10.1176/appi.ps.201800223 PMID:30526340

Gurak, K., & Weisman De Mamani, A. (2017). Caregiver expressed emotion and psychiatric symptoms in African-Americans with schizophrenia: An attempt to understand the paradoxical relationship. *Family Process*, *56*(2), 476–486. https://onlinelibrary-wiley-com.proxy.tamuc.edu/doi/pdfdirect/10.1111/famp.12188. doi:10.1111/famp.12188 PMID:26498273

Hall, J. C. (2018). It is tough being a Black woman: Intergenerational stress and coping. *Journal of Black Studies*, *49*(5), 481–501. doi:10.1177/0021934718766817

Hooley, J. M. (2007). *Expressed emotion and relapse of psychopathology*. Annual Review of Clinical Psychology. doi:10.1146/annurev.clinpsy.2.022305.095236

Hooley, J. M., & Gotlib, I. H. (2000). A diathesis-stress conceptualization of expressed emotion and clinical outcome. *Applied & Preventive Psychology*, *9*(3), 135–151. doi:10.1016/S0962-1849(05)80001-0

Kane, C. M. (2000). African American family dynamics as perceived by family members. *Journal of Black Studies*, *30*(5), 691–702. doi:10.1177/002193470003000504

Kang, E., Wen, Z., Song, H., Christian, K. M., & Ming, G. (2016). Adult neurogenesis and psychiatric disorders. *Cold Spring Harbor Perspectives in Biology*, *8*(9), a019026. doi:10.1101/cshperspect.a019026 PMID:26801682

Kim, M. (2016). Understanding the etiology and treatment approaches of schizophrenia: Theoretical perspectives and their critique. *Journal of Psychiatry*, *6*, 1–9.

Kopelowicz, A., Zarate, R., Gonzalez, V., Lopez, S. R., Ortega, P., Obregon, N., & Mintz, J. (2002). Evaluation of expressed emotion in schizophrenia: A comparison of Caucasians and Mexican-Americans. *Schizophrenia Research*, *55*(1-2), 179–186. doi:10.1016/S0920-9964(01)00193-1 PMID:11955977

Kymalainen, J. A., Weisman, A. G., Rosales, G. A., & Armesto, J. C. (2006). Ethnicity expressed emotion and communication deviance in family members of patients with schizophrenia. *The Journal of Nervous and Mental Disease*, *194*(6), 391–396. doi:10.1097/01.nmd.0000221171.42027.5a PMID:16772854

Kymalainen, J. A., & Weisman de Mamani, A. G. (2008). Expressed emotion, communication deviance, and culture in families of patients with schizophrenia: A review of the literature. *Cultural Diversity & Ethnic Minority Psychology*, *14*(2), 85–91. doi:10.1037/1099-9809.14.2.85 PMID:18426280

Lincoln, T. M., Lullman, E., & Rief, W. (2007). Correlates and long-term consequences of poor insight in patients with schizophrenia: A systematic review. *Schizophrenia Bulletin*, *33*(6), 1324–1342. doi:10.1093chbulbm002 PMID:17289653

Linszen, D. H., Dingemans, P. M., Nugter, M. A., Van der Does, J. W., Scholte, W. F., & Lenior, M. A. (1997). Patient attributes and expressed emotion as risk factors for psychotic relapse. *Schizophrenia Bulletin*, *23*(1), 119–130. doi:10.1093chbul/23.1.119 PMID:9050118

Mallinger, J., Fisher, S., Brown, T., & Lamberti, J. A. (2006). Racial disparities in the use of second-generation antipsychotics for the treatment of schizophrenia. *Psychiatric Services (Washington, D.C.)*, *57*(1), 133–136. https://www.researchgate.net/profile/J-Lamberti/publication/7371795_Racial_Disparities_in_the_Use_of_Second-Generation_Antipsychotics_for_the_Treatment_of_Schizophrenia/links/56c39c0f08ae60234250a2d0/Racial-Disparities-in-the-Use-of-Second-Generation-Antipsychotics-for-the-Treatment-of-Schizophrenia.pdf. doi:10.1176/appi.ps.57.1.133 PMID:16399976

Mazza, C., Formica, F., Ferracuti, S., Ricci, E., Colasanti, M., Biondi, S., Di Domenico, A., & Roma, P. (2022). High expressed emotion (HEE), assessed using the Five-Minute Speech Sample (FMSS), as a predictor of psychiatric relapse in patients with schizophrenia and major depressive disorder: A meta-analysis and meta-regression. *Journal of Clinical Medicine*, *11*(21), 6533. doi:10.3390/jcm11216533 PMID:36362760

McCutcheon, R., Marques, T., & Howes, O. (2020). Schizophrenia-an overview. *JAMA Psychiatry*. https://jamanetwork.com/journals/jamapsychiatry/article-abstract/2753514

Metzl, J. M. (2009). *The protest psychosis: How schizophrenia became a Black disease*. Beacon Press.

Nagendra, A., Black, C., & Penn, D. (2022). Black Americans and schizophrenia: Racism as a driver of inequities in psychosis diagnosis, assessment, and treatment. *Schizophrenia Research*. doi:10.1016/j.schres.2022.10.007 PMID:36396493

Nagendra, A., Weiss, D., Merritt, C., Cather, C., Sosoo, E., Mueser, K., & Penn, D. (2023). Clinical and psychosocial outcomes of Black Americans in the Recovery After an Initial Schizophrenia Episode Early Treatment Program (RAISE-ETP) study. *Social Psychiatry and Psychiatric Epidemiology*, *58*(1), 77–89. doi:10.100700127-022-02297-9 PMID:35932309

National Alliance on Mental Illness. (2020a). *Mental health in Black communities: Challenges, resources, community voices*. NAMICA. https://namica.org/mental-health-challenges-in-african-american-communities/

National Alliance on Mental Illness. (2020b). *The annual state of the communities' reports with diverse communities*. NAMICA. https://namica.org/wp-content/uploads/2019/12/nca_Diverse-Communities-ASoCR-Summary-18-19_Final.test_.pdf

National Alliance on Mental Illness. (2022). *Black/African American*. NAMI. https://www.nami.org/Your-Journey/Identity-and-Cultural-Dimensions/Black-African-American

National Institute of Mental Health. (2021). *Schizophrenia*. NIMH. https://www.nimh.nih.gov/health/publications/schizophrenia

Neighbors, H. W., Jackson, J. S., Campbell, L., & Williams, D. (1989). The influence of racial factors on psychiatric diagnosis: A review and suggestions for research. *Community Mental Health Journal*, *25*(4), 301–311. doi:10.1007/BF00755677 PMID:2697490

Office of Minority Mental Health, U.S. Department of Health and Human Services. (2017). Mental health and African Americans. *Minority Health*. https://minorityhealth.hhs.gov/omh/browse.aspx?lvl=4&lvlid=24

Olbert, C. M., Nagendra, A., & Buck, B. (2018). Meta-analysis of Black vs. White racial disparity in schizophrenia diagnosis in the United States: Do structured assessments attenuate racial disparities? *Journal of Abnormal Psychology*, *127*(1), 104–115. doi:10.1037/abn0000309 PMID:29094963

Pate, K., Cherian, J., Gohil, K., & Atkinson, D. (2014). Schizophrenia: Overview and treatment options. *Journal of Pharmacy and Therapeutics*, *39*(9), 638–645. PMID:25210417

Roffman, J. L., Weiss, A. P., Goff, D. C., Rauch, S. L., & Weinberger, D. R. (2005). Neuroimaging-Genetic Paradigms: A new approach to investigate the pathophysiology and treatment of cognitive deficits in schizophrenia. *Harvard Review of Psychiatry*, *14*(2), 78–91. doi:10.1080/10673220600642945 PMID:16603474

Rogan, R. G., & Hammer, M. R. (1998). An exploratory study of message affect behavior: A comparison between African Americans and Euro-Americans. *Journal of Language and Social Psychology*, *17*, 449–464.

Rosenfarb, I. S., Bellack, A. S., & Aziz, N. (2006). Family interactions and the course of schizophrenia in African American and White patients. *Journal of Abnormal Psychology*, *115*(1), 112–120. doi:10.1037/0021-843X.115.1.112 PMID:16492102

Schwartz, R. C., & Blankenship, D. M. (2014). Racial disparities in psychotic disorder diagnosis: A review of the empirical literature. *World Journal of Psychiatry*, *4*(4), 133–140. doi:10.5498/wjp.v4.i4.133 PMID:25540728

Snowden, L. R. (2003). Bias in mental health assessment and intervention. *American Journal of Public Health*, *93*(2), 239–243. doi:10.2105/AJPH.93.2.239 PMID:12554576

Substance Abuse and Mental Health Services Administration. (2015). *Racial/ethnic differences in mental health service use among adults*. SAMHSA. https://www.integration.samhsa.gov/MHServicesUseAmongAdults.pdf

U.S. Department of Health and Human Services Office of Minority Health. (2021). *Mental and Behavioral Health – African Americans*. US DOHH. https://minorityhealth.hhs.gov/omh/browse.aspx?lvl=4&lvlid=24

Usher, K. (2001). Taking neuroleptic medications as the treatment for schizophrenia: A phenomenological study. *The Australian and New Zealand Journal of Mental Health Nursing*, *10*(1), 145–155. doi:10.1046/j.1440-0979.2001.00205.x PMID:11493286

van Manen, M. (1990). *Researching lived experience: Human science for an action sensitive pedagogy*. State University of New York Press.

van Manen, M. (1997). *Researching the lived experience: Human science for an action sensitive pedagogy* (2nd ed., rev.). Althouse.

Varcarolis, E. M., & Halter, M. J. (2010). *Foundations of psychiatric mental health nursing: A clinical approach* (6th ed.). Saunders.

Whaley, A. L. (2001). Cultural mistrust: An important psychological construct for diagnosis and treatment of African Americans. *Professional Psychology, Research and Practice, 32*(6), 555–562. https://psycnet.apa.org/doi/10.1037/0735-7028.32.6.555. doi:10.1037/0735-7028.32.6.555

Wolny, J., Moussa-Tooks, A. B., Bailey, A. J., O'Donnell, B. F., & Hetrick, W. P. (2022). Race and self-reported paranoia: Increased item endorsement on subscales of the SPQ. *Schizophrenia Research.* Advance online publication. doi:10.1016/j.schres.2021.11.034 PMID:34895794

World Health Organization. (2023). *Schizophrenia.* WHO. https://www.who.int/news-room/fact-sheets/detail/schizophrenia

Chapter 12 The Neurodevelopment of the Brain

Marcus Karltonian Bills
Best Alcohol & Drug Services, USA

ABSTRACT

The pleasure pathway is a form of the limbic part of the brain that is responsible for behaviors. The brain is a very interesting phenomenon. It is comprised of various parts that consist of neurotransmitters (serotonin, dopamine, and norepinephrine, just to name a few). Serotonin's chemical function is to carry messages between nerve cells in the brain and throughout your body. Serotonin plays a key role in such body functions as mood, sleep, digestion, nausea, wound healing, bone health, blood clotting, and sexual desire; in essence, sending signals of the state of well-being. The dopamine neurotransmitter sends signals of pleasure or euphoria to the nerves cells that your body makes. Norepinephrine sends chemicals of adrenaline; it is also known as the fight or flight neurotransmitter. It increases the breathing rate, relaxes the intestinal muscles, increases the heart rate, and increases the blood sugar levels. As a neurotransmitter in your brain and spinal cord, it increases alertness, arousal, and attention for the individual to protect themselves from harm.

INTRODUCTION

The brain is an incredibly fascinating phenomenon. It is comprised of various parts that consist of neurotransmitters (serotonin, dopamine, and norepinephrine) just to name a few. Serotonin's chemical function is to carry messages between nerve cells in the brain and throughout your body. Serotonin plays a key role in such body functions as mood, sleep, digestion, nausea, wound healing, bone health, blood

DOI: 10.4018/978-1-6684-8918-5.ch012

clotting, and sexual desire, in essence, sends signals of the state of well-being. The dopamine neurotransmitter sends signals of pleasure or euphoria to the nerve cells that your body makes. Norepinephrine sends chemicals of adrenaline; it is also known as the fight or flight neurotransmitter. It increases the breathing rate, relaxes the intestinal muscles, increases the heart rate, and increases the blood sugar levels. As a neurotransmitter in your brain and spinal cord, it increases alertness, arousal, and attention for the individual to protect themselves from harm. These three neurotransmitters are in the prefrontal lobe of the brain and this area of the brain is also known as the pleasure pathway. The pleasure pathway is a form of the limbic part of the Brain that is responsible for behaviors.

There are other parts of the brain that have a major responsibility like the occipital lobe which is where the motor functioning of an individual occurs. The way a person speaks, and the gait of the individual is regulated in this portion of the brain. The amygdala is a small part of your brain, but it has a big job. It is a major processing center for emotions. It also links your emotions to many other brain abilities, especially memories, learning, and your senses. When it does not work as it should, it can cause or contribute to disruptive feelings and symptoms.

The autonomic nervous system is a component of the peripheral nervous system that regulates involuntary physiologic processes including heart rate, blood pressure, respiration, digestion, and sexual arousal. It contains three anatomically distinct divisions: sympathetic, parasympathetic, and enteric (Cacioppo, & Berntson, 2011).

The brain functions systematically the same for everyone, but there are some factors that contribute to the way individual behaviors vary from race to race. There are cultural factors that weigh in on an individual's behavior based on values, thoughts, attitudes, and beliefs. As far as Black and African American community and Mental Health go overall, mental health conditions occur in Black and African American (B/AA) people in America at about the same or less frequency than in White Americans. However, the historically Black and African American experience in America has and continues to be characterized by trauma and violence more often than for their White counterparts and impacts the emotional and mental health of both youth and adults.

Historical dehumanization, oppression, and violence against Black and African American people has evolved into present-day racism - structural, institutional, and individual – and cultivates a uniquely mistrustful and less affluent community experience, characterized by a myriad of disparities including inadequate access to and delivery of care in the health system. Processing and dealing with layers of individual trauma on top of new mass traumas from COVID-19 (uncertainty, isolation, grief from financial or human losses), police brutality and its fetishization in news media, and divisive political rhetoric adds compounding layers of complexity for individuals to responsibly manage.

Help-seeking behavior is affected by mistrust of the medical system and often begins with faith-based outreach. However, MHA screening data shows that Black and African American people who screen positive for depression self-identify as planning to seek help at higher rates than the general population say they will seek help. Unfortunately, Black and African American providers, who are known to give more appropriate and effective care to Black and African American help-seekers, make up a very small portion of the behavioral health provider workforce (see treatment statistics below). Because of these factors and more, Black and African American people are more likely to experience chronic and persistent, rather than episodic, mental health conditions. Yet, hope for recovery should remain, as light is shed on these issues - and the public holds accountable policymakers and health systems to evolve better systems that eliminate inequities in mental health services.

BLACK AND AFRICAN AMERICAN COMMUNITIES AND MENTAL HEALTH

The Origin of the Concept of Neurodevelopmental Disorder

"Developmental disorders" were included for the first time in *DSM-III*, for the category that comprised autistic disorder. "Neurodevelopmental disorders" (NDDs) were introduced as an overarching disorder category in *DSM-5*. 2 This new section replaced a previous chapter that was termed "Disorders usually first diagnosed in infancy, childhood, or adolescence." In *ICD-11*, the latest revision of the International Classification of Diseases published by the WHO, NDDs gained even more prominence by becoming an integral part of the title of the chapter on psychiatry: "Mental, behavioral or neurodevelopmental disorders." *Figure 1* outlines the main categories comprising neurodevelopmental disorders in *DSM-5*, their historical background, and the hypothesis of the genetic spectrum of neurodevelopmental disorders that will be discussed later in this article.

In *DSM-5*, NDDs are defined as a group of conditions with onset in the developmental period, inducing deficits that produce impairments of functioning. NDDs comprise intellectual disability (ID); Communication Disorders; Autism Spectrum Disorder (ASD); Attention-Deficit/Hyperactivity Disorder (ADHD); Neurodevelopmental Motor Disorders, including Tic Disorders; and Specific Learning Disorders. The classification of NDDs in *ICD-11* does not diverge significantly from that in *DSM-5*. Importantly, all NDDs in *DSM-5* may include the specifier "associated with a known medical or genetic condition or environmental factor." This specifier offers the clinician the possibility to document etiological factors, such as fragile X syndrome, and is a harbinger of the fact that this disorder category will probably be transformed in the coming decades by new data emerging from genetics research.

The validity of NDDs as a construct is supported by the high rates of comorbidity between various disorders within this diagnostic grouping. For instance, various studies showed that 22% to 83% of children with ASD have symptoms that satisfy the *DSM-IV* criteria for ADHD, and vice versa, 30% to 65% of children with ADHD have clinically significant symptoms of ASD. 3 Also, although not part of the criteria of ASD, accompanying intellectual or language impairments are frequent in ASD and their presence must be specified. NDDs share the characteristic of being diagnosed more often in males than females; *DSM-5* mentions male-to-female ratios of 4:1 for the diagnosis of ASD, 2:1 for the diagnosis of ADHD in children, and 1.6:1 and 1.2:1 for mild and severe ID, respectively. The idea of gathering these various disorders into one single diagnostic group came with *DSM-5*. As late as in the 10th editions of Kaplan & Sadock's comprehensive textbook of psychiatry (2017), ADD, ASD, and ID were distinct disorders whose only commonality was being part of child psychiatry. According to Berrios (year?), 4 the historian of psychiatry, the concept of developmental disorder in psychiatry appeared for the first time in 1820 in a textbook by Étienne Jean Georget (1795-1828), a student of Philippe Pinel (1745-1826) and Jean-Étienne Esquirol (1772-1840), the pioneers of a modern psychiatric nosology based on mental symptoms instead of humoral concepts. Pinel translated William Cullen's nosology into French in 1785 and published his own classification of mental illnesses in 1801; in his nosography, idiocy was a psychiatric disorder, along with mania, melancholia, and dementia. Correcting Pinel's nosography to further delineate the field of mental illness, Georget 5 wrote (p 102) that Idiocy is " *a lack of development of intellectual faculties,* " (emphasis added) and he added in a footnote that "a *developmental defect* is not, strictly speaking, a *disease*, " and that "idiots should be classified among *monsters* ." At a distance of two centuries, the word "monster" should not be read anachronistically as an insult, but as a reference to a genetic abnormality in the human body. Within the larger group of idiots, Georget included a subtype of "imbeciles," with higher cognitive abilities. Georget died at the early age of 33, and Berrios suggests that Esquirol later adopted Georget's developmental view, without quoting him. Esquirol 6 criticized Pinel for having differentiated dementia and idiocy on the sole basis of the degree of impairment of intelligence—Pinel considered idiocy as the most severe degree of dementia—and for admitting the existence of both acquired and innate idiocy. Instead, Esquirol stated that idiocy was not an illness, but a condition in which intellectual faculties could not achieve sufficient *development*. This statement by Esquirol has often been quoted in various textbooks over the following two centuries. Esquirol stated that there were innumerable degrees of severity, and, like Georget, he distinguished two main categories: idiocy per se, a severe intellectual impairment, and imbecility, a mild or moderate impairment. In Georget's suggestive words, imbeciles "have memory, can judge simple acts of life … are clean, know how to appreciate the difference between the sexes," whereas "the idiots urinate and defecate wherever they are and are often very prone to masturbation" (p 104).

Early Descriptions of ADHD, Intellectual Disabilities, and ASD

ADHD

The first known description of attention deficit was published in 1775 by the German physician Melchior Adam Weikard, under the name Mangel der Aufmerksamkeit/ Attentio volubilis, in a book entitled *Der philosophische Arzt.* 7 This work was the subject of several editions. Weikard (1742-1803) began his medical career in 1764 in Bavaria, near his birthplace, as a doctor at the Bad Brückenau spa. In 1784 he was appointed doctor at the court of Empress Catherine II of Russia. He was known as a scholar and a prolific author. In an edition of his book published in 1799, 8 Weikard devoted six pages to the description of attention deficit. He describes how sensory stimuli capture the patient's attention and diverts him from his thoughts: "... it is easier to perceive impressions through the sense organs than to form or retain ideas, to recover memories or to do other reflective operations. Each sense can disturb us in our thoughts or thinking, distract us from our object, and draw our attention to something else. Of all the senses, this occurs most often with hearing and sight. The result is a distraction, lack of attention, inattention." The Latin term "volubilis" comes from the verb "volvere" (to turn). The literal meaning of Volubilis is "easily rotating," and by extension "fickle" or "changing." This image of a permanent rotation of ideas is sometimes used by some patients who relate to the subjective feeling that their attention does not hold in place but twirls.

Separating ASD From Mental Retardation

The terms "idiocy" and "imbecility" are attested to by the Oxford English Dictionary as early as the 16th century. Also, behaviors consistent with autism were described long before that diagnostic category was named and defined by Leo Kanner 9 in 1943 and Hans Asperger 10 in 1944. Russian specialists 11 suppose that many of the "holy fools," or Orthodox church ascetics (yuródivïe) who roamed ancient Russia displayed autistic behaviors, being notoriously nonverbal, impervious to social conventions, and indifferent to cold weather or pain. Famous cases showed that some "idiots" had specific problems in social communication—consistent with autism—rather than a mere global mental deficiency. One such case is Victor, the Wild Boy of Aveyron (c 1788-1828), a feral child who was discovered when he was about 12. Victor was taken to Paris, and his case was taken up by a young physician, Jean Étard, who tried to instruct him and repeatedly assessed his sensory, intellectual, and affective progress over 5 years. Edouard Seguin 12 (1812-1880), a pioneer of the education of children with intellectual disability, first in France and afterward in the United States, recounted the various diagnostic hypotheses discussed at the time. According to Seguin, Pinel had declared Victor "idiotic" and therefore uneducable; Étard, on the other hand, asserted that the child was wild and entirely untaught. Étard's observations over the following years suggest that both diagnoses might have been erroneous and that Victor might have been a child with autism, abandoned by his parents. As Étard reports, Victor demonstrated aberrant requesting strategies like the use of hand-over-hand (e.g., Victor once seized Étard's hand and directed it to a locked door to ask him to open it), he was using others as tools to satisfy his needs, a hallmark of the clinical picture was his difficulty initiating and maintaining social relationships, and even though he learned letters and some spelling, he could not use this knowledge in regular interaction with others.

Dr. J. Langdon Down (1828-1896) is best known for having described Down's syndrome (trisomy 21). In a series of lectures delivered before the Medical Society of London in 1887, 13 he also described 10 cases of "idiots savants," patients with exceptional abilities in an extremely narrow field, such as calendar calculating. While these cases were not all autistic, most of them would now satisfy Criterion B for ASD in DSM-5 (i.e., restricted and repetitive patterns of behavior, interest, or activities). In papers published after these lectures, 14 Down based himself on three decades of clinical experience to propose a classification of mental retardation into (i) "congenital;" (ii) "accidental;" and (iii) a third kind which he termed "developmental." The latter type occurred in children who did not have the usual "physical aspects" of retardation. Some of these children had developed normally "until the period of second dentition," and then suddenly regressed, lost their "wanted brightness" and speech, lived "in a world of their own," spoke "in the third person," had "rhythmical and automatic movements" and "lessened responsiveness to all endearments of friends." Treffert 15 comments on Down's interesting choice of the term "developmental retardation" for this category which probably corresponds to cases of both early-onset and late-onset regressive autism.

We have described the history of diagnostic categories for NDDs in DSM-5. We will now discuss how these psychopathological concepts can fare in the era of neurosciences. **The history and future of a diagnostic concept.**

Case Studies

African Americans and other underrepresented minorities make up only about 5% of the people in genetics research studies.

Mental illness can run in families. And Dr. Kafui Dzirasa grew up in one of these families. His close relatives include people with schizophrenia, bipolar disorder and depression. As a medical student, he learned about the ones who'd been committed to psychiatric hospitals or who "went missing" and were discovered in alleyways.

Dzirasa decided to dedicate his career to "figuring out how to make science relevant to ultimately help my own family." He became a psychiatrist and researcher at Duke University and began to study the links between genes and brain disorders. Then Dzirasa realized something: "I was studying genes that were specifically related to illness in folks of European ancestry." His family had migrated from West Africa, which meant anything he discovered might not apply to them. Dzirasa also realized that people with his ancestry were missing not only from genetics research but from the entire field of brain science.

"It was a really crushing moment for me," Dzirasa s stated. So, when a group in Baltimore asked Dzirasa to help do something about the problem, he said yes. The group is the African Ancestry Neuroscience Research Initiative. It's a partnership between community leaders and the T Lieber Institute for Brain Development. an independent, nonprofit research organization on the medical campus of Johns Hopkins University.

The Lieber Institute's goals include reducing health-care disparities and ensuring that brain research includes individuals from all populations.

A History of Exclusion

Early genetics studies were often limited to people of European ancestry. Scientists reasoned that focusing on this population made it easier to link a particular gene with a specific disease. Now that genetic tools have become less expensive and more powerful, studies are including other groups. Even so, most large genomic data sets come from people of European descent. Also, African Americans and other underrepresented minorities make up only about 5% of the people in genetics research studies. These disparities are especially troubling when it comes to brain disorders that are more prevalent in people of African ancestry, says Dr. Daniel Weinberger, the Lieber Institute's CEO.

African Americans are about 20% more likely than other people to experience a serious mental health problem and perhaps twice as likely to develop Alzheimer's disease.

To understand how genetics and the environment are interacting to cause these high rates of disease, "you have to study brains," Weinberger says.

And that's where the Lieber Institute had something to offer. Over the past decade, it has received more than 700 brains from African American families who chose to donate the brain of a relative who died. As part of the African ancestry initiative, "we have produced molecular data — detailed molecular data — on about 300 brains of African Americans, plus about 1,000 brains of people of European ancestry," Weinberger says. By 2 comparing these brains, scientists hope to figure out why Alzheimer's occurs more often in African Americans. They also hope to learn why having African ancestry can sometimes protect a person from the disease. For example, Weinberger says, there's a gene mutation that greatly increases the risk of Alzheimer's in people whose ancestors came from Europe. "If you're of African ancestry, the risk from inheriting that gene from both your parents is about a fourth of what it is if you're of European ancestry," he says. Figuring out why that might lead to a drug that would protect all people, Weinberger says.

A Matter of Trust

This sort of research is tricky in a nation that has often mixed science with racism.

Baltimore was home to Henrietta Lacks, an African American woman whose cancerous cells were taken and grown in the lab without her consent or knowledge. Those cells, which had the ability to divide without aging, became one of the most important discoveries in medical research. And research suggesting a link between race and intelligence continues to fuel social debates, though most scientists dismiss the idea. "When you begin to talk about the brain, you begin to talk about the genomic data set — immediately within the community that triggers all kinds of suspicions," says the Rev. Alvin Hathaway Sr., the pastor of Union Baptist Church in Baltimore and a participant in the neuroscience research initiative.

Hathaway has worked to ensure that the effort is transparent and inclusive For example, he wanted to involve Morgan State University a public, historically black school in Baltimore. Therefore, he approached the Lieber Institute with a big request: "That I should have persons from Morgan at every step of this process, from technicians to principal investigators to researchers," he says. "And there was overwhelming acceptance of that."

Mental Health has existed since the beginning of time and has crossed all racial lines. People from all over the world suffer from some form of mental health problems. For all intent and purposes for this chapter, Sade Thompson Bell states that more than 20% (9 million) of 45 million blacks in the United States are more likely to have mental health illness (Narkhede, 2020) Narkhede). However, how they choose to deal with mental health issues may differ from other cultures. These differences exist due to mental health barriers. According to the National Alliance of Mental Illness (2023), there are social economic disparities, stigma, provider bias and inequality of care that prevents many from seeking the care needed to assist with mental health concerns.

As it relates to socioeconomic disparities, socioeconomic factors can make treatment options less available. According to NAMI (2023), in 2020, 10.4% of black adults in the United States had no form of medical coverage. Resulting in socioeconomic disparities such as exclusion from health, educational, social and economic resources. These disparities may contribute to worse mental health outcomes NAMI (2023).

Then there are the stigmas mentioned in NAMI (2023) that contribute to Blacks not seeking help for mental health issues. Research shows that many Black adults – especially older adults – view mental health conditions because of personal weakness. This results in people experiencing shame because of their condition and them feeling discriminated against. For many, it can be incredibly challenging to discuss the topic of mental health in fear of how others may perceive them NAMI (2023). This fear could prevent people from seeking mental health care when they really need help.

Many Blacks find solace in using their faith-based community for their mental health care. Because faith and spirituality can help in the recovery process and be an important part of a treatment plan, this is the route many from the black community utilize rather than seek help from other resources NAMI (2023). Although faith-based communities are good for support and to prevent one from feeling isolated, it should not be the only option for people whose daily functioning is impaired by mental health symptoms according to NAMI (2023).

Other factors that contribute to blacks not seeking mental health care is due to provider bias and inequality of care (NAMI, 2023). Blacks have been negatively affected by prejudice and discrimination in the health care system in the U.S. for years. Unfortunately, according to NAMI blacks still have these negative experiences when they seek treatment today. They go on to state that provider bias, both conscious and unconscious, and a lack of cultural competency can result in misdiagnosis and inadequate treatment. Resulting in mistrust of mental health professionals and creating a barrier for many to engage in treatment (NAMI, 2023). Another interesting fact connoted by NAMI is that black people may also be more likely to identify and describe physical symptoms related to mental health problems. An example they provided is that blacks may describe bodily aches and pains when talking about depression. Whereas NAMI states that a healthcare provider who is not culturally competent may not recognize these as symptoms of a mental health condition. In turn, allowing a mental health condition to go untreated. Other factors that contribute to blacks not receiving mental health care is according to Dr. Racine Henry in Pyscom (2022), "Not all clinicians are trained to be aware or curious about how culture, race, and ethnicity impact a person's mental and emotional wellbeing."

In conclusion, it is essential for Black/African Americans dealing with mental health disorders as a result of a childhood trauma or an inherited mental disorder, to seek the help they need in order to live productive lives. Overcoming undiagnosed mental health disorders within marginalized races requires education to build trust and knowledge.

REFERENCES

Black and African American Communities and Mental Health. (n.d.). MHA. https://www.mhanational.org/issues/black-and-african-american-communities-and-mental-health

Bryant, T. (2022, February 9). 10 Biggest Barriers To Black Mental Health. *Psycom.* https://www.psycom.net/black-mental-health-barriers

Narkhede, A. (2020, August 14). *Barriers to Mental Health Treatment in the Black Community.* Cleveland Clinic.

National Alliance of Mental Illness. (n.d.). *Black/African American.* NAMI. https://www.nami.org/Your-Journey/Identity-and-Cultural-Dimensions/Black-African-American

Waxenbaum, J., Reddy, V., & Varacallo, M. (2020). *Anatomy, Autonomic Nervous System.* NCBI. https://www.ncbi.nlm.nih.gov/books/NBK539845/#:~:text=The%20autonomic%20nervous%20system%20is,sympathetic%2C%20parasympathetic%2C%20and%20enteric

Chapter 13
Drug and Alcohol Use Among Blacks:
Mental Health Implications

Gracie Brownell
Texas A&M University, Commerce, USA

ABSTRACT

Drugs and alcohol abuse is a global social problem with negative consequences on personal, community, and societal levels. Earlier research has shown that Blacks use drugs and alcohol less than their white and Hispanic counterparts. However, evidence also shows that there are more negative and severe drugs and alcohol-induced consequences among Blacks in the United States. This disconnect between the low prevalence and higher negative outcomes is worsened by lack of culturally appropriate and timely interventions. This chapter has four main sections. The first part begins with a case study and covers the causes of drugs and alcohol use among Black and the factors that contribute to drug use and abuse, the second part is devoted to the consequences or outcomes that result from drug and alcohol abuse, while the third and fourth sections address treatment options available to this population and mental health perceptions.

INTRODUCTION

Drugs and alcohol abuse is a global social problem with negative consequences on the personal, community, and societal levels. Earlier research has shown that Blacks use drugs and alcohol less than their white and Hispanic counterpart. However, evidence also shows that there are more negative and severe drug and

DOI: 10.4018/978-1-6684-8918-5.ch013

alcohol-induced consequences among Blacks in the United States. This disconnect between the low prevalence and higher negative outcomes is worsened by a lack of culturally appropriate and timely interventions. This chapter has four main sections. The first part begins with a case study and covers the causes of drug and alcohol use among Black and the factors that contribute to drug use and abuse, the second part is devoted to the consequences or outcomes that result from drug and alcohol abuse, while the third and fourth sections address treatment options available to this population and mental health perceptions.

DRUG AND ALCOHOL USE AMONG BLACKS: MENTAL HEALTH IMPLICATIONS

Wonder Freeman, age 22 is an African American male and a senior majoring in Kinesiology. Wonder was referred to the Student Advocacy and Support services by his professor who checked in with him about the sudden drop in his grades, attendance, and engagement in class. Since Mr. Freeman considered the professor his favorite professor, he confided in her about his recent unemployment, food shortage, and fears concerning his grades, mental state, and his future after graduation. Wonder disclosed an increase in his social activities which centered on partying and substance abuse. According to him, he went from partying occasionally to about 2-3 times a week and from experimenting with weed in high school and drinking occasionally in college to using substances almost daily. This has cost him the two part-time jobs he had (on and off campus), some friends, and his grades. He admitted that he is often hungry and with what little money he had left from saving, he always spends it on his preferred substances because they make him feel better.

Wonder is a first-generation college student who was raised by a single parent. He grew up as an only child although he has 2 half siblings through his biological father with whom he has a nonexistent relationship. His mother passed away suddenly due to cancer and since then, his life spiraled out of control. Wonder described his relationship with his remaining family (maternal grandparents and cousins) as strained, admitting that he cut communications with them. He also admitted pushing his old friends away after his mother passed away though they tried reaching out to him. Wonder described feeling sad, down, and disinterested in the activities he enjoyed doing such as hanging out with his friends, playing basketball, video games etc. He reconnected with some old friends who invited him out a few times and since then has continued to party non-stop. According to him, although he enjoys hanging out with his party friends because it provides him a means of escape from his worries when they party; however, he does not have any meaningful connections with them. He also reported that he stopped attending church after his mom died but still believes in God. Prior to the death of his mother, Wonder had no mental health concerns, substance use,and criminal justice history. He, however, experienced child abuse and neglect before the age of 10 by his biological father. This led to his parent's divorce and his nonexistent relationship with his father. Wonder does not remember receiving any counseling for child abuse. He was recently arrested at a party and shares that his race played a role in his arrest since his white friends were let go. He said he feels traumatized and scared since other Black men died during their arrests. While this was his first arrest, he said he was worried that it could happen again. He is now worried about his upcoming court date and the possible effects on this record and future. At the Student Advocacy and Support Services, Wonder met with a case manager who assessed his concerns and at once referred him to the campus food pantry and the campus counseling center. As needed, the campus counseling center provides students with crisis intervention, individual and group counseling etc.

Drugs refer to habit-forming substance that affects human behavior through their effects on the brain, nervous system, moods, perceptions, consciousness, and body functions. Drug abuse or substance abuse occurs when drugs are used excessively resulting in harmful outcomes on the abusers' health, relationship with others,and society. Drugs and alcohol use have serious social and health implications across the world including the United States. Drug and alcohol consumption have become an integral part of some recreational social scenes or coping mechanisms which often yield negative health and social consequences for its users. Globally, 270 million use drugs yearly about 35 million are affected by drug disorders while alcohol consumption led to approximately 3 deaths and alcohol-induced disabilities and health problems (World Health Organization, 2022 & 2023). More people consume alcohol worldwide (76 million people), and even moderate consumption has a significant association with a substantial number of chronic diseases and causes harm not only to the user but the people around them; therefore; alcohol abuse is considered more harmful for public health and society than illicit drug use (van Amsterdam & van den Brink, 2013). Without adequate interventions, alcohol abuse can strain global healthcare with outcomes ranging from diseases to premature mortality, especially among 15 to 49-year-olds. Similarly, drug use disorders without adequate interventions not only lead to individuals being more at risk for morbidity and mortality, but it significantly diminish their functioning on the personal, family, social, educational,and occupational levels. Marginalized populations who abuse drugs and alcohol tend to have higher rates of deaths and hospitalization (WHO, 2022).

This chapter explores drug and alcohol use among African Americans, a subpopulation with a history of disenfranchisement in the United States. It provides an overview of the causes of drug and alcohol use among Blacks including the risk and protective factors, how it affects Blacks, the coping methods users and caregivers practice,and treatment available to the Black community. It is important to understand the characteristics of this problem within the black community because this information is critical in setting up innovative culturally appropriate treatment that seeks to address social injustices resulting from drug and alcohol use.

In the United States, 46.3 million people (about twice the population of New York) 12 or older had a substance abuse disorder (29.5 million with alcohol use disorder, 24 million with drug disorder,and 7.3 million people (about twice the population of Oklahoma) with both alcohol use disorder and drug use disorder alcohol in 2023 (Substance Abuse and Mental Health Services Administration, 2023). The prevalence, effects,and treatment of drugs and alcohol use, vary across subsects of the Black population in the United States based on age, gender, education, socioeconomic status,and health. Blacks have lower than expected alcohol use disorder risk although they experience more alcohol use risk factors (socioeconomic difficulty, stressor exposures, and individual stress) as compared with non-Hispanic Whites (Ransome, & Gilman, 2016). According to the Substance Abuse and Mental Health Services Administration (2023), Blacks were more likely to use illicit drugs (marijuana and crack) in the past year compared with Hispanic or Asian people. Additionally, more blacks had a drug use disorder and marijuana use disorder than their white counterparts. A high percentage of blacks (96.7%) who were diagnosed with an illicit drug or alcohol use disorder in the past year did not receive substance abuse treatment facility or feel like they needed treatment (The Substance Abuse and Mental Health Services Administration, 2023) and were thus, less likely to receive inpatient, outpatient, prescription medication and virtual treatment.

A few studies investigated substance abuse across ethnic groups and other subpopulations within the black community. Black Americans and U.S. Caribbean blacks reported higher rates of substance abuse while Blacks living in Jamaica and Guyana reported lower rates of substance abuse (Lacey, Mouzon, Govia, Matusko, Forsythe-Brown, Abelson, & Jackson, 2016). Additionally, the study also found higher substance abuse was higher among Blacks between the ages of 45 and 59 and men who were separated, divorced,or widowed. Forsythe-Brown, Abelson, & Jackson, 2016). In another study, researchers found evidence of methamphetamine use among Black men who have sex with other men in New City who were in danger of not meeting their basic needs since they reported using other substances on an income of $20,00 or less while spending $159 a month on methamphetamine (Jerome, Halkitis, Coley, & The Hope Team, 2009).Causes and Consequences of Drugs and Alcohol

It is important to understand the factors that increase the likelihood of drug and alcohol abuse among African Americans although it is difficult to establish causality in research. The factors that help decide why and how many substances people use or abuse have been categorized as biological, socioeconomic, demographic (age, gender religion), environmental,and cultural (Mooney, Knox & Schacht, 2015).

Risk Factors. The literature recognizes substance abuse addiction as a family disease since it runs in families leading to the highest risk of future substance abuse among children of substance abusers (Kumpfer, 2014). Risk factors that determine the age of first alcohol use and heavy drinking are biological, social, economic,and cultural (Lo, Howell, & Cheng, 2012) which may be present as early as childhood. African Americans who have a history of underage drinking are more likely to experience alcohol-related problems or be diagnosed with alcohol use disorder as compared to their non-African American counterparts (Delker, Brown, & Hasin, 2016). Similarly, Horseman (2018) found that African Americans with a history of underage drinking are 4 times more likely to experience alcohol use disorder than African Americans without a history of underage drinking. Some of the risk factors that contribute to alcohol use among underage children include parents' alcohol use disorder, parenting styles, lack of parental connection and support, and failure to promote cultural values (Horseman, 2018). These findings were supported by a later study that found a significant relationship between parenting behaviors and recent alcohol use among African American adolescents (Vidourek, King, Burbage, & Okuley, 2018).

Regardless of the setting, negative experiences during childhood appeared to factor into their use of alcohol as children and later as adults. One study in particular assessed associations of child sexual abuse, alcohol use, and drug use problems among adult black sexual minority men and found a high prevalence of child sexual abuse and positive correlations between a history of child abuse and alcohol and drug use problems (Shangani, van den Berg, Dyer, Mayer, & Operario, 2022). In addition to family dynamics during childhood, stress related to specific family situations during adulthood also appears to contribute to the use of drugs and alcohol among African Americans. This phenomenon is clear among African American women who played the role of caregivers to older relatives 65 years and older,and had a low religious attendance use alcohol to cope with the burden of being a caregiver (Pickard, Williams Woodson, & Johnson, 2021).

Low Socioeconomic Status. Low socioeconomic status during childhood and later are also prominent risk factors that promote a pathway to undesirable socioeconomic and school experiences which leads to lower educational attainment and, eventually, greater heavy drinking at midlife among African Americans (Mulia, Witbrodt, Karriker, Lui, & Zapolski, 2022). Low-income African American men are the most at risk for alcoholism and problems associated with alcoholism (Zapolski, Pedersen, McCarthy, & Smith, 2014). Risk factors have the tendency to lead to other risk factors and the same could be said about protective factors. An example of this is seen in the literature which shows how substance use is linked to unsafe sexual behavior, such as having unprotected sex (Browne, Wechsberg, White, Middlesteadt Ellerson, Raiford, Carry, & Herbst, 2014). While socioeconomic status has been documented as a protective factor against substance abuse, one study claims that regardless of socioeconomic status, Blacks have a shorter and sicker life span than their White counterparts (DeAngelis, 2022).

Adversity and Stress. Despite the well-publicized health risks associated with drugs and alcohol, some adults resort to drugs and alcohol to cope with stress and mental health symptoms (Lo, Howell, & Cheng, 2012). Lo, Howell,and Cheng (2012) found a high prevalence of chronic mental illness among US-born Blacks while foreign-born Blacks showed extremely low levels. There was a high prevalence of frequent binge drinking among Blacks who experienced chronic mental health problems in the past year pointing to the possibility that Whites address their mental health problems through mental health services rather than alcohol (Lo, Howell, & Cheng, 2012). However, this may not be the same for all groups within the Black community, in particular Black women. While trauma exposure significantly predicts mental health outcomes like depression and anxiety among African American women, it does not predict the use of alcohol and drugs among them (Staton-Tindall, Duvall, Stevens-Watkins, & Oser, (2013). Loneliness within a relationship is another source of stress linked to illicit drug use and heavy drinking which is especially true for black women (Whitehead, 2016).

Despite lower levels of stress, blacks living in higher socioeconomic areas experience more perceived stress which manifests through chronic pain, elevated stress hormones, high blood pressure related to stress, and fear from striving to achieve while fearing goals achieving obstacles or failures (DeAngelis, 2022). Goal-striving stress is defined as psychological outcomes that result from seeking but not achieving socioeconomic mobility, otherwise known as intergenerational mobility (Mouzon, Watkins, Perry, Simpson, & Mitchell, 2019). It is important not to lump the Black population into one category because stress and other experiences may be unique depending on ethnicity and nativity (Mouzon, Watkins, Perry, Simpson, & Mitchell, 2019). Within the black population in the United States, the relationship between intergenerational mobility and goal-striving stress is different for U.S. born blacks as compared to foreign-born Blacks. Research found that among U.S. born Blacks and Caribbean, intergenerational mobility was linked to lower goal-striving stress as compared to their foreign-born Caribbean counterparts who experienced relatively high goal-striving stress irrespective of achieved intergenerational mobility and education (Mouzon, Watkins, Perry, Simpson, & Mitchell, 2019). Understanding the unique experiences and needs of Blacks in America are crucial factors to consider when developing and implementing culturally appropriate substance interventions.

Chronic stress is linked to increased susceptibility to drug use and inevitably drug induced health disparities in the African American community (Cavanagh, &

Obasi, 2022). According to McNeil Smith and Taylor (2015), African Americans are more exposed to stress and adversity in the United States and thus. Some of the adversities and ensuing impacts members of the Black community experience are linked to discrimination related to their race. Black Americans and Caribbean Americans who report elevated levels of discrimination are more at risk for mood and substance use disorder (Clark, Salas-Wright, Vaughn, & Whitfield, 2014). In the case of black college women, racism increased their engagement in risky drinking (Pittman & Kaur, 2018). For others struggling with poverty, unfair treatment,and depressive symptoms were linked to heavy drinking (Mulia, Yu Ye, Zemore, & Greenfield, 2008). This suggests that black youths have an increased risk of drug and alcohol use since they are still developing their identities and learning coping skills amid uncontrollable factors impacting their socioeconomic status. Van Gundy, Howerton-Orcutt,and Mills (2015) state, as compared to White you adults, African American young adults show lower problem-focused coping, and higher avoidance-oriented coping. They also found that African Americans who used problem-focused coping were less likely to use illicit drugs (excluding marijuana), while those who used avoidance-oriented coping had lower odds of marijuana use disorder (Van Gundy, Howerton-Orcutt, & Mills, 2015).

There is an established link between drug use and sexual experiences. Alcohol and drugs can affect sexual responses at the low end by reducing inhibitions and anxiety and improving sexual functioning and at the high end, it acts as a depressant, reduces arousal,and leads to sexual dysfunction (Hyde & DeLamater, 2017). Therefore, some users are motivated to use substances for their potential sexual benefit. For instance, in one study, African American young adults reported using MMDA (ecstasy/molly) for several reasons including wanting to alter the effects of marijuana and alcohol, prolong their sexual experience, enhance sexual pleasure, and aid them in achieving "freaky" sexual experience (Rigg, 2017). Similarly, young Black women with education ranging from no college education to college-educated disclosed the use of alcohol and other drugs just before or during their last sex activity as compared to their less educated counterparts (Browne, Bonner, Kline, Cox, Gichane, & Wechsberg, 2023).

Protective Factors

Education. Education attainment is an important protective factor against alcohol that not only increases users' knowledge about potential negative social and health consequences but also their earning ability allowing individuals to afford healthier methods of coping with stress or boredom rather than engaging in drug and alcohol use. An example of this is seen in Skalamera and Hummer (2016) study where college-educated young adults reported less binge drinking and marijuana use.

However, contrasting findings from a more recent study revealed heavy alcohol use (four or more drinks per day) in the past 30 days among African American women who completed some or more college (Browne, Bonner, Kline, Cox, Gichane, & Wechsberg, 2023). On the other hand, some college or more attainment emerged as a protective factor for using cocaine and reporting unprotected sex (Browne et al., 2014). Other factors that protect African American women who experience traumatic and mental health life events from using cocaine include spirituality as measured by existential well-being on the spiritual well-being scale (Staton-Tindall, Duvall, Stevens-Watkins, & Oser, (2013).

Environment. A longitudinal study involving a 172 African American adult cohort of mostly substance users showed an association between moving to neighborhoods with better economic and social conditions and less risky drug-alcohol networks. (Linton, Cooper, Luo, Karnes, Renneker, Haley, Hunter-Jones, Ross, Bonney, & Rothenberg, 2016). For Blacks living in higher advantaged states and mostly white neighborhoods, the research found lower neuroendocrine stress hormones as compared to other Blacks living in disadvantaged neighborhoods (DeAngelis, 2022). Zapolski, et. al. (2014) named family and culture as two dual-acting environmental factors that protect African Americans against drug and alcohol use; however, the researchers noted that they may also serve as risk factors as well. Norms within African American culture discourage heavy use of alcohol; however, on the other side, it encourages disapproval from community members especially since members of the African American community recognize their susceptibility to more alcohol-related legal problems as compared to their white counterparts.

Consequences

Physical Consequences. In the United States, the death attributed to alcohol consumption grew from approximately 88,000 deaths (70% male and 30% female) in 2018 (Centers for Disease Control and Prevention [CDC], 2018) to 140,000 people (CDC, 2023). Not only does alcohol consumption shorten lives by 26 years on average, (Centers for Disease Control and Prevention, 2023), but it also created an economic cost of more than 249 billion in 2010 (Sacks, Gonzales, Bouchery, Tomedi, & Brewer, 2010). Excessive drinking is defined as binge drinking, heavy drinking,or drinking by underage or pregnant individuals (The Centers for Disease Control and Prevention, 2022). The Centers for Disease Control and Prevention (2022) distinguishes binge drinking (4 or more drinks during a single occasion for women and 5 or more drinks for men) from heavy drinking which refers to women drinking 8 or more drinks per week while men 15 or more drinks per week. The consequences of binge drinking tend to be short-term including injuries from accidents (vehicular, falls, drownings, etc.), violence against self (suicide) or other (homicide, sexual assault, and intimate partner violence), alcohol poisoning, risky sexual behaviors resulting in sexually transmitted diseases or unwanted pregnancies and pregnancy loss (miscarriage and stillbirth) and fetal alcohol syndrome. Furthermore, excessive drinking is related to suicides (Mooney & Schacht, 2015). The outcomes of excessive drinking, on the other hand, are more long-term in nature resulting in chronic health problems that develop over time including problems with high blood pressure, the heart, liver, and digestive system which can lead to cancer in various body parts, a weakened immune system, weakened memory, mental health and social problems related to family or work (The Centers for Disease Control and Prevention, 2022).

Social Consequences. Historically, African Americans were not knowledgeable about the negative consequences of alcohol and drug abuse (Williams, Newby, & Kanitz, 1993) despite the early and alarming severity of alcohol-related health and social problems among African Americans including but not limited to high death rates due to liver cirrhosis (Mosley, Atkins, & Klein, 1988) and higher alcohol-related homicide death (Harper & Dawkins, 1977). Researchers criticized seminal studies for their flawed generalizations of heavy alcohol use among Black college students resulting from design and sampling methods design. In contrast to historical findings, later findings showed that black college students experience fewer negative consequences including problems with class attendance, fewer problems with the opposite sex, and a source of regret (Williams, Newby, & Kanitz, 1993).

Generally, African Americans experience higher levels of social problems despite having later initiation and lower rates of alcohol use (Zapolski, Pedersen, McCarthy, & Smith, 2014). Studies showed differences in the level of alcohol consumption and the result of alcohol and drugs among subpopulations in the United States. For instance, one study found the highest prevalence of alcohol use among Whites, the most abuse and dependence among Native Americans but Native Americans and Blacks as the most vulnerable to alcohol-related health problems (Delker, Brown, & Hasin, 2016). Drug and alcohol abuse problems extend beyond the individual abuser to members of their family and community. For instance, past research found a positive association between the use of illicit drugs and partner problem drinking with intimate partner violence among blacks (Caetano, Cunradi, Alter, Mair, Yau, & Gerson, 2019).

At least one study examined the role racism plays in risky drinking behavior among Black college women and found that general life stress and perceived racism are associated with alcohol use among Black college women while increased experiences of racism increase Black college women's engagement in risky drinking (Pittman, & Kaur, 2018). Amaro et al. (2005) found a prevalence of disadvantaged economic and social life conditions including community violence among Black and Hispanic women as compared to White women, yet they did not show more severe clinical symptoms of co-occurring mental health and substance abuse disorders.

Violent experiences can lead to trauma which the literature links to substance use. Among Black college students, researchers found a link between the severity of post-traumatic stress disorder and alcohol use which they resorted to while trying to cope with heightened emotional regulation difficulties (McGrew, Raines, Walker, Leonard, & Vujanovic, 2023).

Treatment Options for Substance Abuse Within the African American Community

Throughout the years, helping professionals have used many diverse types of interventions to aid African Americans in addressing drug and alcohol-related problems. These interventions range from micro-level interventions including rehab and therapy, mezzo-level interventions like educational and therapeutic groups to macro-level interventions like advocacy for policies and programs. A search of the literature uncovers several examples of micro-level drug and alcohol interventions. At least one study explored spiritually based treatment with substance abusing and violent African American men and found that substance abuse points to a spiritual thirst for power, control, or a desire to escape and bring balanceto a spiritually imbalanced life that can only be mitigated in a therapeutic setting that facilitates substance abusers' quest for wholeness and balance (Freeman, 2006). Most notably, forms of response to alcohol and drug abuse within the African American communities stemmed from church denominations that are instrumental in addressing the needs of alcohol and substance abusers and their families.

Treatment Methods. Evidence of effective treatment methods is available in the literature though African Americans' experiences vary across treatment methods. Cognitive behavioral therapy, motivational interviewing, motivational enhancement therapy, and multisystemic therapy are effective evidence-based substance use disorder treatment interventions (Windsor, Jemal, & Alessi, 2015; Pederson, Curley, & Collins, 2021; Randall, Cunningham, & Henggeler, 2018). Multisystemic therapy-substance abuse is an effective treatment designed for adolescents with substance use disorders. It is based on a reward system wherein adolescents can earn incentives from a thorough list for negative drug screens and clean living (Randall, Cunningham, & Henggeler, 2018). At least one meta-analysis investigated Cognitive based therapy's impact on substance use between studies with predominantly non-Hispanic whites and studies with predominantly black and or Hispanics and found a significantly stronger impact among Black and Hispanic studies (Windsor, Jemal, & Alessi, 2015). The outcome for blacks is comparable to their white counterpart. For instance, past research found a relationship between receiving formal treatment and abstaining from alcohol for 30 days the same among Whites and Blacks (Avalos and Mulia, 2012). To prevent lifelong substance abuse disorder, helping professionals must recognize and address substance misuse early through screening, followed by a brief intervention, and a subsequent referral to a long-term intervention (Haughwout, Harford, Castle, & Grant, 2016). However, little research exists about the effectiveness of these interventions as well as the processes needed to guide prevention measures such as substance abuse and dependence awareness and prevention in African American communities (Clark, McGovern, Mgbeokwere, Wooten, Owusu, & McGraw, 2014).

There are some unique treatment options available by and for members of the African American community. Sanders (2002) described what he termed as five indigenous recovery movements including Glide Memorial Methodist Church which empowers about 80% of its congregation who are in recovery; One church-one addict, which provides long-term care support; Free-N-One which provides Christian-based support for addicts and their families; the Nation of Islam which helps African American substance abusers in the criminal justice system; and the African American Survivors organization which addresses racism in the context of recovery. Sanders (2002) urged helping professionals to recognize, learn, partner, and build relationships with recovery movements like the ones listed above with the goal of supplying joint service delivery models because they are a part of recovery support services within the African American community. Racial and ethnic differences must be factored into the design and delivery of alcohol and drug interventions (Amaro, Larson, Gampel, Richardson, Savage, & Wagler, 2005).

Without effective treatment, African Americans are more likely to experience alcohol-related social problems (Williams et al., 2016). However, in the United States, African Americans experience more barriers to treatment and significant disparities in the quality of care they receive for alcohol and drug use (Wong, Derose, Miles, & Litt, 2018). To find potential points for early interventions, researchers conducted a longitudinal study that estimated pathways from childhood socio-economic position (SEP) to educational attainment and mid-life heavy drinking in black Americans and argued for earlier interventions rather than mid-life timed interventions (Mulia, Witbrodt, Karriker, Lui, & Zapolski, 2022). Early interventions can begin as early as childhood, with the parents as the primary targets. Since past research confirmed the importance of parenting behaviors in youth alcohol use, there is a need for alcohol prevention and reduction interventions to teach positive parenting behaviors (Vidourek, King, Burbage, & Okuley, 2018) strengthen current parenting skills, and nurture the mother-adolescent relationship (Clark, Belgrave, & Abell, 2012). Substance use interventions should also include child abuse awareness and prevention components since some users report a history of child abuse (Shangani, van den Berg, Dyer, Mayer, & Operario, 2022).

Providers who design and implement substance abuse treatment programs must also consider the gender-related differences among users. Mannes, Burrell, Bryant,

Dunne, Hearn, and Whitehead (2016) advocated for gender-specific interventions that address interpersonal relationship problems linked to illicit drug use and heavy drinking. Earlier research found that regardless of race and ethnicity, women needed and received more services targeted to their needs and reported more positive relations with service providers. (Guerrero, Marsh, Cao, Shin, & Andrews, 2014).

Barriers to Treatment. Despite some treatment options, members of the Black community experience barriers to accessing and completing substance abuse treatment. A systematic review of studies between 1995 and 2018 found African American women are likely to experience treatment readiness barriers such as guilt or shame, little or no motivation for treatment, not believing in the necessity of treatment, and the possible impact on interpersonal relationships with family and childcare (Redmond, Smith, & Collins, 2020). The relationship between readiness to change and retention was investigated among 194 African women and men and results showed a strong relationship between retention and readiness to change (RTC) over time for men more than women. These findings have important implications for the development and implementation of substance use interventions because it highlightthe need for pre-intervention strategies that will enhance female substance users' readiness by providing resources to incentivize participation and address feelings, child care, and interpersonal strain among family members (Redmond, Smith, & Collins, 2020) and during intervention strategy that will increase readiness to change over time for men (Montgomery, Burlew, & Korte, 2017). To address the socioeconomic and cultural barriers and increase the completion rate of alcohol and drug treatment among Blacks, Saloner and Lê Cook (2013) called for increased Medicaid funding for residential treatment and better cultural competence training for providers.

Blacks and Hispanics are significantly less likely to use specialty treatment and complete treatment for alcohol and drugs due to problem severity, perceived treatment need, and low socioeconomic status marred by greater unemployment and housing instability as compared to Whites and Asians. (Pinedo, 2019 & Saloner and Lê Cook, 2013). Past research revealed that Blacks were least likely to start treatment and when they did, it was done mostly in facilities with mixed substance abuse and mental health focus rather than a substance abuse-focused facility as compared to their White and Native American counterparts (Acevedo, Garnick, Lee, Horgan, Ritter, Panas, Davis, Leeper, Moore, & Reynolds, 2012). Similarly, Montgomery, Burlew, and Korte (2017) reported that as compared to other races, African Americans have low engagement and completion of outpatient substance abuse treatment.

According to Pickard, et al., (2021) helping professionals can use the strengths perspective to help minority caregivers increase their personal power, develop strong coping skills, and improve their social support system. The social support team within the African American community often includes religious leaders. For example, one study revealed that after receiving formal treatment, Blacks who did not attend Alcoholics Anonymous meetings were likely to abstain largely due to their religious practices and a drier drinking culture within their network (Avalos and Mulia, 2012). For those with a history of child sexual abuse, it is imperative that substance use interventions address their psychological health needs related to sexual abuse (Shangani, van den Berg, Dyer, Mayer, & Operario, 2022). Substance abuse treatment programs can also teach African American problem-focused coping skills (Van Gundy, Howerton-Orcutt, & Mills, 2015) to address problems appropriately.

However, stigma or the fear of being labeled as a substance abuser and lack of perceived social support or the fear of being gossiped about once news of their treatment gets out are barriers that prevent more blacks than whites from pursuing substance use treatment (Pinedo, Zemore, & Mulia, 2022). Although developed to address substance abuse-related problems, policies can be unintended sources of stigmatization. For those recovering from substance abuse and wanting to rebuild their lives, the language used to label them, their behaviors, and treatment act as obstacles that discourage access to health care, policy, employment, and insurance policies (Zwick, Appleseth, & Arndt, 2020). Therefore, scholars have suggested that efforts be made to destigmatize language that describes substance use behaviors, substance users, and substance use treatment (Zwick, Appleseth, & Arndt, 2020).

Environmental Interventions. The person in the environment is an approach often used in social work that acknowledges the individuals' multiple environments as a forceful interactive system with a concurrent impact on human behavior (Hare, 2004). To understand an individual, it must be done within the context of the individual and his or her environment which forms the ecosystem that encompasses the individual and various systems the individual has mutual relationships. In short, the individual influences and is influenced by his or her environment (Weiss-Gal, 2008). This approach is useful in understanding the cause, consequences, and potential interventions used to address substance abuse among Blacks. Thus, former drugs and alcohol users looking to make a change weaken or end their connection with the substance use community by relocating to a new environment (Linton, Cooper, Luo, Karnes, Renneker, Haley, Hunter-Jones, Ross, Bonney, & Rothenberg, 2016). Evidence shows an association between moving to areas with improved economic and social conditions and to less risky drug/alcohol networks among African American adults (Linton et. al., 2016, because they will build new social connections with non-alcohol or drug users. Van Gundy, Howerton-Orcutt, & Mills (2015) recommended helping professionals contextualize alcohol and substance abuse policies and interventions using sociocultural stress and coping styles. McNeil Smith& Taylor (2015) assert the need for substance abuse prevention interventions to target environmental and social structures related to adolescent drug use.

African Americans Views on Mental Health

How Blacks Perceive Mental Health. African Americans' negative perception and distrust of the mental health system can be traced back to America's history of slavery, racism, and discriminatory practices in the areas of healthcare and research. Examples of these unethical practices include experimenting on slaves, carrying out family planning sterilization without victims' consent,and most notably, the federally funded Tuskegee Syphilis study which withheld syphilis medication to African American men despite its availability (Washington, 2006). Evidence of this is seen in past studies when Hispanics and Blacks reported more concerns about the breach of personal privacy and the possibility of being included in harmful experimentation (Boulware, Cooper, Ratner, LaVeist, & Powe, 2003).

The negative feelings about mental health and the mental health system are known barriers to service use among African Americans (Gaston, Earl, Nisanci, & Glomb, 2016). Negative perceptions of the mental health system may be attributed to past discrimination which inevitably leads to uncertainty or distrust of the mental health system overall (Copeland, & Snyder, 2011).

According to Gaston, Earl, Nisanci, & Glomb (2016) there are four barriers that prevent African Americans from pursuing mental health namely, poverty, racism, discrimination, reliance on other coping mechanisms, and fear. As reported by African American women, some structural barriers that discourage mental health service use are low education, unemployment, lack of health insurance, and housing issues (Ward, & Heidrich, 2009). Uninsured patients are more likely to report discrimination in mental health/substance abuse visits (Mays, Jones, Delany-Brumsey, Coles, & Cochran, 2017). Blacks credited discrimination based on race/ethnicity as the main reason behind health care discrimination they experience and their perceived discrimination in mental health/substance abuse visits were associated with early treatment termination (Mays, Jones, Delany-Brumsey, Coles & Cochran, 2017). While most of the literature points to discrimination from external sources, Yu, Matlin, Crusto, Hunter, & Tebes, (2022) emphasized the role of internalized self-stigma and racial play in preventing Black adults diagnosed with mental illness or addiction from seeking help.

Researchers surveyed Black undergraduate and graduate students across the United States and found a significant association between positive perception of mental health climate, higher levels of positive mental health and sense of belonging,and lower levels of depression (Peoples, Butler-Barnes, Stafford, Williams, & Smith, 2023). This means that institutions with Black students and employees play a significant role in Blacks' mental health and should therefore encourage organizational culture and practice that promote belonging and mental health care.

Culturally, African Americans perceived depression as normal, themselves as "strong" and therefore using mental health services was not "normal" and a sign of being weak (Conner et al., 2010). Rather than depending on mental health services, Blacks tend to rely on themselves, their families, or their support system including community and religion. For example, one study found that among foreign-born Blacks, Haitian immigrants relied on family members instead of mental health workers (Schwartz et al., 2014). Similar findings showed similar practices among African immigrants who reported dealing with mental health issues within their families first before relying on their faith (Piwowarczyk et al., 2014). This is also partly due to the negative perceptions of the mental health care services they received (Cai, & Robst, 2016) in the past. Structural and interpersonal factors are sources of vulnerability, stigma,and expected discrimination for African Americans with substance use disorders and comorbid mental illness (Jegede, Muvvala, Katehis, Paul, Soipe, & Jolayemi, 2021).

The relationship between interpersonal relationships and perceived mental health is underscored in the literature. Research suggests an association between social support from friends, and church members, and better perceived mental health, regardless of race. However, mental health perception varied between black men and women. The study showed weak perceived mental health among affluent Black women, the association between family support and better mental health among low-income black women, and lower subjective mental health among affluent Black men with high family support (Roxburgh, & MacArthur, 2020).

Stress among Black Immigrants. Although Blacks experience stress in the United States more than their white counterparts which suggest a higher need for mental health service, the level of stress varies among subsect of the Black population including immigrants. For instance, Black Africans who originated from racially mixed or majority Black contexts reported less severe psychological distress as compared to U.S.-born Black Americans from majority white contexts (Marquez-Velarde, Miller, Ma, & Keith, 2022). Similarly, first and second-generation immigrant men from Africa reported lower depression and anxiety symptoms, while gender and marital status affected immigrant women's depression and anxiety symptoms,and loneliness and discrimination negatively impacted immigrants' mental health regardless of gender (Escamilla, & Saasa, 2020).

There are several circumstances when Blacks were more likely to access mental health services. For example, Blacks reported willingness to use mental health services when the interventions included knowledge-building components like psychoeducation that extend beyond general knowledge to provide specific knowledge that helps them identify specific mental illnesses including schizophrenia (Pederson, Tsai, Hawkins, Moskowitz, & Dixon, 2023). The support of a religious/spiritual leader is also a principal factor that motivates African American emerging adults to use substance abuse treatment services (Williams & Cabrera-Nguyen, 2016). Factors that contributed to treatment utilization among adolescents with substance use disorders included involvement with the criminal justice system, and perceived need for treatment while those with substance use disorder other than alcohol use, older, and in communication with parents were more likely to use treatment (Haughwout, Harford, Castle, & Grant, 2016).

There are several comorbid conditions including untreated psychiatric disorders, lower income, and criminal justice problems that make substance abuse treatment harder for African Americans (Jacobson, Robinson, & Bluthenthal, 2007). The conditions and quality of the treatment centers that Blacks use also complicate the services they receive. Past research shows that Blacks often use lower-quality treatment centers with less trained, less educated clinicians with fewer licenses and training opportunities (Wheeler, & Nahra, 2000). This is extremely dangerous since clinical professionals are the gatekeepers to alcohol and substance use disorder treatment. Therefore, there is a need for competent providers with adequate education and training (Van Boekel, Brouwers, Van Weeghel, Garretsen, 2013). Evidence suggests that substance use disorder treatment centers that accept federal funding and are in predominantly Black communities are less likely to use empirically supported treatment (van den Berk-Clark, Patterson Silver Wolf, & Williams, 2017).

Barriers to mental health treatment. There are personal and organizational barriers to implementing empirically supported treatment. Often influenced by personal characteristics, providers' attitudes toward new or evidence backed clinical practices serve as personal barriers that can aid or impede the treatment (Patterson, Dulmus, & Maguin, 2013). Some of these notable characteristics are educational level, race, gender,and substance abuse history. For instance, positive attitudes are more prevalent among highly educated providers (Ogborne, Wild, Braun, & Newton-Taylor, 1998). Additionally, professional identity formulated by providers' attributes, beliefs, values, motives, preferences,and past experiences (Watkins-Hayes, 2009) plays a vital role in the facilitation of empirically supported treatment. This means that providers who are recovering addicts and are biased toward the 12-step model might be less enthused about using cognitive behavior or trauma therapies (Miller, Sorensen, Selzer, & Brigham, 2006) based upon what they believed worked in their own personal sobriety experience. Some health professionals might hold negative attitudes and beliefs that view substance use disorder patients as manipulative, violent, and unmotivated which in turn reduce patients' feelings of empowerment and overall healthcare treatment (Van Boekel, Brouwers, Van Weeghel, Garretsen, 2013).

In their quest to hire providers who represent the population they serve, employers higher more Black practitioners in community mental health organizations and substance use treatment centers that provide services within highly Black populated areas (Hewitt, 2004). This practice is important because Black employees can use their race as a foundation for commonality which they can draw upon to develop rapport, and show solidarity and support for clients of the same race (Watkins-Hayes, 2011). Personal characteristics such as race and past experiences are integral components of one's identity which affects their judgment, actions,and inevitably the services they provide in the workplace. Therefore, black providers have more potential when it comes to connecting with and building trust and rapport with other Blacks seeking substance abuse treatment as compared to white providers.

On one hand, professional identity encompasses the providers' attributes, beliefs, values, motives, preferences, and past experiences outside of the organization,and on the other, providers' professional roles are decided within the organization and given based on leadership and professional identity (Watkins-Hayes, 2011). Both professional identities are influenced by the organizational culture defined as shared beliefs, norms,and expected behaviors valued and encouraged (Altaf, 2011). Organizational culture is instrumental in the employees' performance, strategic implementation of goals, and job satisfaction (Van-Eerven Ludolf et al., 2017). Organizational cultural values drive many aspects of the organization including the organizations' accreditations and affiliations, employees' training provided, the value of employees' education and training (van den Berk-Clark, Patterson Silver Wolf, & Williams, 2017),and employees' attitude toward evidence supported treatments (Patterson, Ramsey, & van den Berk-Clark, 2015). Another important organizational barrier related to values is the type of business model they adopt. Substance abuse treatment organizations using the not-for-profit business models have different goals and sources of funding thus prioritizing clients' well-being even when they cannot afford the service. However, substance abuse treatment under the for-profit model goals tends to be more profit-related. They are more likely to charge for services, thereby marginalizing subsects of the population including Blacks who evidence shows are significantly more likely to live in low-income households (Roxburgh, & MacArthur, 2020).

Racial inequalities exist at the macro level through advocacy for distinct types of drug policies depending on the legislator or their constituents. For example, Jin Woo Kim, Morgan, and Nyhan, (2020) investigated longitudinal data from the House of Representatives on the co-sponsorship of legislation on drug abuse over the past four decades. Findings revealed that legislators advocated for more punitive drug-related bills during the crack scare as compared to the treatment-oriented bills introduced during the opioid crisis. Between 1983 and 2016, lawmakers sponsored more treatment-oriented legislation in response to district-level opioid-related deaths of white victims as compared to cocaine-related deaths of black victims (Jin Woo Kim, Morgan, and Nyhan, 2020). To improve access to mental health services, Gaston, Earl, Nisanci, & Glomb, (2016) highlights the importance of addressing mental health barriers through specific cultural practice.

The Application of the Person in Environment Approach to Case Study

To identify Wonder's needs and the services needed to address them, he would be assessed informally and formally. During the formal assessment, a clinical interview/ assessment will be conducted to examine his mental status and rate his symptoms subjectively. A life event chart would be useful in collecting information about his history and the major events he experienced. During the formal assessment, Wonder could be screened using the drug abuse screening test. Subsequently, the interventions will include the counselor or social worker building a rapport with Wonder, providing supportive psychotherapy, psychoeducation, relaxation techniques, or even family therapy with his estranged family members if he wants to rebuild those relationships.

The person-in-environment approach is suggested because it will facilitate a holistic understanding of his current behaviors and concerns to determine needed interventions. The first task for Wonder is to take responsibility for his own behaviors including partying, experimenting with drugs, and the aftermath (missing school, and work, losing his job, and getting arrested for a DUI). With the help of the counselor or social worker, he needs to recognize substance abuse and depression as his primary problems considering everything he felt and did shortly after he lost his mother. Using the person-in-environment approach, the counselor or social worker can assess how his environment affects him (partying buddies who enable his substance use) and his impact on his environment (school, loss of job, and criminal justice system). His perceptions of mental health and receiving mental health intervention can be addressed. It would be helpful to help him process his arrest experience and any related trauma he might have as a result of it. His fears surrounding his upcoming court date and implications for his future will also be explored.

CONCLUSION

This chapter provided an overview of drug and alcohol abuse in the Black or African American population. It identified influential factors that contribute to the causes and consequences of substance use including biological, socioeconomic, demographic (age, gender religion), environmental and cultural factors. The discussion also covered treatment methods available to members of the Black community, placing careful emphasis on recovery movement interventions that exclusively target the Black community namely: Glide Memorial Methodist church, One church- one addict, Free-N-One, the Nation of Islam, and the African American Survivors organization. It also underscored the importance of addressing barriers that discourage Blacks from seeking and completing treatment as well as the perceptions of mental health and mental health treatment taking into consideration unique adversities that members of the Black community endure. It concluded with an application of the person-in-environment approach and chapter material to the case study of Wonder Freeman introduced at the beginning of the chapter.

REFERENCES

Acevedo, A., Garnick, D. W., Lee, M. T., Horgan, C. M., Ritter, G., Panas, L., Davis, S., Leeper, T., Moore, R., & Reynolds, M. (2012). Racial and ethnic differences in substance abuse treatment initiation and engagement. *Journal of Ethnicity in Substance Abuse*, *11*(1), 1–21. https://doi-org.proxy.tamuc.edu/10.1080/15332640.2012.652516. doi:10.1080/15332640.2012.652516 PMID:22381120

Altaf, A. (2011). The Impact of Organizational Culture on Organizational Effectiveness: Implication of Hofstede Cultural Model as Organizational Effectiveness Model. *The International Journal of Interdisciplinary Social Sciences: Annual Review*, *6*(1), 161–174. doi:10.18848/1833-1882/CGP/v06i01/51996

Amaro, H., Larson, M. J., Gampel, J., Richardson, E., Savage, A., & Wagler, D. (2005). Racial/Ethnic Differences in Social Vulnerability among Women with Co-Occurring Mental Health and Substance Abuse Disorders: Implications for Treatment Services. *Journal of Community Psychology*, *33*(4), 495–511. doi:10.1002/jcop.20065

Avalos, L. A., & Mulia, N. (2012). Formal and informal substance use treatment utilization and alcohol abstinence over seven years: Is the relationship different for blacks and whites? *Drug & Alcohol Dependence*, *121*(1/2), 73–80. https://doi doi:org.proxy.tamuc.edu/10.1016/j.drugalcdep.2011.08.018

Boulware, L. E., Cooper, L. A., Ratner, L. E., LaVeist, T. A., & Powe, N. R. (2003). Race and trust in the health care system. *Public Health Reports*, *118*(4), 358–365. doi:10.1016/S0033-3549(04)50262-5 PMID:12815085

Browne, F. A., Bonner, C. P., Kline, T. L., Cox, E. N., Gichane, M. W., & Wechsberg, W. M. (2023). Alcohol, drug use, and sexual risk among young African American women in North Carolina: Is educational attainment protective? *Vulnerable Children and Youth Studies*, *18*(2), 149–155. https://doi-org.proxy.tamuc.edu/10.1080/17450128.2022.2089794. doi:10.1080/17450128.2022.2089794

Browne, F. A., Wechsberg, W. M., White, V. M., Middlesteadt Ellerson, R., Raiford, J. L., Carry, M. G., & Herbst, J. H. (2014). The influence of social determinants on sexual risk among out-of-school African American female adolescents. *Vulnerable Children and Youth Studies*, *9*(2), 139–150. doi:10.1080/17450128.2013.832828 PMID:26692886

Caetano, R., Cunradi, C. B., Alter, H. J., Mair, C., Yau, R. K., & Gerson, L. W. (2019). Drinking and Intimate Partner Violence Severity Levels Among U.S. Ethnic Groups in an Urban Emergency Department. *Academic Emergency Medicine*, *26*(8), 897–907. https://doi-. doi:10.1111/acem.13706 PMID:30706610

Cai, A., & Robst, J. (2016). The relationship between race/ethnicity and the perceived experience of mental health care. *The American Journal of Orthopsychiatry*, *86*(5), 508–518. https://doi-. doi:10.1037/ort0000119 PMID:26460698

Cavanagh, L., & Obasi, E. M. (2022). Chronic Stress, Autonomic Dysregulation and Prospective Drug Use Among African American Emerging Adults. *Cultural Diversity & Ethnic Minority Psychology*, *28*(1), 91–102. https://doi-org.proxy.tamuc.edu/10.1037/cdp0000364. doi:10.1037/cdp0000364 PMID:34672646

Centers for Disease Control and Prevention. (2016). *Fact sheets: Underage drinking*. CDC. https://www.cdc.gov/alcohol/fact-sheets/underage-drinking.htm

Centers for Disease Control and Prevention. (2018). *Fact sheets –alcohol use and your health*. CDC.

Centers for Disease Control and Prevention. (2022). *Alcohol Use and your heath*. CDC. https://www.cdc.gov/alcohol/fact-sheets/alcohol-use.htm

Centers for Disease Control and Prevention. (2022). Alcohol-Related Disease Impact Application (ARDI) Application. Accessed April 19, 2022. https://nccd.cdc.gov/DPH_ARDI/defaul/default.aspx

Centers for Disease Control and Prevention. (2023). *Addressing Excessive Alcohol Use: State Fact Sheet*. CDC. https://www.cdc.gov/alcohol/fact-sheets/states/excessive-alcohol-use-united-states.html

Clark, T. T., Belgrave, F. Z., & Abell, M. (2012). The Mediating and Moderating Effects of Parent and Peer Influences upon Drug Use among African American Adolescents. *The Journal of Black Psychology*, *38*(1), 52–80. doi:10.1177/0095798411403617

Clark, T. T., McGovern, P., Mgbeokwere, D., Wooten, N., Owusu, H., & McGraw, K. A. (2014). Systematic review: The nature and extent of social work research on substance use disorders treatment interventions among African Americans. *Journal of Social Work, 14*(5), 451–472. https://doi-org.proxy.tamuc.edu/10.1177/1468017313479858. doi:10.1177/1468017313479858

Clark, T. T., Salas-Wright, C. P., Vaughn, M. G., & Whitfield, K. E. (2014). Everyday discrimination and mood and substance use disorders: A latent profile analysis with African Americans and Caribbean blacks. *Addictive Behaviors, 40*(1), 119–125. PMID:25254321

Conner, K. O., Copeland, V. C., Grote, N. K., Rosen, D., Albert, S., McMurray, M. L., & Koeske, G. (2010). Barriers to treatment and culturally endorsed coping strategies among depressed African American older adults. *Aging & Mental Health, 14*(8), 971–983. doi:10.1080/13607863.2010.501061 PMID:21069603

Copeland, V. C., & Snyder, K. (2011). Barriers to mental health treatment services for low-income African American women whose children receive behavioral health services: An ethnographic investigation. *Social Work in Public Health, 26*(1), 78–95. doi:10.1080/10911350903341036 PMID:21213189

DeAngelis, R. T. (2022). Moving on Up? Neighborhood Status and Racism-Related Distress among Black Americans. *Social Forces, 100*(4), 1503–1532. https://doi-org.proxy.tamuc.edu/10.1093/sf/soab075. doi:10.1093foab075 PMID:35847476

Delker, E., Brown, Q., & Hasin, D. S. (2016). Alcohol Consumption in Demographic Subpopulations An Epidemiologic Overview. *Alcohol Research: Current Reviews, 38*(1), 7–15. http://0-www jstor org library ualr edu/stable/42659795 PMID:27159807

Escamilla, S., & Saasa, S. (2020). Gendered Patterns in Depression and Anxiety among African Immigrants in the United States. *Journal of Evidence-Based Social Work (2640-8066), 17*(4), 392–405. https://doi-org.proxy.tamuc.edu/10.1080/2640 8066.2020.1748153

Freeman, D. R. (2006). Spirituality in Violent and Substance-Abusing African American Men: An Untapped Resource for Healing. *Journal of Religion & Spirituality in Social Work, 25*(1), 3–22. https://doi-org.proxy.tamuc.edu/10.1300/J377v25n01_02. doi:10.1300/J377v25n01_02

Gaston, G. B., Earl, T. R., Nisanci, A., & Glomb, B. (2016). Perception of mental health services among Black Americans. *Social Work in Mental Health, 14*(6), 676–695. https://doi-org.proxy.tamuc.edu/10.1080/15332985.2015.1137257. doi: 10.1080/15332985.2015.1137257

Gaston, G. B., Earl, T. R., Nisanci, A., & Glomb, B. (2016). Perception of mental health services among Black Americans. *Social Work in Mental Health, 14*(6), 676–695. https://doi-org.proxy.tamuc.edu/10.1080/15332985.2015.1137257. doi: 10.1080/15332985.2015.1137257

Guerrero, E. G., Marsh, J. C., Cao, D., Shin, H.-C., & Andrews, C. (2014). Gender disparities in utilization and outcome of comprehensive substance abuse treatment among racial/ethnic groups. *Journal of Substance Abuse Treatment, 46*(5), 584–591. https://doi-org.proxy.tamuc.edu/10.1016/j.jsat.2013.12.008. doi:10.1016/j.jsat.2013.12.008 PMID:24560127

Hare, I. (2004). Defining social work for the 21st century. The International Federation of Social Workers' revised definition of social work. *International Social Work, 47*(3), 407–424. doi:10.1177/0020872804043973

Harper, F. D., & Dawkins, M. P. (1977). Alcohol abuse in the Black community. *The Black Scholar, 8*(6), 23–31. doi:10.1080/00064246.1977.11658635

Haughwout, S. P., Harford, T. C., Castle, I.-J. P., & Grant, B. F. (2016). Treatment Utilization Among Adolescent Substance Users: Findings from the 2002 to 2013 National Survey on Drug Use and Health. *Alcoholism, Clinical and Experimental Research, 40*(8), 1717–1727. https://doi-org.proxy.tamuc.edu/10.1111/acer.13137. doi:10.1111/acer.13137 PMID:27427179

Hewitt, C. M. (2004). African-American concentration in jobs the political economy of job segregation and contestation in Atlanta. *Urban Affairs Review, 39*(3), 318–341. doi:10.1177/1078087403253416

Horsman, E. N. (2018). Underage drinking as a predictor of alcohol use disorder among African Americans. *Journal of Psychology in Africa, 28*(4), 323–329. doi: 10.1080/14330237.2018.1507097

Hyde, J. S., & DeLamater, J. D. (2017). Understanding Human Sexuality (13ed.). New York: McGraw-Hill.

Jacobson, J. O., Robinson, P., & Bluthenthal, R. N. (2007). A multilevel decomposition approach to estimate the role of program location and neighborhood disadvantage in racial disparities in alcohol treatment completion. *Social Science & Medicine, 64*(2), 462–476. doi:10.1016/j.socscimed.2006.08.032 PMID:17055634

Jegede, O., Muvvala, S., Katehis, E., Paul, S., Soipe, A., & Jolayemi, A. (2021). Perceived barriers to access care, anticipated discrimination and structural vulnerability among African Americans with substance use disorders. *The International Journal of Social Psychiatry*, *67*(2), 136–143. https://doi-org.proxy.tamuc.edu/10.1177/0020764020934512. doi:10.1177/0020764020934512 PMID:32666877

Jerome, R., Halkitis, P., & Coley, M.The Hope Team. (2009). Methamphetamine use patterns among urban Black men who have sex with men. *Culture, Health & Sexuality*, *11*(4), 399–413. https://doi-org.proxy.tamuc.edu/10.1080/13691050902780768. doi:10.1080/13691050902780768 PMID:19301167

Jin, W. K., Morgan, E., & Nyhan, B. (2020). Treatment versus Punishment: Undersdanding Racial Inequalities in Drug Policy. *Journal of Health Politics, Policy & Law*, *45*(2), 177–209. https://doi-org.proxy.tamuc.edu/10.1215/03616878-8004850

Kanny, D., Liu, Y., & Drewer, R. D. (2009). Binge drinking—United States, 2009. Morbidity and Mortality Weekly Report. National Center for Chronic Disease Prevention and Health Promotion.

Lacey, K. K., Mouzon, D. M., Govia, I. O., Matusko, N., Forsythe-Brown, I., Abelson, J. M., & Jackson, J. S. (2016). Substance Abuse Among Blacks Across the Diaspora. *Substance Use & Misuse*, *51*(9), 1147–1158. https://doi-org.proxy.tamuc.edu/10.3109/10826084.2016.1160124. doi:10.3109/10826084.2016.1160124 PMID:27191862

Latendresse, S. J., Ye, F., Chung, T., Hipwell, A., & Sartor, C. E. (2017). Parental monitoring and alcohol use across adolescence in Black and White girls: A cross-lagged panel mixture model. *Alcoholism, Clinical and Experimental Research*, *41*(6), 1144–1153 https://doi-org/10 1111/acer 13386 PMID:28391598

Linton, S. L., Cooper, H. L. F., Luo, R., Karnes, C., Renneker, K., Haley, D. F., Hunter-Jones, J., Ross, Z., Bonney, L., & Rothenberg, R. (2016). People and places: Relocating to neighborhoods with better economic and social conditions is associated with less risky drug/alcohol network characteristics among African American adults in Atlanta, GA. *Drug and Alcohol Dependence*, *160*, 30–41. https://doi-org.proxy.tamuc.edu/10.1016/j.drugalcdep.2015.11.036. doi:10.1016/j.drugalcdep.2015.11.036 PMID:26781062

Lo, C. C., Howell, R. J., & Cheng, T. C. (2012). Problem drinking by race and nativity: What is learned from social structural and mental health-related data of US-born and immigrant respondents? *The American Journal on Addictions*, *21*, S77–S87. https://doi-org.proxy.tamuc.edu/10.1111/j.1521-0391.2012.00292.x. doi:10.1111/j.1521-0391.2012.00292.x PMID:23786515

Mannes, Z. L., Burrell, L. E., Bryant, V. E., Dunne, E. M., Hearn, L. E., & Whitehead, N. E. (2016). Loneliness and substance use: The influence of gender among HIV+ Black/African American adults 50+. *AIDS Care*, *28*(5), 598–602. https://doi-org.proxy.tamuc.edu/10.1080/09540121.2015.1120269. doi:10.1080/09540121.2015.1120269 PMID:26654243

Marquez-Velarde, G., Miller, G. H., Ma, G., & Keith, V. M. (2022). Psychological Distress among Black Immigrants by Region of Birth. *Journal of Immigrant and Minority Health*, *24*(2), 368–375. https://doi-org.proxy.tamuc.edu/10.1007/s10903-021-01203-w. doi:10.100710903-021-01203-w PMID:33905047

Mays, V. M., Jones, A. L., Delany-Brumsey, A., Coles, C., & Cochran, S. D. (2017). Perceived Discrimination in Health Care and Mental Health/Substance Abuse Treatment Among Blacks, Latinos, and Whites. *Medical Care*, *55*(2), 173–181. https://doi-org.proxy.tamuc.edu/10.1097/MLR.0000000000000638. doi:10.1097/MLR.0000000000000638 PMID:27753743

McGrew, S. J., Raines, A. M., Walker, R. L., Leonard, S. J., & Vujanovic, A. A. (2023). Posttraumatic Stress, Alcohol Use, and Alcohol Use Motives among Non-Hispanic Black/African American College Students: The Role of Emotion Regulation. *Journal of Dual Diagnosis*, *19*(1), 3–15. https://doi-org.proxy.tamuc.edu/10.1080/15504263.2022.2160037. doi:10.1080/15504263.2022.2160037 PMID:36583682

McNeil Smith, S., & Taylor, J. (2015). The Relationship Between Social Stress and Substance Use Among Black Youths Residing in South Florida. *Journal of Child & Adolescent Substance Abuse*, *24*(6), 372–378. https://doi-org.proxy.tamuc.edu/10.1080/1067828X.2013.872062. doi:10.1080/1067828X.2013.872062

Miller, W. R., Sorensen, J. L., Selzer, J. A., & Brigham, G. S. (2006). Disseminating evidence-based practices in substance abuse treatment: A review with suggestions. *Journal of Substance Abuse Treatment*, *31*(1), 25–39. doi:10.1016/j.jsat.2006.03.005 PMID:16814008

Montgomery, L., Burlew, A. K., & Korte, J. E. (2017). Does change in readiness influence retention among African American women and men in substance abuse treatment? *Journal of Ethnicity in Substance Abuse*, *16*(4), 420–431. https://doi-. doi:10.1080/15332640.2017.1300553 PMID:28368681

Mooney, L. A., Knox, D., & Schacht, C. (2015). Understanding Social Problems (9thed.). Standford, CT: Cengage Learning.

Mosley, B., Atkins, B. J., & Klein, M. (1988). Alcoholism and Blacks. *Journal of Alcohol and Drug Education*, *33*(4), 51–58.

Mouzon, D. M., Watkins, D. C., Perry, R., Simpson, T. M., & Mitchell, J. A. (2019). Intergenerational Mobility and Goal-Striving Stress Among Black Americans: The Roles of Ethnicity and Nativity Status. *Journal of Immigrant and Minority Health*, *21*(2), 393–400. https://doi-org.proxy.tamuc.edu/10.1007/s10903-018-0735-4. doi:10.100710903-018-0735-4 PMID:29611019

Mulia, N., Witbrodt, J., Karriker, J. K. J., Li, L., Lui, C. K., & Zapolski, T. (2022). Education matters: Longitudinal pathways to mid-life heavy drinking in a national cohort of black Americans. *Addiction (Abingdon, England)*, *117*(8), 2225–2234. https://doi-org.proxy.tamuc.edu/10.1111/add.15882. doi:10.1111/add.15882 PMID:35320593

Mulia, N., Ye, Y., Zemore, S. E., & Greenfield, T. K. (2008). Social Disadvantage, Stress, and Alcohol Use Among Black, Hispanic, and White Americans: Findings From the 2005 U.S. National Alcohol Survey. *Journal of Studies on Alcohol and Drugs*, *69*(6), 824–833. https://doi-org.proxy.tamuc.edu/10.15288/jsad.2008.69.824. doi:10.15288/jsad.2008.69.824 PMID:18925340

National Institute on Alcohol Abuse and Alcoholism. (1990). *Seventh special report to the U.S. congress on alcohol and health Rockville*. U. S. Department of Health and Human Services.

Ogborne, A. C., Wild, T. C., Braun, K., & Newton-Taylor, B. (1998). Measuring treatment process beliefs among staff of specialized addiction treatment services. *Journal of Substance Abuse Treatment*, *15*(4), 301–312. doi:10.1016/S0740-5472(97)00196-7 PMID:9650138

Patterson, D. A., Dulmus, C. N., & Maguin, E. (2013). Is openness to using empirically supported treatments related to organizational culture and climate? *Journal of Social Service Research*, *39*(4), 562–571. doi:10.1080/01488376.2013.804023 PMID:24159247

Patterson, D. A., Ramsey, A. T., & van den Berk-Clark, C. (2015). Implementing outside the box: Community-based social service provider experiences with using an alcohol screening and intervention. *Journal of Social Service Research*, *41*, 233–245. doi:10.1080/01488376.2014.980963 PMID:25798019

Pederson, A. B., Tsai, A. C., Hawkins, D., Moskowitz, J. T., & Dixon, L. (2023). Understanding the Association Between Mental Health Knowledge and Mental Health Service Utilization Among Black Adults. *Community Mental Health Journal*, *59*(1), 57–67. https://doi-org.proxy.tamuc.edu/10.1007/s10597-022-00988-w. doi:10.100710597-022-00988-w PMID:35794413

Pederson, S. D., Curley, E. J., & Collins, C. J. (2021). A Systematic Review of Motivational Interviewing to Address Substance Use with Justice-Involved Adults. *Substance Use & Misuse*, *56*(5), 639–649. https://doi-org.proxy.tamuc.edu/10.1080/10826084.2021.1887247. doi:10.1080/10826084.2021.1887247 PMID:33726607

Peoples, J. E., Butler-Barnes, S. T., Stafford, J. D., Williams, S.-L., & Smith, I. (2023). Exploring the association between mental health climate and depression: the protective role of positive mental health and sense of belonging among Black college students. *Journal of American College Health*, 1–11. https://doi-org.proxy.tamuc.edu/10.1080/07448481.2022.2155466

Pickard, J. G., Williams Woodson, S.-L., & Johnson, S. D. (2021). The relationship of public and private religiosity to African American women caregivers' use of alcohol for coping with caregiving burden. *Aging & Mental Health*, *25*(3), 551–558. https://doi-org.proxy.tamuc.edu/10.1080/13607863.2019.1699020. doi:10.1080/13607863.2019.1699020 PMID:31809587

Pinedo, M. (2019). A current re-examination of racial/ethnic disparities in the use of substance abuse treatment: Do disparities persist? *Drug and Alcohol Dependence*, *202*, 162–167. https://doi-org.proxy.tamuc.edu/10.1016/j.drugalcdep.2019.05.017. doi:10.1016/j.drugalcdep.2019.05.017 PMID:31352305

Pinedo, M., Zemore, S., & Mulia, N. (2022). Black-White differences in barriers to specialty alcohol and drug treatment: Findings from a qualitative study. *Journal of Ethnicity in Substance Abuse*, *21*(1), 112–126. https://doi-org.proxy.tamuc.edu/10.1080/15332640.2020.1713954. doi:10.1080/15332640.2020.1713954 PMID:31961283

Piowowarczyk, L., Bishop, H., Yusuf, A., Mudymba, F., & Raj, A. (2014). Congolese and Somali beliefs about mental health services. *The Journal of Nervous and Mental Disease*, *202*(3), 209–216. doi:10.1097/NMD.0000000000000087 PMID:24566506

Pittman, D. M., & Kaur, P. (2018). Examining the role of racism in the risky alcohol use behaviors of black female college students. *Journal of American College Health*, *66*(4), 310–316. https://doi-org.proxy.tamuc.edu/10.1080/07448481.2018.1440581. doi:10.1080/07448481.2018.1440581 PMID:29448892

Randall, J., Cunningham, P. B., & Henggeler, S. W. (2018). The Development and Transportability of Multisystemic Therapy-Substance Abuse: A Treatment for Adolescents with Substance Use Disorders. *Journal of Child & Adolescent Substance Abuse*, *27*(2), 59–66. https://doi-org.proxy.tamuc.edu/10.1080/1067828X.2017.1411301. doi:10.1080/1067828X.2017.1411301

Ransome, Y., & Gilman, S. E. (2016). The role of religious involvement in black-white differences in alcohol use severity. *Journal of Studies on Alcohol and Drugs*, *77*(5), 792–801. doi:10.15288/jsad.2016.77.792 PMID:27588538

Redmond, M. L., Smith, S., & Collins, T. C. (2020). Exploring African-American womens' experiences with substance use treatment: A review of the literature. *Journal of Community Psychology*, *48*(2), 337–350. https://doi-org.proxy.tamuc.edu/10.1002/jcop.22241. doi:10.1002/jcop.22241 PMID:31609461

Rigg, K. K. (2017). Motivations for Using MDMA (Ecstasy/Molly) among African Americans: Implications for Prevention and Harm-Reduction Programs. *Journal of Psychoactive Drugs*, *49*(3), 192–200. https://doi-org.proxy.tamuc.edu/10.1080/02791072.2017.1305518. doi:10.1080/02791072.2017.1305518 PMID:28406348

Roxburgh, S., & MacArthur, K. R. (2020). Racial Differences in the Salience of Social Support for Mental Health: An Intersectional Approach. *Michigan Sociological Review*, *34*, 46–72.

Sacks, J. J., Gonzales, K.R., Bouchery, E.E., Tomedi, L,E., & Brewer, R.D. (2010) National and State Costs of Excessive Alcohol Consumption. *American Journal Preventative Medicine, 49*(5), e73–e79.

Saloner, B., & Lê Cook, B. (2013). Blacks And Hispanics Are Less Likely Than Whites To Complete Addiction Treatment, Largely Due To Socioeconomic Factors. *Health Affairs*, *32*(1), 135–145. https://doi-org.proxy.tamuc.edu/10.1377/hlthaff.2011.0983. doi:10.1377/hlthaff.2011.0983 PMID:23297281

Sanders, M. (2002). The Response of African American Communities to Alcohol and Other Drug Problems: An Opportunity for Treatment Providers. *Alcoholism Treatment Quarterly*, *20*(3/4), 167–174. https://doi-org.proxy.tamuc.edu/10.1300/J020v20n03_11. doi:10.1300/J020v20n03_11

Schwartz, B., Bernal, D., Smith, L., & Nicolas, G. (2014). Pathways to understand help-seeking behaviors among Haitians. *Journal of Immigrant and Minority Health*, *16*(2), 239–243. doi:10.100710903-012-9751-y PMID:23192378

Shangani, S., van den Berg, J. J., Dyer, T. V., Mayer, K. H., & Operario, D. (2022). Childhood sexual abuse, alcohol and drug use problems among Black sexual minority men in six US Cities: Findings from the HPTN 061 study. *PLoS One*, *17*(12), 1–13. https://doi-org.proxy.tamuc.edu/10.1371/journal.pone.0279238. doi:10.1371/journal.pone.0279238 PMID:36548261

Skalamera, J., & Hummer, R. A. (2016). Educational attainment and the clustering of health-related behavior among US young adults. *Preventive Medicine*, *84*, 83–89. doi:10.1016/j.ypmed.2015.12.011 PMID:26740348

Staton-Tindall, M., Duvall, J., Stevens-Watkins, D., & Oser, C. B. (2013). The Roles of Spirituality in the Relationship Between Traumatic Life Events, Mental Health, and Drug Use Among African American Women from One Southern State. *Substance Use & Misuse, 48*(12), 1246–1257. https://doi doi:org.proxy.tamuc.edu /10.3109/10826084.2013.799023

Substance Abuse and Mental Health Services Administration. (2023). *Key Substance Use and Mental Health Indicators in the United States: Results from the 2021 National Survey on Drug Use and Health.* SAMHSA. https://www.samhsa.gov/data/sites/default/files/reports/rpt39443/2021NSDUHFFRRev010323.pdf

van Amsterdam, J., & van den Brink, W. (2013). The high harm score of alcohol. Time for drug policy to be revisited? *Journal of Psychopharmacology (Oxford, England)*, *27*(3), 248–255. https://doi-org.proxy.tamuc.edu/10.1177/0269881112472559. doi:10.1177/0269881112472559 PMID:23325370

Van Boekel, B. & Van Weeghel, G. (2013). Stigma among health professionals towards patients with substance use disorders and its consequences for healthcare delivery: systematic review. *Drug Alcohol Depend*, *131,* 23-35. doi:10.1016/j.drugalcdep.2013.02.018

van den Berk-Clark, C., Patterson Silver Wolf, A. U. W. D. A., & Williams, S.-L. (2017). Impact of Race on the Implementation of Empirically Supported Treatments in Substance Abuse Treatment. *Journal of Social Work Practice in the Addictions*, *17*(1/2), 36–56. https://doi-org.proxy.tamuc.edu/10.1080/1533256X.2017.1302883. doi:10.1080/1533256X.2017.1302883

Van-Eerven Ludolf, N., do Carmo Silva, M., Simões Gomes, C. F., & Oliveira, V. M. (2017). The Organizational Culture and Values Alignment Management Importance for Successful Business. *Brazilian Journal of Operations & Production Management*, *14*(2), 272–280. https://doi-org.proxy.tamuc.edu/10.14488/BJOPM.2017.v14.n2.a15. doi:10.14488/BJOPM.2017.v14.n2.a15

Van Gundy, K. T., Howerton-Orcutt, A., & Mills, M. L. (2015). Race, Coping Style, and Substance Use Disorder Among Non-Hispanic African American and White Young Adults in South Florida. *Substance Use & Misuse*, *50*(11), 1459–1469. https://doi-org.proxy.tamuc.edu/10.3109/10826084.2015.1018544. doi:10.3109/10826084.2015.1018544 PMID:26549159

Vidourek, R. A., King, K. A., Burbage, M., & Okuley, B. (2018). Impact of Parenting Behaviors on Recent Alcohol Use Among African American Students. *Child & Adolescent Social Work Journal*, *35*(3), 271–282. https://doi-org.proxy.tamuc.edu/10.1007/s10560-017-0524-2. doi:10.100710560-017-0524-2

Ward, E. C., & Heidrich, S. M. (2009). African American women's beliefs about mental illness, stigma, and preferred coping behaviors. *Research in Nursing & Health*, *32*(5), 480–492. doi:10.1002/nur.20344 PMID:19650070

Washington, H. (2006). *Medical apartheid: The dark history of medical experimentation on black Americans from colonial times to the present*. Random House.

Watkins-Hayes, C. (2009). Raceing the bootstrap climb: Black and Latino bureaucrats in post-reform welfare offices. *Social Problems*, *56*(2), 285–310. doi:10.1525p.2009.56.2.285

Watkins-Hayes, C. (2011). Race, respect, and red tape: Inside the black box of racially representative bureaucracies. *Journal of Public Administration: Research and Theory*, *21*(Suppl. 2), i233–i251. doi:10.1093/jopart/muq096

Weiss-Gal, I. (2008). The Person-in-Environment Approach: Professional Ideology and Practice of Social Workers in Israel. *Social Work*, *53*(1), 65–75. https://doi-org.proxy.tamuc.edu/10.1093/sw/53.1.65. doi:10.1093w/53.1.65 PMID:18610822

Wheeler, J. R., & Nahra, T. A. (2000). Private and public ownership in outpatient substance abuse treatment: Do we have a two-tiered system? *Administration and Policy in Mental Health*, *27*(4), 197–209. doi:10.1023/A:1021357318246 PMID:10911669

Williams, E. C., Gupta, S., Rubinsky, A. D., Jones-Webb, R., Bensley, K. M., Young, J. P., & Harris, A. H. S. (2016) Racial/ethnic differences in the prevalence of clinically recognized alcohol use disorders among patients from the U S Veterans Health Administration Alcoholism. *Clinical and Experimental Research*, *40*(2), 359–366 https://doi 12950 PMID:26842254 doi:org/101111/acer

Williams, J. E., Newby, R. G., & Kanitz, H. E. (1993). Assessing the Need for Alcohol Abuse Programs for African-American College Students. *Journal of Multicultural Counseling and Development*, *21*(3), 155–167. https://doi-org.proxy.tamuc.edu/10.1002/j.2161-1912.1993.tb00595.x. doi:10.1002/j.2161-1912.1993.tb00595.x

Williams, S.-L. L., & Cabrera-Nguyen, E. P. (2016). Impact of lifetime evaluated need on mental health service use among African American emerging adults. *Cultural Diversity & Ethnic Minority Psychology*, *22*(2), 205–214. https://doi-org.proxy.tamuc.edu/10.1037/cdp0000040. doi:10.1037/cdp0000040 PMID:25844566

Windsor, L. C., Jemal, A., & Alessi, E. J. (2015). Cognitive Behavioral Therapy: A Meta-Analysis of Race and Substance Use Outcomes. *Cultural Diversity & Ethnic Minority Psychology*, *21*(2), 300–313. https://doi-org.proxy.tamuc.edu/10.1037/a0037929. doi:10.1037/a0037929 PMID:25285527

Wong, E. C., Derose, K. P., Miles, J. N. V., & Litt, P. (2018). Sources of Care for Alcohol and Other Drug Problems: The Role of the African American Church. *Journal of Religion and Health*, *57*(4), 1200–1210. https://doi-org.proxy.tamuc.edu/10.1007/s10943-017-0412-2. doi:10.100710943-017-0412-2 PMID:28502023

World Health Organization. (2022). *Drugs Impact*. WHO. https://www.who.int/health-topics/drugs-psychoactive#tab=tab_2

World Health Organization. (2023). *Alcohol Overview*. WHO. https://www.who.int/health-topics/alcohol#tab=tab_1

Yu, Y., Matlin, S. L., Crusto, C. A., Hunter, B., & Tebes, J. K. (2022). Double Stigma and Help-Seeking Barriers Among Blacks With a Behavioral Health Disorder. *Psychiatric Rehabilitation Journal*, *45*(2), 183–191. https://doi doi:org.proxy.tamuc.edu/10.1037/prj0000507

Zapolski, T. C. B., Pedersen, S. L., McCarthy, D. M., & Smith, G. T. (2014). Less Drinking, Yet More Problems: Understanding African American Drinking and Related Problems. *Psychological Bulletin*, *140*(1), 188–223. https://doi-org.proxy.tamuc.edu/10.1037/a0032113. doi:10.1037/a0032113 PMID:23477449

Zemore, S. E., Mulia, N., Williams, E., & Gilbert, P. A. (2017). Job loss and alcohol dependence among Blacks and Whites in a National Longitudinal Survey. *Journal of Ethnicity in Substance Abuse*, *16*(3), 314–327. https://doi-org.proxy.tamuc.edu/10.1080/15332640.2016.1209144. doi:10.1080/15332640.2016.1209144 PMID:27594166

Zwick, J., Appleseth, H., & Arndt, S. (2020). Stigma: How it affects the substance use disorder patient. *Substance Abuse Treatment, Prevention, and Policy*, *15*(1), 1–4. https://doi-org.proxy.tamuc.edu/10.1186/s13011-020-00288-0. doi:10.118613011-020-00288-0 PMID:32718328

Chapter 14
The Impact of the Psychoeducational Approach:
Changing the Stigma of Mental Health

Sindu Padmanabhan
https://orcid.org/0000-0001-8267-1112
Bharathiar University, India

ABSTRACT

People who suffer from mental diseases may encounter stigma; they could be treated differently, judged negatively, or made to feel undeserving or lower than others. Stigma can lead to discrimination, which can make mental illness worse. It arises as a result of misunderstandings and false information about mental illness, as well as some people's unfavorable opinions or beliefs (prejudice). This could lead to discrimination against people who have mental illnesses. The lives of many people can be changed by helping to understand what emotions are, how to detect them, what they mean, and how to cope with them healthily with the help of psychoeducation. The initial step is to educate oneself on the basics of mental illness. Make sure there is a safe space where individuals feel appreciated, where they can be honest about their struggles, and where they can express their emotions. Ask them if they feel that receiving treatment for a mental disorder will harm them. If necessary, add counseling and other forms of support services to the medical care.

DOI: 10.4018/978-1-6684-8918-5.ch014

INTRODUCTION

Stigma

Stigma is a social phenomenon characterized by negative attitudes, beliefs, stereotypes, or discrimination directed towards a particular group or individuals with certain characteristics, attributes, or circumstances that are perceived as different or deviating from what is considered "normal" or socially accepted. Stigma can be experienced by individuals or groups in various contexts, such as mental health, physical health, race, gender, sexual orientation, disability, and more. Stigmatized individuals often face prejudice, bias, and exclusion due to the stigma associated with their identity or situation.

Key Aspects of Stigma

Stigmatized individuals may be labeled or categorized based on certain characteristics, leading to the perception that they are somehow inferior, flawed, or less deserving of respect. Stereotypes are oversimplified and often inaccurate beliefs about a particular group. These stereotypes contribute to stigma by reinforcing negative assumptions and generalizations.

Prejudice involves negative feelings or attitudes towards individuals based on their stigmatized characteristics. Prejudiced beliefs can lead to discriminatory actions. Discrimination is the unjust or differential treatment of individuals or groups based on their stigmatized attributes. This can manifest in various ways, such as unequal opportunities, exclusion, or denial of rights.

Stigma can have significant emotional, psychological, and social effects on individuals. It can lead to feelings of shame, isolation, and low self-esteem. Stigmatized individuals may be less likely to seek help, participate in social activities, or access necessary services. Refers to the negative attitudes and beliefs held by the broader society about a specific group. Public stigma can contribute to social exclusion and reinforce the cycle of discrimination. This occurs when individuals internalize the negative beliefs and stereotypes directed at their stigmatized attributes, leading to feelings of self-blame, reduced self-worth, and diminished self-efficacy.

Addressing stigma requires education, awareness, challenging stereotypes, promoting empathy, and creating inclusive environments. Efforts to combat stigma can be targeted at both the individual level (changing attitudes) and the systemic level (changing policies and structures). Understanding and challenging stigma is crucial for building a more inclusive, empathetic, and equitable society. It involves recognizing the harmful effects of stigma and working to create environments that value diversity and treat all individuals with dignity and respect.

MENTAL HEALTH STIGMA

Mental health stigma refers to the negative attitudes, beliefs, stereotypes, and discrimination that individuals with mental health conditions often face from others. This stigma can manifest in various ways, including social exclusion, labeling, or misunderstanding. Stigma is a significant barrier that can prevent individuals from seeking help, support, and treatment for their mental health issues.

Key Aspects of Mental Health Stigma

Public stigma refers to the general attitudes and beliefs that the public holds about mental illness. Negative stereotypes, misconceptions, and the perception that individuals with mental health conditions are dangerous or unpredictable contribute to public stigma. People with mental health conditions may internalize negative stereotypes and beliefs about mental illness, leading to self-stigma. This self-judgment can reduce self-esteem, hinder recovery, and discourage help-seeking. Structural Stigma exists in societal institutions, policies, and systems. It can manifest as unequal access to healthcare, limited resources for mental health services, and discriminatory practices in areas such as education or employment. Stigma can have profound effects on individuals' lives. It may lead to isolation, reluctance to disclose their condition, reduced opportunities for education and employment, and decreased quality of life. Stigma is a significant factor that prevents many individuals from seeking professional help for mental health issues. The fear of judgment, labeling, or being treated differently can discourage people from accessing the care they need.

The portrayal of mental health in the media can contribute to stigma by perpetuating stereotypes or sensationalizing mental health issues. Accurate and sensitive representation in the media is crucial in combating stigma. Education and awareness campaigns play a vital role in challenging stigma. Providing accurate information about mental health conditions, sharing personal stories, and promoting empathy can help reduce stigma. Creating a supportive and inclusive environment in communities, schools, workplaces, and healthcare settings can help reduce stigma. Encouraging open conversations about mental health and providing resources for support can make a positive difference.

Advocating for laws and policies that protect the rights of individuals with mental health conditions and promote equal access to healthcare and opportunities can help address structural stigma. Reducing mental health stigma is essential for creating a society where individuals feel safe, supported, and empowered to seek help and lead fulfilling lives regardless of their mental health status.

MENTAL HEALTH STIGMA AND ITS CONSEQUENCES

Mental health stigma refers to the negative attitudes, stereotypes, and discriminatory beliefs that society holds towards individuals with mental health conditions. These stigmatizing attitudes can have severe consequences for both individuals experiencing mental health challenges and the broader community.

Key Consequences of Mental Health Stigma

Stigma often leads individuals to avoid seeking professional help for mental health issues. Fear of being judged, labeled, or ostracized can prevent people from accessing necessary mental health services, resulting in delayed treatment and potentially worsened outcomes. Stigmatized individuals may feel isolated and alienated from their social networks. Friends, family, and colleagues may distance themselves due to a lack of understanding or fear, leading to feelings of loneliness and disconnection.

Internalized stigma occurs when individuals with mental health conditions internalize negative stereotypes, leading to lowered self-esteem, shame, and a negative self-image. This can hinder their ability to cope effectively. Stigma can affect various life domains, including employment, housing, relationships, and education. Discrimination in these areas can limit opportunities, leading to a reduced quality of life.

Stigma can undermine individuals' belief in their capacity to recover from mental health challenges. This lack of confidence may affect adherence to treatment plans and contribute to a longer and more difficult recovery process. Stigma may create barriers to education for individuals with mental health conditions. These barriers can include bullying, lack of accommodations, and decreased access to educational opportunities.

Mental health stigma can lead to chronic stress, which can have detrimental effects on physical health. The physiological toll of stigma-related stress can increase the risk of various health issues. Stigma-related employment discrimination can result in job loss or underemployment, contributing to financial instability for individuals with mental health conditions. This economic impact affects not only individuals but also their families.

Stigma can lead to reduced public investment in mental health services, research, and public awareness campaigns. This underfunding hinders efforts to provide effective mental health care and education. Stigma infringes upon the human rights and dignity of individuals with mental health conditions. It perpetuates inequality, hampers access to basic rights, and reinforces social injustice.

Addressing mental health stigma is essential for creating a more compassionate and supportive society. This requires raising awareness, promoting education, encouraging open dialogue, and advocating for policies that protect the rights and well-being of individuals with mental health conditions. Reducing stigma benefits individuals, families, communities, and public health as a whole.

Figure 1. The vicious cycle of stigma

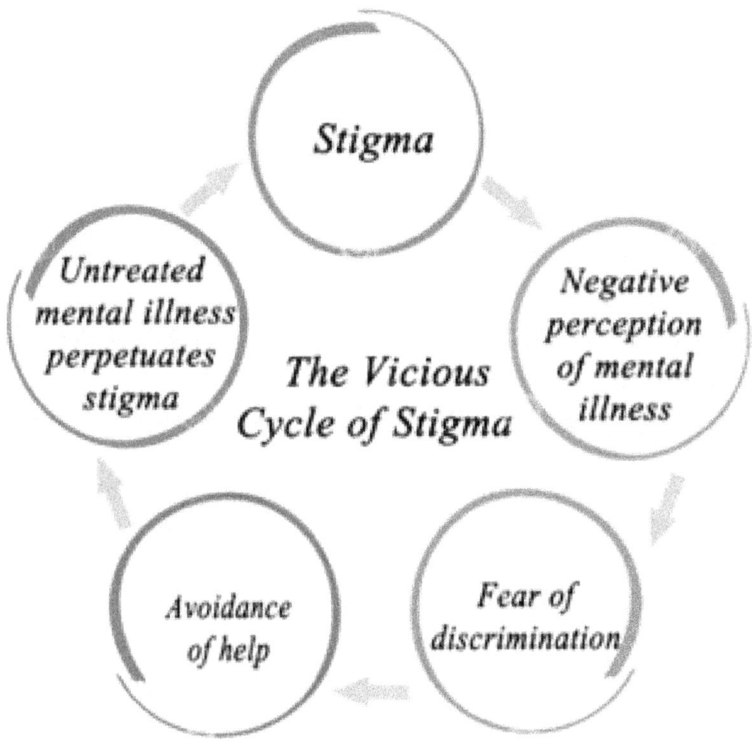
Stigma
Negative perception of mental illness
Fear of discrimination
Avoidance of help
Untreated mental illness perpetuates stigma
The Vicious Cycle of Stigma

The perception of mental health services among Black Americans is influenced by a complex interplay of historical, cultural, systemic, and socio-economic factors. Understanding these factors is crucial for improving mental health services accessibility and effectiveness for this population. It's essential to recognize that the experiences and perceptions of mental health services among Black Americans are diverse, and any strategies to improve services should consider this diversity and address the unique needs of individuals within the community. Black Americans have experienced significant historical traumas, including slavery, systemic racism, and discrimination. These historical experiences can impact trust in institutions, including mental health services provided by predominantly white systems (Gaston et al. (2016).

African Americans living in the rural South often have unique perspectives shaped by a combination of historical, cultural, social, economic, and geographic factors. It's crucial to approach the perspectives of African Americans in the rural South with cultural sensitivity and an understanding of the historical context. Recognizing the strengths and resilience of these communities, addressing systemic disparities, and supporting community-based initiatives can help improve the quality of life and opportunities for African Americans in rural areas while honoring their unique experiences and perspectives (Hayes et al. 2017). Mental health disparities among college students of color are a significant concern that highlights the intersection of mental health, race, and higher education. These disparities reflect a complex interplay of cultural, social, systemic, and institutional factors that can impact the mental well-being of students from diverse racial and ethnic backgrounds (Lipson et al. 2018).

Perceived and personal mental health stigma in Latino and African American college students can have significant implications for their mental well-being, help-seeking behaviors, and overall college experiences. Understanding the dynamics of stigma within these communities is essential for providing appropriate support and reducing barriers to mental health care (DeFreitas et al., 2018). Barriers to the utilization of mental health services on college campuses by African-American students can be complex and multifaceted, stemming from a combination of cultural, systemic, and institutional factors. Recognizing and addressing these barriers is crucial for improving the mental health and well-being of African American students (Anderson et al., 2018) The relationship between skin tone, life satisfaction, psychological distress, and stigma consciousness among African Americans is a complex and important area of study. This topic explores how perceived skin tone affects well-being and the potential mediating role of stigma consciousness (Gaddy et al., 2020).

Diagnostic labeling and mental illness stigma among Black Americans are significant issues with far-reaching implications for mental health care and overall well-being. Understanding how diagnostic labels interact with stigma is crucial for promoting equitable and effective mental health support within this community Abdullah et al., (2020). It is essential to note that stigma can vary across regions, communities, and cultural backgrounds. Additionally, the ongoing evolution of public attitudes toward mental health is influenced by current events, advocacy efforts, and ongoing education. By addressing stigma, understanding the unique challenges faced by African American male college students, and providing culturally competent support, colleges can foster an environment where these students feel comfortable seeking help and accessing the counseling services they need to thrive academically and personally. (Shannon, et al., 2022).

Anxiety-related disorders in the context of racism are a significant concern, particularly for individuals who experience racial discrimination or belong to marginalized racial or ethnic groups. Racism can contribute to heightened stress, anxiety, and the development of various anxiety disorders (MacIntyre et al., 2023).

IMPACT OF PSYCHOEDUCATIONAL APPROACH: CHANGING THE STIGMA OF MENTAL HEALTH

The psychoeducational approach can have a significant impact on changing the stigma surrounding mental health. Stigma is a major barrier that prevents many individuals from seeking help for their mental health issues. Psychoeducation helps people understand that mental health issues are common and affect a significant portion of the population. This awareness alone can reduce the perception that mental health problems are rare or that individuals experiencing them are somehow abnormal. The psychoeducational approach provides accurate information about mental health, its causes, symptoms, and available treatments. Dispelling myths and misconceptions through education can counteract stigmatizing beliefs and foster a more informed and empathetic perspective. By sharing personal stories, experiences, and insights, psychoeducational programs can humanize mental health issues. When individuals understand that mental health challenges can happen to anyone and that they are not indicative of a person's character or worth, it helps break down stigma.

Learning about the struggles that individuals with mental health issues face encourages empathy and compassion. Understanding the emotional and psychological pain associated with these challenges can lead to more supportive attitudes. One of the primary consequences of stigma is the reluctance to seek help for mental health concerns. Psychoeducation can empower individuals to seek support early, reducing the negative impact of untreated mental health issues. Group-based psychoeducational programs create a sense of community among participants. When individuals share their experiences and support each other, it fosters a sense of belonging and reduces feelings of isolation, which can be particularly beneficial in combating stigma.

Psychoeducation challenges stereotypes about mental health and those who experience it. It encourages individuals to view mental health issues as medical conditions that deserve understanding and appropriate care, just like physical health conditions. The more widespread the understanding of mental health becomes, the more likely it is that public discourse and policies will shift to be more supportive and inclusive. This can lead to improved access to mental health services and resources.

Psychoeducation, which involves providing individuals with knowledge and understanding about their mental health condition, treatment options, coping strategies, and available resources, can have several positive effects on Korean Americans with chronic mental illness. To maximize the effectiveness of psychoeducation for Korean Americans with chronic mental illness, it's crucial to collaborate with mental health professionals who understand cultural nuances, provide materials in the Korean language, and involve community leaders or organizations to ensure that the program is culturally appropriate. By addressing the specific needs and challenges faced by Korean Americans, psychoeducation can play a vital role in improving mental health outcomes within this community (Sun-Kyung Shin et al., 2002).

Neurobiology-based psychoeducation is a powerful approach for reducing the stigma associated with depression and promoting a better understanding of the condition. By providing individuals with accurate information about the underlying biological factors contributing to depression, this form of education helps challenge misconceptions, normalize the experience, and foster empathy (Han et al., 2014).

A brief psychoeducational program targeting stigma in Malaysian pre-clinical medical students can have several important effects. Addressing stigma early in medical education is crucial to fostering more empathetic and effective healthcare professionals (Fernandez et al.,2016). A psychoeducational intervention aimed at reducing internalized stigma among psychosocial rehabilitation clients can have several positive outcomes. Internalized stigma, which involves individuals adopting negative beliefs about themselves due to societal stereotypes and prejudices related to mental illness, can be a significant barrier to recovery and well-being (Lucksted et al., 2017). A group psychoeducation program targeting self-stigma, empowerment, and perceived discrimination of individuals with schizophrenia can have significant positive effects on their well-being, self-perception, and overall quality of life (Ivezi, 2017).

Brief, passive psychoeducation targeting suicide literacy, stigma reduction, and attitudes toward help-seeking among Latino immigrants in the United States can have important and positive effects. These outcomes are crucial, as suicide prevention and mental health support are essential for this population (Dueweke et al., 2017). Randomized controlled trials (RCTs) examining various psychoeducation modalities in the management of bipolar disorder have yielded valuable insights into the effectiveness of these interventions. Psychoeducation is an essential component of bipolar disorder treatment, providing individuals and their families with knowledge, skills, and support to better understand and manage the condition(Soo et al., 2018).

The effects of mindfulness-based psychoeducation on the internalized stigmatization level of patients with schizophrenia can be highly beneficial. Addressing internalized stigma, where individuals with schizophrenia may adopt negative beliefs about themselves due to societal stereotypes, is important for their mental well-being and recovery(Yilmaz et al., 2018). Psychoeducation is a valuable opportunity for patients, psychiatrists, and psychiatric educators, offering benefits that extend beyond traditional clinical interactions. This approach focuses on educating patients about their mental health condition, treatment options, coping strategies, and overall well-being (Motlova et al., 2017).

The effect of psychoeducation on the internalized stigma of hospitalized patients with bipolar disorder can be significant and beneficial. Addressing internalized stigma in a hospital setting is essential for the well-being and recovery of individuals with bipolar disorder(Keshavarzpir et al., 2020). A psychoeducational mental health promotion intervention in comprehensive schools with a focus on recognizing problems and reducing stigma can have significant positive effects on students' well-being, awareness, and attitudes toward mental health. This type of intervention is essential for fostering a supportive and inclusive school environment(Onnela et al., **2021).**

Overall, the psychoeducational approach plays a vital role in changing the stigma of mental health by increasing awareness, promoting empathy, encouraging help-seeking behavior, and fostering a more informed and compassionate society.

DEFINITION OF TERMS

The Seven Types of Stigmas

Public Stigma -Public stigma, also known as social stigma, refers to the negative attitudes, beliefs, and stereotypes that society holds about certain individuals or groups based on characteristics such as their race, ethnicity, gender, sexual orientation, disability, mental health condition, or any other distinguishing feature. This stigma can lead to discrimination, exclusion, and unequal treatment, ultimately harming the well-being and opportunities of the stigmatized individuals.

Self-Stigma- Self-stigma, also known as internalized stigma or self-shame, refers to the process by which individuals with a stigmatized condition or identity (such as mental illness, HIV/AIDS, substance abuse, or other marginalized characteristics) internalize the negative attitudes, stereotypes, and judgments that society holds about them. It involves individuals adopting these negative perceptions as part of their self-concept, leading to feelings of shame, low self-esteem, and a reduced sense of self-worth.

Perceived Stigma - Perceived stigma refers to the subjective experience of individuals who feel that they are being judged, devalued, or socially excluded due to certain characteristics, behaviors, or conditions that society considers deviant or undesirable. This feeling of stigma can arise from real or imagined societal attitudes and beliefs, leading individuals to anticipate negative reactions or discrimination from others.

Label Avoidance - "Label avoidance" typically refers to the practice of avoiding or rejecting certain labels or categorizations in the context of personal identity, social identity, or group affiliation. It can be a response to the perceived limitations or stereotypes associated with specific labels, or it may reflect an individual's desire to maintain a more nuanced or complex understanding of themselves or their identity.

Stigma by Association- "Stigma by association" refers to a situation in which an individual or group is stigmatized or judged negatively based on their perceived connection or association with another individual or group that is itself stigmatized or negatively viewed by society. This concept is rooted in the idea that people can face discrimination or bias simply because of their affiliation with a stigmatized person, group, or identity, even if they do not possess the characteristics or behaviors that society finds stigmatizing.

Structural stigma- Structural stigma refers to the societal-level conditions, institutions, and policies that create and perpetuate discrimination, prejudice, and disadvantage for certain groups of people based on their characteristics or identities. Unlike interpersonal or individual-level stigma, which involves biased attitudes and behaviors from individuals, structural stigma operates at a broader level, embedded within social, economic, and political systems.

Health Practitioner Stigma- Health practitioner stigma refers to the negative attitudes, beliefs, and stereotypes that are directed towards individuals who work in healthcare professions. This stigma can come from various sources, including the general public, patients, other healthcare professionals, and even the practitioners themselves.

REFERENCES

Anderson, M. S. (2018). Barriers to the Utilization of Mental Health Services on College Campuses by African-American Students. *McNair Scholars Research Journal, 11*(3). https://commons.emich.edu/mcnair/vol11/iss1/3

DeFreitas, S., Crone, T., DeLeon, M., & Ajayi, A. (2018). Perceived and Personal Mental Health Stigma in Latino and African American College Students. *Frontiers in Public Health, 6*, 49–. doi:10.3389/fpubh.2018.00049

Dueweke, A. R., & Bridges, A. J. (2017). *Stigma and Health: The effects of brief, passive psychoeducation on suicide literacy, stigma, and attitudes toward help-seeking among Latino immigrants living in the United States*. APA. psycnet.apa.org

Fernandez, A., Tan, K.-A., Knaak, S., Chew, B. H., & Ghazali, S. S. (2016). Effects of Brief Psychoeducational Program on Stigma in Malaysian Pre-clinical Medical Students: A Randomized Controlled Trial. *Academic Psychiatry*, *40*(6), 905–911. doi:10.100740596-016-0592-1 PMID:27527730

Gina, B. (2016, November). Gaston Ph.D., LCSW, Tara R. Earl MSW, Ph.D., Aslihan Nisanci MSW, MA & Blake Glomb BA (2016): Perception of Mental Health Services among Black Americans. *Social Work in Mental Health, 14*(6), 676–695. doi:10.1080/15332985.2015.1137257

Grappone, G. (2018). Overcoming Stigma. *National Alliance on Mental Illness (NAMI)*. https://www.nami.org/Blogs/NAMI-Blog/October-2018/Overcoming-Stigma

Haddad, P. & Haddad, I. (2015). Mental Health Stigma. *British Association for Psychopharmacology (BAP)* Articles [online]. https://www.bap.org.uk/articles/mental-health-stigma/

Han, D.-Y., & Chen, S.-H. (2014). Reducing the stigma of depression through neurobiology-based psychoeducation: A randomized controlled trial. *Psychiatry and Clinical Neurosciences*, *68*(9), 666–673. doi:10.1111/pcn.12174 PMID:24521323

Ivezić, S. Š., Sesar, M. A., & Mužinić, L. (2017) Effects of a group psychoeducation program on self-stigma, empowerment and perceived discrimination of persons with schizophrenia. Psychiatria Danubina, 29(1), pp 66-73.

Keshavarzpir, Z., Seyedfatemi, N., Mardani-Hamooleh, M., Esmaeeli, N., & Boyd, J. E. (2020). The Effect of Psychoeducation on Internalized Stigma of the Hospitalized Patients with Bipolar Disorder: A Quasi-Experimental Study. *Issues in Mental Health Nursing*, 1–8. doi:10.1080/01612840.2020.1779881 PMID:32881602

Lipson, S. K., Kern, A., Eisenberg, D., & Breland-Noble, A. M. (2018). Mental Health Disparities Among College Students of Color. *The Journal of Adolescent Health*, *63*(3), 348–356. doi:10.1016/j.jadohealth.2018.04.014 PMID:30237000

Lucksted, A., Drapalski, A. L., Brown, C. H., Wilson, C., Charlotte, M., Mullane, A., & Fang, L. J. (2017). Outcomes of a Psychoeducational Intervention to Reduce Internalized Stigma Among Psychosocial Rehabilitation Clients. *Psychiatric Services (Washington, D.C.)*, *68*(4), 360–367. doi:10.1176/appi.ps.201600037 PMID:27903136

MacIntyre, M. M., Zare, M., & Williams, M. (2023). Anxiety-Related Disorders in the Context of Racism. *Current Psychiatry Reports*, *25*(2), 31–43. doi:10.100711920-022-01408-2 PMID:36645562

McCleary-Gaddy, A. T. & James, D. (2020). Skin tone, life satisfaction, and psychological distress among African Americans: The mediating effect of stigma consciousness. *Journal of Health Psychology*. doi:10.1177/1359105320954251

Motlova, L. B., Balon, R., Beresin, E. V., Brenner, A. M., Coverdale, J. H., Guerrero, A. P. S., Louie, A. K., & Roberts, L. W. (2017). Psychoeducation as an Opportunity for Patients, Psychiatrists, and Psychiatric Educators: Why Do We Ignore It? *Academic Psychiatry, 41*(4), 447–451. doi:10.100740596-017-0728-y PMID:28536990

Onnela, A., Hurtig, T., & Ebeling, H. (2021). A psychoeducational mental health promotion intervention in comprehensive schools: Recognising problems and reducing stigma. *Health Education Journal, 80*(5), 554–566. doi:10.1177/0017896921994134

Pescosolido, B., Halpern-Manners, A., & Luo, L. (2021). Trends in public stigma of mental illness in the US, 1996-2018. *JAMA Netw Open*. doi:10.1001/jamanetworkopen.2021.40202 PMID:34932103

Shannon, J., Seward, D. X., Liu, Y., & Stigma, M. L. (2022, October). help-seeking, and counseling with African American male college students. *Journal of Counseling and Development, 100*(4), 421–432. Advance online publication. doi:10.1002/jcad.12435

Soo, S., Zhang, Z., Jia, S., & Khong, E. (2018). Randomized Controlled Trials of Psychoeducation Modalities in the Management of Bipolar Disorder: A Systematic Review. *Journal of Clinical Psychiatry*.

Sun-Kyung Shin, M. S. W. (2002). Effects of Psychoeducation for Korean Americans with Chronic Mental Illness. *Psychiatric Services*. doi:10.1176/appi.ps.53.9.1125

Yılmaz, E., & Kavak, F. (2018). Effects of Mindfulness-Based Psychoeducation on the Internalized Stigmatization Level of Patients with Schizophrenia. *Clinical Nursing Research*, 105477381879787–. https://www.bap.org.uk/articles/mental-health-stigma/ https://www.nami.org/Blogs/NAMI-Blog/October-2018/Overcoming-Stigma doi:10.1177/1054773818797871

Compilation of References

Abdullah, T., & Brown, T. L. (2020). Diagnostic labeling and mental illness stigma among Black Americans: An experimental vignette study. *Stigma and Health*, *5*(1), 11–21. doi:10.1037ah0000162

Abdullah, T., Graham-LoPresti, J. R., Tahirkheli, N. N., Hughley, S. M., & Watson, L. J. (2021). Microaggressions and posttraumatic stress disorder symptom scores among Black Americans: Exploring the link. *Traumatology*, *27*(3), 244–253. doi:10.1037/trm0000259

Abuse, S. (2019). *Mental Health Services Administration. (2019). Key substance use and mental health indicators in the United States: Results from the 2018 National Survey on Drug Use and Health (HHS Publication No. PEP19-5068, NSDUH Series H-54).* Rockville, MD: Center for Behavioral Health Statistics and Quality. Substance Abuse and Mental Health Services Administration. https://www. samhsa. gov/data

Acevedo, A., Garnick, D. W., Lee, M. T., Horgan, C. M., Ritter, G., Panas, L., Davis, S., Leeper, T., Moore, R., & Reynolds, M. (2012). Racial and ethnic differences in substance abuse treatment initiation and engagement. *Journal of Ethnicity in Substance Abuse*, *11*(1), 1–21. https://doi-org.proxy.tamuc.edu/10.1080/15332640.2012.652516. doi:10.1080/15332640.2012.652516 PMID:22381120

Ackermann, G., Haugke, C., Schaumann, R., von Salis-Soglio, G., & Rodloff, A. C. (2000). Chronic factitious illness presenting as Munchausen's gonarthritis. *European Journal of Clinical Microbiology & Infectious Diseases*, *19*(1), 70–71. doi:10.1007100960050016 PMID:10706187

Adamus-Leach, H. J., Wilson, P. L., O'Connor, D. P., Rhode, P. C., Mama, S. K., & Lee, R. E. (2013). Depression, stress and body fat are associated with binge eating in a community sample of African American and Hispanic women. *Eating and Weight Disorders*, *18*(2), 221–227. doi:10.100740519-013-0021-3 PMID:23760851

Addis, M. E., & Mahalik, J. R. (2003). Men, masculinity, and the contexts of help seeking. *The American Psychologist*, *58*(1), 5–14. doi:10.1037/0003-066X.58.1.5 PMID:12674814

Addison, T. E., & Talan, K. H. (1974). Letter: Jet-set Münchausen syndrome. *The New England Journal of Medicine*, *291*(22), 1195. doi:10.1056/NEJM197411282912225 PMID:4419976

Adewale, V., Ritchie, D., & Everhart Skeels, S. (2016). African American and African perspectives on mental health: A pilot study of the pre and post colonial and slavery influences and their implications on mental health. *Journal of Communication in Healthcare*, *9*(2), 78–89. doi:10.1080/17538068.2016.1170316

Aduan, R. P., Fauci, A. S., Dale, D. C., Herzberg, J. C., & Wolff, S. M. (1979). Factitious fever and self-induced infection: A report of 32 cases and review of the literature. *Annals of Internal Medicine*, *90*(2), 230–242. doi:10.7326/0003-4819-90-2-230 PMID:443658

Affleck, W., Carmichael, V., & Whitley, R. (2018). Men's mental health: Social determinants and implications for services. *Canadian Journal of Psychiatry*, *63*(9), 581–589. doi:10.1177/0706743718762388 PMID:29673270

Algeria, M., Chatterji, P., Wells, K., Cao, Z., Chen, C. N., Takeuchi, D., & Meng, X. L. (2008). Disparity in depression treatment among racial and ethnic minority populations in the United States. *Psychiatric Services (Washington, D.C.)*, *59*(11), 1264–1272. doi:10.1176/ps.2008.59.11.1264 PMID:18971402

Ali, A., Caplan, P. J., & Fagnant, R. (2010). Gender stereotypes in diagnostic criteria. In *Handbook of gender research in psychology* (pp. 91–109). Springer., doi:10.1007/978-1-4419-1467-5_5

Alicandri-Ciufelli, M., Moretti, V., Ruberto, M., Monzani, D., Chiarini, L., & Presutti, L. (2012). Otolaryngology fantastica: The ear, nose, and throat manifestations of Munchausen's syndrome. *The Laryngoscope*, *122*(1), 51–57. doi:10.1002/lary.22373 PMID:22095880

Almenara, C. A. (2022). 40 years of research on eating disorders in domain-specific journals: Bibliometrics, network analysis, and topic modeling. *PLoS One*, *17*(12), 1–21. doi:10.1371/journal.pone.0278981 PMID:36520823

Altaf, A. (2011). The Impact of Organizational Culture on Organizational Effectiveness: Implication of Hofstede Cultural Model as Organizational Effectiveness Model. *The International Journal of Interdisciplinary Social Sciences: Annual Review*, *6*(1), 161–174. doi:10.18848/1833-1882/CGP/v06i01/51996

Amaro, H., Larson, M. J., Gampel, J., Richardson, E., Savage, A., & Wagler, D. (2005). Racial/Ethnic Differences in Social Vulnerability among Women with Co-Occurring Mental Health and Substance Abuse Disorders: Implications for Treatment Services. *Journal of Community Psychology*, *33*(4), 495–511. doi:10.1002/jcop.20065

Ameh, V., & Speak, N. (2008). Factitious hypoglycaemia in a nondiabetic patient. *European Journal of Emergency Medicine*, *15*(1), 59–60. doi:10.1097/MEJ.0b013e3282aa3f70 PMID:18180671

American Association for Marriage and Family Therapy (AAMFT). (2015). *Code of ethics*. AAMFT. https://www.aamft.org/Legal_Ethics/Code_of_Ethics.aspx

American Psychiatric Association. (1994). *Diagnostic and Statistical Manual of Mental Disorders: DSM-4*. American Psychiatric Association.

American Psychiatric Association. (2000). *Diagnostic and Statistical Manual of Mental Disorders Text Revision: DSM-4-TR*. American Psychiatric Association.

American Psychiatric Association. (2013). *Feeding and eating disorders. In Diagnostic and statistical manual of mental disorders (5th ed.)*. APA. https://doiorg.libproxy.lib.unc.edu/10.1176

American Psychiatric Association. (2017). *Mental health disparities: African Americans*. APA. https://www.psychiatry.org/File%20Library/Psychiatrists/Cultural-Competency/Mental-Health-Disparities/Mental-Health-Facts-for-African-Americans.pdf

American Psychiatric Association. (2022). Personality disorders. In Diagnostic and statistical manual of mental disorders (5th ed., text rev.). APA.

American Psychological Association. (2015). *Demographic characteristics of division 12 members by membership status, 2015*. APA. http://www.apa.org/about/division/officers/services/div-12-2015.pdf

American Psychological Association. (2017). *Mental health disparities: African Americans*. APA. *https://www.psychiatry.org/File%20Library/Psychiatrists/Cultural-Competency/Mental-Health-Disparities/Mental-Health-Facts-for-African-Americans.pdf*

American Psychological Association. (2022). *Demographics of U.S. Psychology Workforce [Interactive data tool]*. APA. https://www.apa.org/workforce/data-tools/demographics

American Psychological Association. (n.d). *APA Dictionary of Psychology*. APA. https://dictionary.apa.org/

Ameringen, M., Patterson, B., & Simpson, W. (2014). Dsm-5 Obsessive-compulsive and related disorders: Clinical implications of new criteria. *Depression & Anxiety (1091-4269), 31*(6), 487–493. doi:10.1002/da.22259

Anders, G. (1993). Machismo: Dead or alive? *Hispanic*, *3*, 14–20.

Anderson, M. S. (2018). Barriers to the Utilization of Mental Health Services on College Campuses by African-American Students. *McNair Scholars Research Journal, 11*(3). https://commons.emich.edu/mcnair/vol11/iss1/3

Anderson, L. B. (2014). African American males diagnosed with Schizophrenia: A phenomenological study. *Issues in Mental Health Nursing*, *35*(1), 580–587. doi:10.3109/01612840.2013.867464 PMID:25072210

Ando, T., Nomura, T., Sejiyama, S. Y., Shin, T., Mori, K. I., Sumino, Y., Sato, F., & Mimata, H. (2014). Munchausen syndrome in the act of creating and enacting macroscopic hematuria. *Urologia Internationalis*, *93*(3), 371–372. doi:10.1159/000357919 PMID:24576852

APA. (2019). *Acta Dermatovenerologica Alpina, Pannonica, et Adriatica*, 13-15.

Arciniega, G. M., Anderson, T. C., Tovar-Blank, Z. G., & Tracey, T. J. (2008). Toward a fuller conception of Machismo: Development of a traditional Machismo and Caballerismo scale. *Journal of Counseling Psychology*, *55*(1), 19–33. doi:10.1037/0022-0167.55.1.19

Arias, I. (2004). Report from the CDC. The legacy of child maltreatment: Long-term health consequences for women. *Journal of Women's Health*, *13*(5), 468–473. doi:10.1089/1540999041280990 PMID:15257839

Arnulf, I., Zeitzer, J. M., File, J., Farber, N., & Mignot, E. (2005). Kleine–Levin syndrome: A systematic review of 186 cases in the literature. *Brain*, *128*(12), 2763–2776. doi:10.1093/brain/awh620 PMID:16230322

Assari, S. (2018). Perceived discrimination and binge eating disorder; gender differences in African Americans. *Journal of Clinical Medicine*, *7*(5), 89. doi:10.3390/jcm7050089 PMID:29695062

Assari, S., & Caldwell, C. H. (2018). High risk of depression in high-income African American boys. *Journal of Racial and Ethnic Health Disparities*, *5*(4), 808–819. doi:10.100740615-017-0426-1 PMID:28842841

Avalos, L. A., & Mulia, N. (2012). Formal and informal substance use treatment utilization and alcohol abstinence over seven years: Is the relationship different for blacks and whites? *Drug & Alcohol Dependence*, *121*(1/2), 73–80. https://doi doi:org.proxy.tamuc.edu/10.1016/j.drugalcdep.2011.08.018

Avent Harris, J. R., Wahesh, E., Barrow, M., & Fripp, J. A. (2021). Demographics, stigma and religious coping and Christian African Americans' help seeking. *Counseling and Values*, *66*(1), 73–91. doi:10.1002/cvj.12145

Avent Harris, J. R., & Wong, C. D. (2018). African American college students, the Black church, and counseling. *Journal of College Counseling*, *21*(1), 15–28. doi:10.1002/jocc.12084

Avent, J. R., & Cashwell, C. S. (2015). The Black Church: Theology and implications for counseling African Americans. *The Professional Counselor*, *5*(1), 81–90. doi:10.15241/jra.5.1.81

Awad, G. H., Norwood, C., Taylor, D. S., Martinez, M., McClain, S., Jones, B., Holman, A., & Chapman-Hilliard, C. (2015). Beauty and body image concerns among African American college women. *The Journal of Black Psychology*, *41*(6), 540–564. doi:10.1177/0095798414550864 PMID:26778866

Baggerly, J., Tan, T. X., Pichotta, D., & Warner, A. (2017). Race, ethnicity, and gender of faculty members in APA-and CACREP-accredited programs: Changes over five decades. *Journal of Multicultural Counseling and Development*, *45*(4), 292–303. doi:10.1002/jmcd.12079

Bahna, S. L., & Oldham, J. (2014). Munchausen stridor — A strong false alarm of anaphylaxis. *Allergy, Asthma & Immunology Research*, *6*(6), 577–579. doi:10.4168/aair.2014.6.6.577 PMID:25374759

Baig, M. R., Levin, T. T., Lichtenthal, W. G., Boland, P. J., & Breitbart, W. S. (2015). Facitious Disorder (Munchausen's Syndrome) in Oncology: Case Report and Literature Review. *Psycho-Oncology*, *25*(6), 707–711. doi:10.1002/pon.3906 PMID:26179957

Baig, M. R., Levin, T. T., Lichtenthal, W. G., Boland, P. J., & Breitbart, W. S. (2015). Factitious disorder (Munchausen's syndrome) in oncology: Case report and literature review. *Psycho-Oncology*, 1. PMID:26179957

Bailey, R. K., Blackmon, H. L., & Stevens, F. L. (2009). Major depressive disorder in the African American population: Meeting the challenges of stigma, misdiagnosis, and treatment disparities. *Journal of the National Medical Association*, *101*(11), 1084–1089. doi:10.1016/S0027-9684(15)31102-0 PMID:19998635

Bailey, R. K., Mokonogho, J., & Kumar, A. (2019). Racial and ethnic differences in depression: Current perspectives. *Neuropsychiatric Disease and Treatment*, *15*, 603–609. doi:10.2147/NDT.S128584 PMID:30863081

Bailey, R. K., Patel, M., Barker, N. C., Ali, S., & Jabeen, S. (2011). Major depressive disorder in the African American population. *Journal of the National Medical Association*, *103*(7), 548–559. doi:10.1016/S0027-9684(15)30380-1 PMID:21999029

Bains, N., & Abdijadid, S. (2022, June 1). Major Depressive Disorder In *StatPearls [Internet]*. StatPearls. https://www.ncbi.nlm.nih.gov/books/NBK559078/

Ballas, S. K. (1996). Factitious sickle cell acute painful episodes: A secondary type of Munchausen syndrome. *American Journal of Hematology*, *53*(4), 254–258. doi:10.1002/(SICI)1096-8652(199612)53:4<254::AID-AJH10>3.0.CO;2-C PMID:8948666

Banks, J. A. & Grambs, J. D. (). Black Self-Concept: Implications for Education and Social Science. McGraw-Hill.

Barkin, J. A., Biagini, T. M., & Barkin, J. S. (2013). Factitious disorder as a cause of gastrointestinal bleeding: Use of a gastroenterologist's "secondary survey". *The American Journal of Gastroenterology*, *108*(3), 456–458. doi:10.1038/ajg.2012.420 PMID:23459058

Barnes, A. (2008). Race and hospital diagnosis of schizophrenia and mood disorders. *Social Work*, *53*(1), 77–83. doi:10.1093w/53.1.77 PMID:18610823

Bartels, S. J. (2003). Improving the United States' system of care for older adults with mental illness: Findings and recommendations for the President's New Freedom Commission on Mental Health. *The American Journal of Geriatric Psychiatry*, *11*(5), 486–497. doi:10.1097/00019442-200309000-00003 PMID:14506082

Bashi, V., & Mcdaniel, A. (2016). A theory of immigration and racial stratification. *Journal of Black Studies*, *27*(5), 668–682. doi:10.1177/002193479702700505

Bass, C., & Halligan, P. (2014). Factitious disorders and malingering: Challenges for clinical assessment and management. *Lancet*, *383*(9926), 1422–1432. doi:10.1016/S0140-6736(13)62186-8 PMID:24612861

Batelaan, K. (2022). It's not the science we distrust; it's the scientists: Reframing the anti-vaccination movement within Black communities. *Global Public Health: An International Journal for Research, Policy and Practice*, *17*(6), 1099–1112. doi:10.1080/17441692.2021.1912809 PMID:33843472

Bauer, M., & Boegner, F. (1996). Neurological syndromes in factitious disorder. *The Journal of Nervous and Mental Disease*, *184*(5), 281–288. doi:10.1097/00005053-199605000-00003 PMID:8627273

Baum, F., MacDougall, C., & Smith, D. (2006). Participatory action research. *Journal of Epidemiology and Community Health*, *60*(10), 854–857. doi:10.1136/jech.2004.028662 PMID:16973531

Baweja, R., Baweja, R., & Hameed, A. (2014). Munchausen's syndrome with rare hematological disorder, systemic mastocytosis: A case report, J Neuropsychiatry Clin Neurosci Bhargava, D., Al-Abri, R., Rizvi, SG, Okbi, MH AL, Bhargava, K. and Al Adawi, S. (2007). Phenomenology and outcome of factitious disorders in otolaryngology clinic in Oman. *International Journal of Psychiatry in Medicine*, *37*(2), 229–240.

Bazargan, M., Bazargan, S., & King, L. (2001). Paranoid ideation among elderly African American persons. *The Gerontologist*, *41*(3), 366–373. doi:10.1093/geront/41.3.366 PMID:11405434

Bazargan, M., Cobb, S., & Assari, S. (2021). Discrimination and medical mistrust in a racially and ethnically diverse sample of California adults. *Annals of Family Medicine*, *19*(1), 4–15. doi:10.1370/afm.2632 PMID:33431385

Becker, C. B., Middlemass, K. M., Gomez, F., & Martinez-Abrego, A. (2019). Eating disorder pathology among individuals living with food insecurity: A replication study. *Clinical Psychological Science*, *7*(5), 1144–1158. doi:10.1177/2167702619851811

Becker, C. B., Middlemass, K., Taylor, B., Johnson, C., & Gomez, F. (2017). Food insecurity and eating disorder pathology. *International Journal of Eating Disorders*, *50*(9), 1031–1040. doi:10.1002/eat.22735 PMID:28626944

Beel, N., Jeffries, C., Brownlow, C., Winterbotham, S., & Du Preez, J. (2018). Recommendations for male-friendly individual counseling with men: A qualitative systematic literature review for the period 1995–2016. *Psychology of Men & Masculinity*, *19*(4), 600–611. doi:10.1037/men0000137

Behary, W. T., & Dieckmann, E. (2011). The art of empathetic confrontation, limit-setting, and leverage. In W. K. Campbell & J. D. Miller (Eds.), *The handbook of narcissism and narcissistic personality disorder: Theoretical approaches, empirical findings, and treatments* (pp. 445–456).

Bell, C. C., Bland, I. J., Houston, E., & Jones, B. E. (1983). Curriculum development implementation: Enhancement of knowledge and skills for the psychiatric treatment of black populations. In J. C. Chunn II, P. J. Dunston, & F. Ross-Sheriff (Eds.), *Mental health & people of color: Curriculum development and change* (pp. 205–238). Howard University Press.

Benjamin, E. J., Virani, S. S., Callaway, C. W., Chamberlain, A. M., Chang, A. R., Cheng, S., Chiuve, S. E., Cushman, M., Delling, F. N., Deo, R., de Ferranti, S. D., Ferguson, J. F., Fornage, M., Gillespie, C., Isasi, C. R., Jiménez, M. C., Jordan, L. C., Judd, S. E., Lackland, D, & Muntner, P. (2018). Heart disease and stroke statistics—2018 update: A report from the American Heart Association. *Circulation, 137*(12), e67–e492. doi:10.1161/CIR.0000000000000558 PMID:29386200

Bennett, D., & Rosenheck, R. (2021). Socioeconomic status and the effectiveness of treatment for first-episode psychosis. *Health Services Research, 56*(3), 409–417. doi:10.1111/1475-6773.13606 PMID:33231881

Berchick, E., Hood, E., & Barnett, J. (2018, September 12). *Health Insurance Coverage in the United States: 2017.* United Stated Cenus Bureau. Retrieved February 28, 2023, from https://www.census.gov/library/publications/2018/demo/p60-264.html

Berman, N. C., Gallegos-Guajardo, J., Reuman, L., Ramirez, M., Valdez, G., & Abramowitz, J. S. (2020). Cross-cultural differences in obsessive-compulsive symptom dimensions across young adults in Mexico and USA. *Mental Health, Religion & Culture, 23*(5), 443–454. doi:10.1080/13674676.2020.1793309

Biarge, M. M., García-Alix, A., Hoyo, M., Alarcón, A., Pipaón, M., & Hernández, F. (2014). Intussusception in a preterm neonate; a very rare, major intestinal problem — Systematic review of cases. *Journal of Perinatal Medicine, 32*(2), 190–194.

Bilsker, D., & White, J. (2011). The silent epidemic of male suicide. *British Columbia Medical Journal, 53*(10).

Bjordahl, K. K., Salgado, D. S., & Johnson, B. (2015, May). *Associations between men's concern for heterosexual self-presentation and attitudes towards psychological help seeking.* Poster session presented at the 95th Annual Convention of the Western Psychological Association, Las Vegas, NV.

Black and African American Communities and Mental Health. (n.d.). MHA. https://www.mhanational.org/issues/black-and-african-american-communities-and-mental-health

Black, D. W., Gaffney, G. R., Schlosser, S., & Gabel, J. (2003). Children of parents with obsessive-compulsive disorder – a 2-year follow-up study. *Acta Psychiatrica Scandinavica, 107*(4), 305–313. doi:10.1034/j.1600-0447.2003.02182.x PMID:12662254

Blank, M. B., Mahmood, M., Fox, J. C., & Guterbock, T. (2002). Alternative mental health services: The role of the Black church in the South. *American Journal of Public Health, 92*(10), 1668–1672. doi:10.2105/AJPH.92.10.1668 PMID:12356619

Blumberg, S. J., Clarke, T. C., & Blackwell, D. L. (2015). Racial and ethnic disparities in men's use of mental health treatments. *National Center for Health Statistics Data Brief No.*, (206), 1–8. PMID:26079520

Blumberg, S., Clarke, T., & Blackwell, D. (2015). Racial and ethnic disparities in men's use of mental health treatments. *NCHS Data Brief, 206*. https://files.eric.ed.gov/fulltext/ED578186.pdf PMID:26079520

Boden, J. M., & Fergusson, D. M. (2011). Alcohol and depression. *Addiction (Abingdon, England), 106*(5), 906–914. doi:10.1111/j.1360-0443.2010.03351.x PMID:21382111

Bohrer, B. K., Carroll, I. A., Forbush, K. T., & Chen, P. Y. (2017). Treatment seeking for eating disorders: Results from a nationally representative study. *International Journal of Eating Disorders, 50*(12), 1341–1349. doi:10.1002/eat.22785 PMID:28963793

Bolden, L., & Wicks, M. (2005). Length of stay, admission types, psychiatric diagnoses, and the implications of stigma in African Americans in the nationwide inpatient sample. *Issues in Mental Health Nursing, 26*(10), 1043–1059. doi:10.1080/01612840500280703 PMID:16283998

Boon, K. A. (2005). Heroes, metanarrative, and the paradox of masculinity in contemporary western culture. *Journal of Men's Studies, 13*(3), 301–312. doi:10.3149/jms.1303.301

Bor, J., Venkataramani, A. S., Williams, D. R., & Tsai, A. C. (2018). Police killings and their spillover effects on the mental health of black Americans: A population-based, quasi-experimental study. *Lancet, 392*(10144), 302–310. doi:10.1016/S0140-6736(18)31130-9 PMID:29937193

Boulware, L. E., Cooper, L. A., Ratner, L. E., LaVeist, T. A., & Powe, N. R. (2003). Race and trust in the health care system. *Public Health Reports, 118*(4), 358–365. doi:10.1016/S0033-3549(04)50262-5 PMID:12815085

Bovasso, G. B. (2014). Cannabis abuse as a risk factor for depressive symptoms. *The American Journal of Psychiatry*, •••, 9. PMID:11729021

Boyd, A. S., Ritchie, C., & Likhari, S. (2014). Munchausen syndrome and Munchausen syndrome by proxy in dermatology. *Journal of the American Academy of Dermatology, 71*(2), 376–381. doi:10.1016/j.jaad.2013.12.028 PMID:24613506

Boyd-Franklin, N. (2003). Black families in therapy: Understanding the African American experience. New York: Guilford.

Branscombe, N. R., Schmitt, M. T., & Harvey, R. D. (1999). Perceiving pervasive discrimination among African Americans: Implications for group identification and well-being. *Journal of Personality and Social Psychology, 77*(1), 135–149. doi:10.1037/0022-3514.77.1.135

Brennan, D. J., Souleymanov, R., George, C., Newman, P. A., Hart, T. A., Asakura, K., & Betancourt, G. (2015). Masculinity, muscularity, and HIV sexual risk among gay and bisexual men of color. *Psychology of Men & Masculinity, 16*(4), 393–403. doi:10.1037/a0038725

Bridges to Recovery. *Types of Borderline Personality Disorder*. Bridges to Recovery. (n.d.). Retrieved February 28, 2023, from https://www.bridgestorecovery.com/

Briere, J., & Gil, E. (1998). Self-mutilation in clinical and general population samples: Prevalence, correlates, and functions. *The American Journal of Orthopsychiatry*, *68*(4), 609–620. doi:10.1037/h0080369 PMID:9809120

Bright, R., Damon, L., & Eisendrath, S. (2001). A case of factitious aplastic anemia. *International Journal of Psychiatry in Medicine*, *31*(4), 433–441. doi:10.2190/TUJB-B2M7-6UPV-XPLV PMID:11949741

British Columbia Vital Statistics Agency. (2011). *Selected vital statistics and health status indicators: Annual Report 2002*. VS Agency. www.vs.gov.bc.ca/ stats/annual/2002/

Brooks Holiday, S., Dubowitz, T., Haas, A., Ghosh-Dastidar, B., DeSantis, A., & Troxel, W. M. (2020). The association between discrimination and PTSD in African Americans: Exploring the role of gender. *Ethnicity & Health*, *25*(5), 717–731. doi:10.1080/13557858.2018.1444150 PMID:29490467

Brooks, J. R., Lebeaut, A., Zegel, M., Walker, R. L., & Vujanovic, A. A. (2021). Anxiety sensitivity and suicide risk: Mindfulness as a psychological buffer for Black adults. *Journal of Affective Disorders*, *289*, 74–80. doi:10.1016/j.jad.2021.04.012 PMID:33945917

Browne, F. A., Bonner, C. P., Kline, T. L., Cox, E. N., Gichane, M. W., & Wechsberg, W. M. (2023). Alcohol, drug use, and sexual risk among young African American women in North Carolina: Is educational attainment protective? *Vulnerable Children and Youth Studies*, *18*(2), 149–155. https://doi-org.proxy.tamuc.edu/10.1080/17450128.2022.2089794. doi:10.1080/17450128.2022.2089794

Browne, F. A., Wechsberg, W. M., White, V. M., Middlesteadt Ellerson, R., Raiford, J. L., Carry, M. G., & Herbst, J. H. (2014). The influence of social determinants on sexual risk among out-of-school African American female adolescents. *Vulnerable Children and Youth Studies*, *9*(2), 139–150. doi:10.1080/17450128.2013.832828 PMID:26692886

Browne, J., & Mohamed, S. (2021). Evaluation of disparities in the impact of mental health intensive case management on 6-month symptoms, functioning, and quality of life between Black and White veterans diagnosed with schizophrenia. *Schizophrenia Research*. doi:10.1016/j.schres.2021.07.002 PMID:34247886

Bryant, T. (2022, February 9). 10 Biggest Barriers To Black Mental Health. *Psycom*. https://www.psycom.net/black-mental-health-barriers

Bryant-Davis, T. (2019). The cultural context of trauma recovery: Considering the posttraumatic stress disorder practice guideline and intersectionality. *Psychotherapy (Chicago, Ill.)*, *56*(3), 400–408. doi:10.1037/pst0000241 PMID:31282715

Bueno-Notivol, J., Gracia-García, P., Olaya, B., Lasheras, I., López-Antón, R., & Santabárbara, J. (2021). Prevalence of depression during the COVID-19 outbreak: A meta-analysis of community-based studies. *International Journal of Clinical and Health Psychology*, *21*(1), 100196. doi:10.1016/j.ijchp.2020.07.007 PMID:32904715

Burroughs, A. D. (2022). Black Market: An Exploration of Black Mental Health in America. *Psychology from the Margins*, *4*(1), 1.

Burström, B., & Tao, W. (2020). Social determinants of health and inequalities in COVID-19. *European Journal of Public Health*, *30*(4), 617–618. doi:10.1093/eurpub/ckaa095 PMID:32638998

Burt, C. H., Lei, M. K., & Simons, R. L. (2017). Racial discrimination, racial socialization, and crime: Understanding mechanisms of resilience. *Social Problems*, *64*(3), 414–438. doi:10.1093ocpropw036

Caetano, R., Cunradi, C. B., Alter, H. J., Mair, C., Yau, R. K., & Gerson, L. W. (2019). Drinking and Intimate Partner Violence Severity Levels Among U.S. Ethnic Groups in an Urban Emergency Department. *Academic Emergency Medicine*, *26*(8), 897–907. https://doi-. doi:10.1111/acem.13706 PMID:30706610

Cai, A., & Robst, J. (2016). The relationship between race/ethnicity and the perceived experience of mental health care. *The American Journal of Orthopsychiatry*, *86*(5), 508–518. https://doi-. doi:10.1037/ort0000119 PMID:26460698

Callaghan, G. M., Summers, C. J., & Weidman, M. (2003). The treatment of histrionic and narcissistic personality disorder behaviors: A single-subject demonstration of clinical improvement using functional analytic psychotherapy. *Journal of Contemporary Psychotherapy*, *33*(4), 321–339. doi:10.1023/B:JOCP.0000004502.55597.81

Calle-Ramirez, X. M., Hernandez, R. M., Saavedra-Lopez, M. A., Esteban, R. F. C., Chaperro, J. E. T., Mamani-Benito, O., & Campos-Ugaz, W. A. (2022). Worldwide scientific production on obsessive-compulsive disorders in time of COVID-19 pandemic. *AVFT, 41*(9), 679-683.

Calloway, A., & Creed, T. A. (2022). Enhancing CBT consultation with multicultural counseling principles. *Cognitive and Behavioral Practice*, *29*(4), 787–795. doi:10.1016/j.cbpra.2021.05.007

Campbell, A. D. (2021). Clergy perceptions of mental illness and confronting stigma in congregations. *Religions*, *12*(12), 1–14. doi:10.3390/rel12121110

Campbell, B. (2019). Past, present, future: A program development project exploring Post Traumatic Stress Syndrome (PTSS) using experiential education and dance/movement therapy informed approaches. *American Journal of Dance Therapy*, *41*(2), 214–233. doi:10.100710465-019-09320-8

Campbell, K. W., & Miller, J. D. (2011). *The handbook of narcissism and narcissistic personality disorder: Theoretical approaches, empirical findings, and treatments*. John Wiley & Sons. doi:10.1002/9781118093108

Campbell, R. D., & Littleton, T. (2018). Mental health counseling in the Black American church: Reflections and recommendations from counselors serving in a counseling ministry. *Mental Health, Religion & Culture*, *21*(4), 336–352. doi:10.1080/13674676.2018.1494704

Campbell, R. D., & Winchester, M. R. (2020). How the Black church can address mental health with Black Americans. *Social Work & Christianity*, *47*(2), 105–122. doi:10.34043wc.v47i2.63

Capraro, R. L. (2000). Why college men drink: Alcohol, adventure, and the paradox of masculinity. *Journal of American College Health*, *48*(6), 307–315. doi:10.1080/07448480009596272 PMID:10863874

Cardoso, A., Almeida, T. C., Ramos, C., Sousa, S., & Brito, J. (2021). Bidirectional relationship between perceived stress and insomnia symptoms: The role of coping and quality of life. *Sleep and Biological Rhythms*, *19*(1), 23–31. doi:10.100741105-020-00284-8

Carnahan, K. T. (2023). *Factitious Disorder*. StatPearls Publishing.

Carney, M. W., & Brown, J. P. (1983). Clinical features and motives among 42 artifactual illness patients. *The British Journal of Medical Psychology*, *56*(1), 57–66. doi:10.1111/j.2044-8341.1983.tb01532.x PMID:6838782

Carroll, A. (2009). Are you looking at me? Understanding and managing paranoid personality disorder. *Advances in Psychiatric Treatment*, *15*(1), 40–48. doi:10.1192/apt.bp.107.005421

Carstensen, L. L. IsAfrican Americancowitz, D. M., & Charles, S. T. (1999). Taking time seriously: A theory of socioemotional selectivity. *American Psychologist*, *54*(3), 165–181. https://doi-org.ezp.twu.edu/10.1037/0003-066X.54.3.165

Casados, A. T. (2017). Reducing the Stigma of Mental Illness: Current Approaches and Future Directions. *Clinical Psychology: Science and Practice*, *24*(3), 306–323. doi:10.1111/cpsp.12206

Casas, J. M., Wagenheim, B. R., Banchero, R., & Mendoza-Romero, J. (1994). Hispanic masculinity: Myth or psychological schema meriting clinical consideration. *Hispanic Journal of Behavioral Sciences*, *16*(3), 315–331. doi:10.1177/07399863940163009

Cavanagh, L., & Obasi, E. M. (2022). Chronic Stress, Autonomic Dysregulation and Prospective Drug Use Among African American Emerging Adults. *Cultural Diversity & Ethnic Minority Psychology*, *28*(1), 91–102. https://doi-org.proxy.tamuc.edu/10.1037/cdp0000364. doi:10.1037/cdp0000364 PMID:34672646

Cazenave, N. A. (1979). Middle-income Black fathers: An analysis of the provider role. *The Family Coordinator*, *28*(4), 583–593. doi:10.2307/583522

Cazenave, N. A. (1984). Race, socioeconomic status, and age: The social context of American masculinity. *Sex Roles*, *11*(7-8), 639–656. doi:10.1007/BF00288117

Centers for Disease and Prevention. (2017). *National Center for Injury Prevention and Control. Web-based Injury Statistics Query and Reporting System*. WISQARS.

Centers for Disease and Prevention. (2019). National Vital Statistics Report, Table 10. [Data set]. CDC. https://www.cdc.gov/nchs/data/nvsr/nvsr68/nvsr68_09.pdf

Centers for Disease and Prevention. (2019). Summary Health Statistics: National Health Interview Survey: 2017. *Table A-7.* [Data set]. CDC. https://www.cdc.gov/nchs/nhis/shs/tables.htm

Centers for Disease Control and Prevention, National Center for Health Statistics. (2022). About Multiple Cause of Death, 1999–2020. CDC WONDER Online Database website. Centers for Disease Control and Prevention., Retrieved February 21, 2022, from.

Centers for Disease Control and Prevention, U.S. Department of Health and Human Services. (2016). Health, United States, 2015: With special feature on racial and ethnic health disparities *DHHS Publication No. 2016-1232.* CDC. https://www.cdc.gov/nchs/data/hus/hus15.pdf

Centers for Disease Control and Prevention. (2016). *Fact sheets: Underage drinking*. CDC. https://www.cdc.gov/alcohol/fact-sheets/underage-drinking.htm

Centers for Disease Control and Prevention. (2018). *Fact sheets –alcohol use and your health.* CDC.

Centers for Disease Control and Prevention. (2019, November 5). Table A-8. *National Health Interview Survey.* CDC. https://www.cdc.gov/nchs/nhis/shs/tables.htm

Centers for Disease Control and Prevention. (2022). *Alcohol Use and your heath.* CDC. https://www.cdc.gov/alcohol/fact-sheets/alcohol-use.htm

Centers for Disease Control and Prevention. (2022). Alcohol-Related Disease Impact Application (ARDI) Application. Accessed April 19, 2022. https://nccd.cdc.gov/DPH_ARDI/defaul/default.aspx

Centers for Disease Control and Prevention. (2022, September 14). *Mental Health Conditions: Depression and Anxiety.* CDC. https://www.cdc.gov/tobacco/campaign/tips/diseases/depression-anxiety.html

Centers for Disease Control and Prevention. (2023). *Addressing Excessive Alcohol Use: State Fact Sheet.* CDC. https://www.cdc.gov/alcohol/fact-sheets/states/excessive-alcohol-use-united-states.html

Chambers, E., Yager, J., Apfeldorf, W., & Camps-Romero, E. (2007). Factitious aortic dissection leading to thoracotomy in a 20-year-old man. *Psychosomatics, 48*(4), 355–358. doi:10.1176/appi.psy.48.4.355 PMID:17600175

Chan, J. W. (2018). School-based karate-do: Supporting the well-being of gay male youth. *Canadian Journal for New Scholars in Education/Revue canadienne des jeunes chercheures et chercheurs en éducation, 9*(1).

Chandra, A., Scott, M. M., Jaycox, L. H., Meredith, L. S., Tanielian, T., & Burnam, A. (2009). Racial/ethnic differences in teen and parent perspectives toward depression treatment. *The Journal of Adolescent Health, 44*(6), 546–553. doi:10.1016/j.jadohealth.2008.10.137 PMID:19465318

Chaney, C. (2009). Boys to men: How perceptions of manhood influence the romantic partnerships of black men. *The Western Journal of Black Studies, 33*, 110–112.

Chapman, J., Fleisher, C., & Jamil, R. (2022, October 25). *Borderline personality disorder.* National Center for Biotechnology Information. Retrieved February 28, 2023, from https://pubmed.ncbi.nlm.nih.gov/28613633/

Chasson, G. S., Williams, M. T., Davis, D. M., & Combs, J. Y. (2017). Missed diagnoses in African Americans with obsessive-compulsive disorder: The structured clinical interview for DSM-IV Axis I disorders (SCID-I). *BMC Psychiatry, 17*(1), 1–10. doi:10.118612888-017-1422-z PMID:28716021

Chatters, L. M., Taylor, R. J., Jackson, J. S., & Lincoln, K. D. (2008). Religious coping among african americans, caribbean blacks and non-hispanic whites. *Journal of Community Psychology, 36*(3), 371–386. doi:10.1002/jcop.20202 PMID:21048887

Cheatham, C. T., Barksdale, D. J., & Rodgers, S. G. (2008). Barriers to health care and health-seeking behaviors faced by Black men. *Journal of the American Academy of Nurse Practitioners, 20*(11), 555–562. doi:10.1111/j.1745-7599.2008.00359.x PMID:19128339

Chen, L. P., Murad, M. H., Paras, M. L., Colbenson, K. M., Sattler, A. L., Goranson, E. N., Elamin, M. B., Seime, R. J., Shinozaki, G., Prokop, L. J., & Zirakzadeh, A. (2010). Sexual abuse and lifetime diagnosis of psychiatric disorders: Systematic review and meta-analysis. *Mayo Clinic Proceedings, 85*(7), 618–629. doi:10.4065/mcp.2009.0583 PMID:20458101

Chetty, R., Friedman, J. N., Hendren, N., Jones, M. R., & Porter, S. R. (2018). *The opportunity atlas: Mapping the childhood roots of social mobility* (No. w25147). National Bureau of Economic Research. doi:10.3386/w25147

Chew, B. H., Pace, K. T., & Honey, R. J. (2002). Munchausen syndrome presenting as gross hematuria in two women. *Urology, 59*(4), 601. doi:10.1016/S0090-4295(01)01608-9 PMID:11927327

Clark, T. T., Belgrave, F. Z., & Abell, M. (2012). The Mediating and Moderating Effects of Parent and Peer Influences upon Drug Use among African American Adolescents. *The Journal of Black Psychology, 38*(1), 52–80. doi:10.1177/0095798411403617

Clark, T. T., McGovern, P., Mgbeokwere, D., Wooten, N., Owusu, H., & McGraw, K. A. (2014). Systematic review: The nature and extent of social work research on substance use disorders treatment interventions among African Americans. *Journal of Social Work, 14*(5), 451–472. https://doi-org.proxy.tamuc.edu/10.1177/1468017313479858. doi:10.1177/1468017313479858

Clark, T. T., Salas-Wright, C. P., Vaughn, M. G., & Whitfield, K. E. (2014). Everyday discrimination and mood and substance use disorders: A latent profile analysis with African Americans and Caribbean blacks. *Addictive Behaviors, 40*(1), 119–125. PMID:25254321

Clauss-Ehlers, C. S., Chiriboga, D. A., Hunter, S. J., Roysircar, G., & Tummala-Narra, P. (2019). APA multicultural guidelines executive summary: Ecological approach to context, identity, and intersectionality. *The American Psychologist, 74*(2), 232–244. doi:10.1037/amp0000382 PMID:30762387

Cobb, S., & Assari, S. (2019). Psychiatric disorders and alcohol consumption among low-income African Americans: Gender differences. *Brain Sciences (2076-3425), 9*(4), 86. doi:10.3390/brainsci9040086

Coffino, J. A., Grilo, C. M., & Udo, T. (2020). Childhood food neglect and adverse experiences associated with DSM-5 eating disorders in U.S. National Sample. *Journal of Psychiatric Research*, *127*, 75–79. doi:10.1016/j.jpsychires.2020.05.011 PMID:32502721

Coleman-Kirumba, L. M., Cornish, M. A., Horton, A. J., & Alvarez, J. C. (2023). Experiences of Black men: Forms of masculinity and effects on psychological help-seeking variables. *The Journal of Black Psychology*, *49*(1), 32–57. doi:10.1177/00957984221098122

Connell, R. W. (1995). *Masculinities*. Routledge.

Connell, R. W., & Messerschmidt, J. W. (2005). Hegemonic masculinity rethinking the concept. *Gender & Society*, *19*(6), 829–859. doi:10.1177/0891243205278639

Conner, K. O., Copeland, V. C., Grote, N. K., Rosen, D., Albert, S., McMurray, M. L., & Koeske, G. (2010). Barriers to treatment and culturally endorsed coping strategies among depressed African American older adults. *Aging & Mental Health*, *14*(8), 971–983. doi:10.1080/13607863.2010.501061 PMID:21069603

Conner, K. O., Lee, B., Mayers, V., Robinson, D., Reynolds, C. F. III, Albert, S., & Brown, C. (2010). Attitudes and beliefs about mental health among African American older adults suffering from depression. *Journal of Aging Studies*, *24*(4), 266–277. doi:10.1016/j.jaging.2010.05.007 PMID:21423819

Conner, K. R., Pinquart, M., & Duberstein, P. R. (2008). Meta-analysis of depression and substance use and impairment among intravenous drug users (IDUs). *Addiction (Abingdon, England)*, *103*(4), 524–534. doi:10.1111/j.1360-0443.2007.02118.x PMID:18261192

Conroy, J., Lin, L., & Stamm, K. (2023). *Center for workforce studies; graduate psychology studies opens doors*. American Psychiatric Association. https://www.apa.org/monitor/2021/09/datapoint-graduate

Constantine, M. G., Myers, L. J., Kindaichi, M., & Moore, J. L. III. (2004). Exploring indigenous mental health practices: The roles of healers and helpers in promoting well-being in people of color. *Counseling and Values*, *48*(2), 110–125. doi:10.1002/j.2161-007X.2004.tb00238.x

Cook, B. L., Zuvekas, S. H., Carson, N., Ferris, G. F., Vesper, A., & McGuire, T. G. (2014). Assessing racial/ethnic disparities in treatment across episodes of mental health care. *Health Services Research*, *49*(1), 206–229. doi:10.1111/1475-6773.12095 PMID:23855750

Cook, E. P. (2015). *Understanding people in context: The ecological perspective in counseling*. John Wiley & Sons., doi:10.1002/9781119222743

Copeland, V. C., & Snyder, K. (2011). Barriers to mental health treatment services for low-income African American women whose children receive behavioral health services: An ethnographic investigation. *Social Work in Public Health*, *26*(1), 78–95. doi:10.1080/10911350903341036 PMID:21213189

Corrigan, P., & Kleinlein, P. (2005). The impact of mental illness stigma. In P. Corrigan (Ed.), *On the stigma of mental illness: Practical strategies for research and social change* (pp. 11–44). American Psychological Association. doi:10.1037/10887-001

Courtenay, W. H. (2000). Constructions of masculinity and their influence on men's well-being: A theory of gender and health. *Social Science & Medicine*, *50*(10), 1385–1401. doi:10.1016/S0277-9536(99)00390-1 PMID:10741575

Courtenay, W. H., McCreary, D. R., & Merighi, J. R. (2002). Gender and ethnic differences in health beliefs and behaviors. *Journal of Health Psychology*, *7*(3), 219–231. doi:10.1177/1359105302007003216 PMID:22114246

Crawford, S. M., Jeyasanger, G., & Wright, M. (2005). A visitor with Munchausen's syndrome. *Clinical Medicine (London, England)*, *5*(4), 400–401. doi:10.7861/clinmedicine.5-4-400 PMID:16138498

Cross Jr, W. E., & Fhagen-Smith, P. (2001). Patterns of African American identity development: A life span perspective. *New perspectives on racial identity development: A theoretical and practical anthology*, 243-270.

Cross, W. E. Jr. (1991). *Shades of Black: Diversity in African-American identity*. Temple University Press.

Cullors, P., & Johnson, M. (2014, August 1). *Impact of disproportionate incarceration of and violence against black ...* Retrieved February 28, 2023, from http://www.antoniocasella.eu/archipsy/Dignity_2014.pdf

Cummings, J. R. (2014). Contextual socioeconomic status and mental health counseling use among US adolescents with depression. *Journal of Youth and Adolescence*, *43*(7), 1151–1162. doi:10.100710964-013-0021-7 PMID:24114588

Cuncic, A. (2022, November 8). *What is quiet borderline personality disorder?* Verywell Mind. Retrieved February 28, 2023, from https://www.verywellmind.com/what-is-quiet-borderline-personality-disorder-5115074

Cutting, L. P., Aakre, J. M., & Docherty, N. M. (2006). *Schizophrenic patients' perceptions of stress, expressed emotion, and sensitivity to criticism*. Schizophrenia Bulletin.

Dahale, A. B., Hatti, S., Thippeswamy, H., & Chaturvedi, S. K. (2014). Factitious disorder — Experience at a neuropsychiatric center in southern India. *Indian Journal of Psychological Medicine*, *36*(1), 62–65. doi:10.4103/0253-7176.127253 PMID:24701013

Davidson, M. N. (2001). *Know the adversary: The impact of race on styles of dealing with conflict*. Sex Roles.

Davis, L. J. (2008). *Obsession: A history*. The University of Chicago Press. doi:10.7208/chicago/9780226137797.001.0001

Day, N. J., Bourke, M. E., Townsend, M. L., & Grenyer, B. F. (2020). Pathological narcissism: A study of burden on partners and family. *Journal of Personality Disorders*, *34*(6), 799–813. doi:10.1521/pedi_2019_33_413 PMID:30730784

de Frias, C. M., & Whyne, E. (2014). Stress on health-related quality of life in older adults: The protective nature of mindfulness. *Aging & Mental Health*, *19*(3), 201–206. doi:10.1080/13607863.2014.924090 PMID:24940847

De Genna, N. M., & Feske, U. (2013, December 1). Phenomenology of borderline personality disorder: The role of race and socioeconomic status. *The Journal of Nervous and Mental Disease*, *201*(12), 1027–1034. doi:10.1097/NMD.0000000000000053 PMID:24284636

Dean. (2016). Anxiety. *Nursing Standard*, *30*(46), 15–15. doi:10.7748/ns.30.46.15.s17

DeAngelis, T. (2021, September 1). Black men's mental health matters. Monitor on Psychology. APA. https://www.apa.org/monitor/2021/09/ce-black-mental-health

DeAngelis, R. T. (2022). Moving on Up? Neighborhood Status and Racism-Related Distress among Black Americans. *Social Forces*, *100*(4), 1503–1532. https://doi-org.proxy.tamuc.edu/10.1093/sf/soab075. doi:10.1093foab075 PMID:35847476

DeFreitas, S. C., Crone, T., DeLeon, M., & Ajayi, A. (2018). Perceived and personal mental health stigma in Latino and African American college students. *Frontiers in Public Health*, *6*, 1–10. doi:10.3389/fpubh.2018.00049 PMID:29536000

Delker, E., Brown, Q., & Hasin, D. S. (2016). Alcohol Consumption in Demographic Subpopulations An Epidemiologic Overview. *Alcohol Research: Current Reviews*, *38*(1), 7–15. http://0-www jstor org library ualr edu/stable/42659795 PMID:27159807

Dempsey, K., Butler, S. K., & Gaither, L. (2016). Black churches and mental health professionals: Can this collaboration work? *Journal of Black Studies*, *47*(1), 73–87. https://www.jstor.org/stable/24572960. doi:10.1177/0021934715613588

DeWitt, D. E., Ward, S. A., Prabhu, S., & Warton, B. (2009). Patient privacy versus protecting the patient and the health system from harm: A case study. *The Medical Journal of Australia*, *191*(4), 213–216. doi:10.5694/j.1326-5377.2009.tb02755.x PMID:19705982

Dhir, V., Arya, V., Chandra Malav, I., Gupta, R., & Dey, A. B. (2007). Idiopathic systemic capillary leak syndrome (SCLS): Case report and systematic review of cases reported in the last 16 years. *Internal Medicine (Tokyo, Japan)*, *46*(12), 899–904. doi:10.2169/internalmedicine.46.6129 PMID:17575386

Diamond, D., & Hersh, R. G. (2020). Transference-focused psychotherapy for narcissistic personality disorder: An object relations approach. *Journal of Personality Disorders*, *34*(Supplement), 159–176. doi:10.1521/pedi.2020.34.supp.159 PMID:32186988

Dolan, T., Taylor, D. J., Bramoweth, A. D., & Rosenthal, L. D. (2010). Cognitive–behavioral therapy of insomnia: A clinical case series study of patients with co-morbid disorders and using hypnotic medications. *Behaviour Research and Therapy*, *48*(4), 321–327. doi:10.1016/j.brat.2009.12.004 PMID:20074701

Donegan, D., Hickey, D. P., & Smith, D. (2012). Hypoglycemia after simultaneous pancreas-kidney transplant: Fact or factitious? *Pancreas*, *41*(6), 974–976. doi:10.1097/MPA.0b013e31823fb6ff PMID:22781913

Douglas, J. G. (2005). Clinical guidelines for the treatment of hypertension in African Americans. *American Journal of Cardiovascular Drugs*, *5*(1), 1–6. doi:10.2165/00129784-200505010-00001 PMID:15631532

Drozek, R. P., & Unruh, B. T. (2020). Mentalization-based treatment for pathological narcissism. *Journal of Personality Disorders*, *34*(Supplement), 177–203. doi:10.1521/pedi.2020.34.supp.177 PMID:32186985

Duck, W. (2009). Black male sexual politics: Avoidance of HIV/AIDS testing as a masculine health practice. *Journal of African American Studies*, *13*(3), 283–306. doi:10.100712111-009-9097-2

Dueweke, A. R., & Bridges, A. J. (2017). *Stigma and Health: The effects of brief, passive psychoeducation on suicide literacy, stigma, and attitudes toward help-seeking among Latino immigrants living in the United States*. APA. psycnet.apa.org

Dufour, R., Novack, K., Picard, L., Chadi, N., & Booij, L. (2022). The use of technology in the treatment of youth with eating disorders: A scoping review. *Journal of Eating Disorders*, *10*(1), 182. doi:10.118640337-022-00697-5 PMID:36434657

Duran, E., Firehammer, J., & Gonzalez, J. (2008). Liberation psychology as the path toward healing cultural soul wounds. *Journal of Counseling and Development*, *86*(3), 288–295. doi:10.1002/j.1556-6678.2008.tb00511.x

Duster, T. (2006). Explaining differential trust of DNA forensic technology: Grounded assessment or inexplicable paranoia? *The Journal of Law, Medicine & Ethics*, *34*(2), 293–300. doi:10.1111/j.1748-720X.2006.00034.x PMID:16789950

Eack, S., Bahorik, A., Newhill, C., Neighbors, H., & Davis, L. (2012). *Interviewer-perceived honesty as a mediator of racial disparities in the diagnosis of schizophrenia*. Psychiatry Online., doi:10.1176/appi.ps.201100388

Eastwood, S., & Bisson, J. L. (2008). Management of factitious disorders: A systematic review. *Psychotherapy and Psychosomatics*, *77*(4), 209–218. doi:10.1159/000126072 PMID:18418027

Edi-Osagie, E. C., Hopkins, R. E., & Edi-Osagie, N. E. (1998). Munchausen's syndrome in obstetrics and gynecology: A review. *Obstetrical & Gynecological Survey*, *53*(1), 45–49. doi:10.1097/00006254-199801000-00023 PMID:9440129

Elliott, M., & Ragsdale, J. M. (2021, September 15). Stress exposure and well-being: Correlates of meeting criteria for bipolar disorder, borderline personality disorder, or both. *Social Psychiatry and Psychiatric Epidemiology, 57*(9), 1885–1896. doi:10.100700127-021-02172-z PMID:34524518

Englar-Carlson, M. (2006). Masculine norms and the therapy process. In M. Englar-Carlson & M. A. Stevens (Eds.), *In the room with men: A casebook of therapeutic change* (pp. 13–47). American Psychological Association., doi:10.1037/11411-002

Englar-Carlson, M., & Kiselica, M. S. (2013). Affirming the strengths in men: A positive masculinity approach to assisting male clients. *Journal of Counseling and Development, 91*(4), 399–409. doi:10.1002/j.1556-6676.2013.00111.x

English, R. A. (1983, November). The challenge for mental health minorities and their world views. *Second Annual Robert L. Sutherland Lecture*. University of Texas at Austin.

Escamilla, S., & Saasa, S. (2020). Gendered Patterns in Depression and Anxiety among African Immigrants in the United States. *Journal of Evidence-Based Social Work (2640-8066), 17*(4), 392–405. https://doi-org.proxy.tamuc.edu/10.1080/26408066.2020.1748153

Espie, P., Pawlecki, B., Waterfield, D., Fitton, K., Radocchia, M., & Luik, A. I. (2018). Insomnia symptoms and their association with workplace productivity: Cross-sectional and pre-post intervention analyses from a large multinational manufacturing company. *Sleep Health, 4*(3), 307–312. doi:10.1016/j.sleh.2018.03.003 PMID:29776626

Facty, N. (2019, April 2). *What is borderline personality disorder - facty health*. Facty Health. Retrieved February 28, 2023, from https://facty.com/conditions/mental-health/what-is-borderline-personality-disorder/

Fain, J. A. (2013). Reading, understanding, and applying nursing research (4th ed.). F. A. Davis.

Falkenstein, M. J., Rogers, K., Malloy, E. J., & Haaga, D. A. F. (2015). Race/Ethnicity and treatment outcome in a randomized controlled trial for trichotillomania (hair-pulling disorder). *Journal of Clinical Psychology, 71*(7), 641–652. doi:10.1002/jclp.22171 PMID:25846982

Farrier, J. N., & Mansel, R. E. (2002). Dermatitis artefacta of the breast: A series of case reports. *European Journal of Surgical Oncology, 28*(2), 189–192. doi:10.1053/ejso.2001.1214 PMID:11884056

Feldman, M. D. Phillips (Ed.), K.A. (2008). Factitious disorder, in somatoform and factitious disorders, American Psychiatric Publishing

Feldman, M. D., & Eisendrath, S. J. (1996). The spectrum of factitious disorders, American Psychiatric Publishing

Feldman, M. D., & Brown, R. M. (2002). Munchausen by proxy in an international context. *Child Abuse & Neglect, 26*(5), 509–524. doi:10.1016/S0145-2134(02)00327-7 PMID:12079087

Felix-Ortiz, M., Abreu, J. M., Briano, M., & Bowen, D. (2001). A critique of machismo measures in psychological research. In F. Columbus (Ed.), *Advances in psychology research* (Vol. III, pp. 63–90). NOVA Science Publishers.

Fernandez, A., Tan, K.-A., Knaak, S., Chew, B. H., & Ghazali, S. S. (2016). Effects of Brief Psychoeducational Program on Stigma in Malaysian Pre-clinical Medical Students: A Randomized Controlled Trial. *Academic Psychiatry*, *40*(6), 905–911. doi:10.100740596-016-0592-1 PMID:27527730

Fleming, P. J., Lee, J. G., & Dworkin, S. L. (2014). "Real men don't": Constructions of masculinity and inadvertent harm in public health interventions. *American Journal of Public Health*, *104*(6), 1029–1035. doi:10.2105/AJPH.2013.301820 PMID:24825202

Fliege, H., Grimm, A., Eckhardt-Henn, A., Gieler, U., Martin, K., & Klapp, B. K. (2007). Frequency of ICD-10 factitious disorder: Survey of senior hospital consultants and physicians in private practice. *Psychosomatics*, *48*(1), 60–64. doi:10.1176/appi.psy.48.1.60 PMID:17209151

Fliege, H., Scholler, G., Rose, M., Willenberg, H., & Klapp, B. F. (2002). Factitious disorders and pathological self-harm in a hospital population: An interdisciplinary challenge. *General Hospital Psychiatry*, *24*(3), 164–171. doi:10.1016/S0163-8343(02)00171-8 PMID:12062141

Floersch, J., Kranke, B., & Munson, M. R. (2011). A qualitative investigation of self-stigma among adolescents taking psychiatric medication. *Psychiatric Services (Washington, D.C.)*, *62*(8), 893–899. doi:10.1176/ps.62.8.pss6208_0893 PMID:21807828

Flowers, K. C., Levesque, M. J., & Fischer, S. (2012). The relationship between maladaptive eating behaviors and racial identity among African American women in college. *The Journal of Black Psychology*, *38*(3), 290–312. doi:10.1177/0095798411416459

Ford, C. V., Friedmann, C. T., & Faguet, R. A. (Eds.), (1982). Munchausen syndrome, in extraordinary disorders of human behaviour. Springer US

Ford, C. V. (1973). The Munchausen syndrome: A report of four new cases and a review of psychodynamic considerations. *International Journal of Psychiatry in Medicine*, *4*(1), 31–45. PMID:4709440

Forrest, L. N., Smith, A. R., & Swanson, S. A. (2017). Characteristics of seeking treatment among U.S. adolescents with eating disorders. *International Journal of Eating Disorders*, *50*(7), 826–833. doi:10.1002/eat.22702 PMID:28323350

Foster, M. D., & Matheson, K. (1998). Perceiving and feeling personal discrimination: Motivation or inhibition for collective action? *Group Processes & Intergroup Relations*, *1*(2), 165–174. doi:10.1177/1368430298012004

Fox, D. (2022, August 3). *Borderline personality disorder and the danger of self-destruction.* Psychology Today. Retrieved February 28, 2023, from https://www.psychologytoday.com/us/blog/the-complex-diagnosis/202208/borderline-personality-disorder-and-the-danger-self-destruction

Fraguas, D., & Breathnach, C. S. (2009). Problems with retrospective studies of the presence of schizophrenia. *History of Psychiatry*, *20*(1), 61–71. doi:10.1177/0957154X08089453 PMID:20617641

Franklin, C. W. (1986). Conceptual and logical issues in theory and research related to Black masculinity. *The Western Journal of Black Studies*, *10*, 161–166.

Franko, D. L., Thompson, D. R., Forbush, K. T., Bryson, S. W., Crow, S. J., Gorin, A. A., & Wilson, G. T. (2012). Racial/Ethnic differences in adults in randomized clinical trials of binge eating disorder. *Journal of Consulting and Clinical Psychology*, *80*(2), 186–195. doi:10.1037/a0026700 PMID:22201327

Frazier, C. (2020). It's more than just news: Print media, the Tuskegee syphilis study and collective memory among African Americans. *Journal of Historical Sociology*, *33*(3), 280–296. doi:10.1111/johs.12281

Frazier, E. F. (1939). *The Negro Family in the United States*. University of Chicago Press., doi:10.2307/2292637

Freeman, D. R. (2006). Spirituality in Violent and Substance-Abusing African American Men: An Untapped Resource for Healing. *Journal of Religion & Spirituality in Social Work*, *25*(1), 3–22. https://doi-org.proxy.tamuc.edu/10.1300/J377v25n01_02. doi:10.1300/J377v25n01_02

French, B. H., Lewis, J. A., Mosley, D. V., Adames, H. Y., Chavez-Dueñas, N. Y., Chen, G. A., & Neville, H. A. (2020). Toward a psychological framework of radical healing in communities of color. *The Counseling Psychologist*, *48*(1), 14–46. doi:10.1177/0011000019843506

Frye, E. M., & Feldman, M. D. (2012). Factitious Disorder by Proxy in Educational Settings: A Review. *Educational Psychology Review*, *24*(1), 47–61. doi:10.100710648-011-9180-9

Fujiwara, T., Kubo, T., Yano, K., & Hosokawa, K. (2008). A case of intractable recurrent abdominal cutaneous ulceration caused by self-injection of menstrual blood. *European Journal of Plastic Surgery*, *30*(6), 303–304. doi:10.100700238-007-0199-6

Gadelkarim, W., Shahper, S., Reid, J., Wikramanayake, M., Kaur, S., Kolli, S., Osman, S., & Fineberg, N. A. (2019). Overlap of obsessive–compulsive personality disorder and autism spectrum disorder traits among OCD outpatients: An exploratory study. *International Journal of Psychiatry in Clinical Practice*, *23*(4), 297–306. doi:10.1080/13651501.2019.1638939 PMID:31375037

Galdas, P. M., Cheater, F., & Marshall, P. (2005). Men and health help-seeking behaviour: Literature review. *Journal of Advanced Nursing*, *49*(6), 616–623. doi:10.1111/j.1365-2648.2004.03331.x PMID:15737222

Galmiche, M., Déchelotte, P., Lambert, G., & Tavolacci, M. P. (2019). Prevalence of eating disorders over the 2000–2018 period: A systematic literature review. *The American Journal of Clinical Nutrition*, *109*(5), 1402–1413. doi:10.1093/ajcn/nqy342 PMID:31051507

Gamble, V. N. (1997). The Tuskegee Syphilis Study and women's health. *Journal of the American Medical Women's Association (1972)*, *52*(4), 195-196.

Gao, J., Li, Y., Cai, Y., Chen, J., Shen, Y., Ni, S., Wei, Y., Qiu, Y., Zhu, X., Liu, Y., Lu, C., Chen, C., Niu, Q., Tang, C., Yang, Y., Wang, Q., Cui, W., Xia, J., Liu, T., & Tao, M. (2012). Perceived parenting and risk for major depression in Chinese women. *Psychological Medicine*, *42*(05), 921–930. doi:10.1017/S0033291711001942 PMID:21943491

Gara, M., Minsky, S., Silverstein, S., Miskimen, T., & Strakowski, S. (2019). A naturalistic study of racial disparities in diagnoses at an outpatient behavioral health clinic. *Psychiatric Services (Washington, D.C.)*, *70*(2), 30–134. doi:10.1176/appi.ps.201800223 PMID:30526340

Garb, H. N. (1997). Race bias, social class bias, and gender bias in clinical judgment. *Clinical Psychology: Science and Practice*, *4*(2), 99–120. doi:10.1111/j.1468-2850.1997.tb00104.x

Garb, H. N. (1998). *Studying the clinician.* American Psychological Association.

Gaston, G. B., Earl, T. R., Nisanci, A., & Glomb, B. (2016). Perception of mental health services among Black Americans. *Social Work in Mental Health*, *14*(6), 676–695. https://doi-org.proxy.tamuc.edu/10.1080/15332985.2015.1137257. doi:10.1080/15332985.2015.1137257

Gatison, Annette Madlock, PhD. (2021). A Woman Approach to Caring for Patients With Empirically Unverifiable Symptoms. *AMA Journal of Ethics*. PMID:34351260

Gavin, H., On the feigned and factitious diseases of soldiers and seamen; with hints for the examination, and rules for the detection of impostors, 1843

Gehlert, S., Sohmer, D., Sacks, T., Mininger, C., McClintock, M., & Olopade, O. (2008). Targeting health disparities: A model linking upstream determinants to downstream interventions. *Health Affairs*, *27*(2), 339–349. doi:10.1377/hlthaff.27.2.339 PMID:18332488

Geller, A., Fagan, J., Tyler, T., & Link, B. G. (2014). Aggressive policing and the mental health of young urban men. *American Journal of Public Health*, *104*(12), 2321–2327. doi:10.2105/AJPH.2014.302046 PMID:25322310

GenPsych PC. (2018). *Signs of Borderline Personality Disorder.* Retrieved February 23, 2023, from https://genpsych.com/

Gerdes, Z. T., & Levant, R. F. (2018). Complex relationships among masculine norms and health/well-being outcomes: Correlation patterns of the conformity to masculine norms inventory subscales. *American Journal of Men's Health*, *12*(2), 229–240. doi:10.1177/1557988317745910 PMID:29219033

Ghafoor, H., Schulz, S. M., & Mohsin, H. (2018). Does religiosity ameliorate the negative impact of obsessive-compulsive disorder on self-esteem? *Mental Health, Religion & Culture*, *21*(2), 171–179. doi:10.1080/13674676.2018.1458082

Giuliodori, K., Campanati, A., Rosa, L., Marconi, B., Cellini, A., & Brandozzi, G. (2014). *Factitious disorders in adults: two cases of unusual skin ulcers.*

Giuliodori, K., Campanati, A., Rosa, L., Marconi, B., Cellini, A., & Brandozzi, G. (2014). Factitious disorders in adults: Two cases of unusual skin ulcers. *Acta Dermatovenerologica Alpina, Panonica, et Adriatica*, *23*(1), 13–15. PMID:24638866

Godbolt, D., Opara, I., & Amutah-Onukagha, N. (2022). Strong Black women: Linking stereotypes, stress, and overeating among a sample of Black female college students. *Journal of Black Studies*, *53*(6), 609–634. doi:10.1177/00219347221087453 PMID:36710718

Goff, P. A., Di Leone, B. A. L., & Kahn, K. B. (2012). Racism leads to pushups: How racial discrimination threatens subordinate men's masculinity. *Journal of Experimental Social Psychology*, *48*(5), 1111–1116. doi:10.1016/j.jesp.2012.03.015

Goode, R. W., Cowell, M. M., Mazzeo, S. E., Cooper-Lewter, C., Forte, A., Olayia, O., & Bulik, C. M. (2019). Binge eating and binge-eating disorder in Black women: A systematic review. *International Journal of Eating Disorders*, *53*(4), 491–507. doi:10.1002/eat.23217 PMID:31922293

Gordon, D. K., & Sansone, R. A. (2013). A relationship between factitious disorder and borderline personality disorder. *Innovations in Clinical Neuroscience*, *10*(11–12), 11. PMID:24563814

Gran-Ruaz, S. M., Taylor, R. J., Jacob, G., & Williams, M. T. (2022). Lifetime trauma exposure and posttraumatic stress disorder among African Americans and Black Caribbeans by sex and ethnicity. *Frontiers in Psychiatry*, *13*, 1–15. doi:10.3389/fpsyt.2022.889060 PMID:35800025

Grappone, G. (2018). Overcoming Stigma. *National Alliance on Mental Illness (NAMI)*. https://www.nami.org/Blogs/NAMI-Blog/October-2018/Overcoming-Stigma

Green, C., & Gaston-Hawkins, L. (2020, July 14). *Racism, policing, and covid-19: How do we justify racial disparities in 2020?* Psychiatric Times. Retrieved February 28, 2023, from https://www.psychiatrictimes.com/view/policing-and-covid-19-disparities-how-do-we-justify-racial-disparities-in-2020

Greer, T. M., & Spalding, A. (2017). The Role of age in understanding the psychological effects of racism for African Americans. *Cultural Diversity & Ethnic Minority Psychology*, *23*(4), 588–594. doi:10.1037/cdp0000148 PMID:28301183

Gregurek-Novak, T., Novak-Bilić, G., & Vučić, M. (2005). Dermatitis artefacta: Unusual appearance in an older woman. *Journal of the European Academy of Dermatology and Venereology*, *19*(2), 223–225. doi:10.1111/j.1468-3083.2005.01022.x PMID:15752297

Grier, W. H., & Cobbs, P. M. (1968). *Black rage*. Basic Books.

Griffith, D. M. (2015). "I AM a Man": Manhood, minority men's health, and health equity. *Ethnicity & Disease*, *25*(3), 287–293. doi:10.18865/ed.25.3.287 PMID:26672674

Griffiths, E. J., Kampa, R., Pearce, C., Sakellariou, A., & Solan, M. C. (2009). Munchausen's syndrome by Google©. *Annals of the Royal College of Surgeons of England*, *91*(2), 159–160. doi:10.1308/003588409X391938 PMID:19317939

Grilo, C. M., White, M. A., Barnes, R. D., & Masheb, R. M. (2012). Posttraumatic stress disorder in women with binge eating disorder in primary care. *Journal of Psychiatric Practice*, *18*(6), 408–412. doi:10.1097/01.pra.0000422738.49377.5e PMID:23160245

Grilo, C. M., White, M. A., Barnes, R. D., & Masheb, R. M. (2013). Psychiatric disorder co-morbidity and correlates in an ethnically diverse sample of obese patients with binge eating disorder in primary care settings. *Comprehensive Psychiatry*, *54*(3), 209–216. doi:10.1016/j.comppsych.2012.07.012 PMID:22943959

Groesz, L. M., McCoy, S., Carl, J., Saslow, L., Stewart, J., Adler, N., Laraia, B., & Epel, E. (2012). What is eating you? Stress and the drive to eat. *Appetite*, *58*(2), 717–721. doi:10.1016/j.appet.2011.11.028 PMID:22166677

Grossmann, I., Karasawa, M., Kan, C., & Kitayama, S. (2014). A cultural perspective on emotional experiences across the life span. *Emotion (Washington, D.C.)*, *14*(4), 679–692. https://doi-org.ezp.twu.edu/10.1037/a0036041. doi:10.1037/a0036041 PMID:24749641

Gross, P. A., Efimoff, I., Patrick, L., Josewski, V., Hau, K., Lambert, S., & Smye, V. (2016). The DUDES Club: A brotherhood for men's health. *Canadian Family Physician Medecin de Famille Canadien*, *62*(6), e311–e318.

Guerrero, E. G., Marsh, J. C., Cao, D., Shin, H.-C., & Andrews, C. (2014). Gender disparities in utilization and outcome of comprehensive substance abuse treatment among racial/ethnic groups. *Journal of Substance Abuse Treatment*, *46*(5), 584–591. https://doi-org.proxy.tamuc.edu/10.1016/j.jsat.2013.12.008. doi:10.1016/j.jsat.2013.12.008 PMID:24560127

Gullestad, F. S., Wilberg, T., Klungsøyr, O., Johansen, M. S., Urnes, O., & Karterud, S. (2011, August 9). Is treatment in a day hospital step-down program superior to outpatient individual psychotherapy for patients with personality disorders? 36 months follow-up of a randomized clinical trial comparing different treatment modalities. *Psychotherapy Research*, *22*(4), 426–441. doi:10.1080/10503307.2012.662608 PMID:22417131

Gurak, K., & Weisman De Mamani, A. (2017). Caregiver expressed emotion and psychiatric symptoms in African-Americans with schizophrenia: An attempt to understand the paradoxical relationship. *Family Process*, *56*(2), 476–486. https://onlinelibrary-wiley-com.proxy.tamuc.edu/doi/pdfdirect/10.1111/famp.12188. doi:10.1111/famp.12188 PMID:26498273

Gutiérrez-Rojas, L., Porras-Segovia, A., Dunne, H., Andrade-González, N., & Cervilla, J. A. (2020). Prevalence and correlates of major depressive disorder: A systematic review. *The British Journal of Psychiatry*, *42*(6), 657–672. doi:10.1590/1516-4446-2020-0650 PMID:32756809

Haddad, P. & Haddad, I. (2015). Mental Health Stigma. *British Association for Psychopharmacology (BAP)* Articles [online]. https://www.bap.org.uk/articles/mental-health-stigma/

Haddad, S. A., Winer, K. K., Gupta, A., Chakrabarti, S., Noel, P., & Klein, H. G. S. A. (2002). A puzzling case of anemia. *Transfusion*, *42*(12), 1610–1613. doi:10.1046/j.1537-2995.2002.00269.x PMID:12473143

Hall, J. C. (2018). It is tough being a Black woman: Intergenerational stress and coping. *Journal of Black Studies*, *49*(5), 481–501. doi:10.1177/0021934718766817

Hambleton, A., Pepin, G., Le, A., Maloney, D., Aouad, P., Barakat, S., Boakes, R., Brennan, L., Bryant, E., Byrne, S., Caldwell, B., Calvert, S., Carroll, B., Castle, D., Caterson, I., Chelius, B., Chiem, L., Clarke, S., Conti, J., & Maguire, S.National Eating Disorder Consortium. (2022). Psychiatric and medical comorbidities of eating disorders: Findings from a rapid review of the literature. *Journal of Eating Disorders*, *10*(132), 1–23. doi:10.118640337-022-00654-2 PMID:36064606

Hammen, C. (2005). Stress and depression. *Annual Review of Clinical Psychology*, *1*(1), 293–319. doi:10.1146/annurev.clinpsy.1.102803.143938 PMID:17716090

Hammer, J. H., & Good, G. E. (2010). Positive psychology: An empirical examination of beneficial aspects of endorsement of masculine norms. *Psychology of Men & Masculinity*, *11*(4), 303–318. doi:10.1037/a0019056

Hammond, W. P. (2010). Psychosocial correlates of medical mistrust among African American men. *American Journal of Community Psychology*, *45*(1-2), 87–106. doi:10.100710464-009-9280-6 PMID:20077134

Hammond, W. P., & Mattis, J. S. (2005). Being a Man About It: Manhood Meaning Among African American Men. *Psychology of Men & Masculinity*, *6*(2), 114–126. doi:10.1037/1524-9220.6.2.114

Han, D.-Y., & Chen, S.-H. (2014). Reducing the stigma of depression through neurobiology-based psychoeducation: A randomized controlled trial. *Psychiatry and Clinical Neurosciences*, *68*(9), 666–673. doi:10.1111/pcn.12174 PMID:24521323

Hankerson, S. H., & Weissman, M. M. (2012). Church-based health programs for mental disorders among African Americans: A review. *Psychiatric Services (Washington, D.C.)*, *63*(3), 243–249. doi:10.1176/appi.ps.201100216 PMID:22388529

Hare, I. (2004). Defining social work for the 21st century. The International Federation of Social Workers' revised definition of social work. *International Social Work*, *47*(3), 407–424. doi:10.1177/0020872804043973

Hariharasubramony, A., Chankramath, S., & Srinivasa, S. (2012). Munchausen syndrome as dermatitis simulate. *Indian Journal of Psychological Medicine*, *34*(1), 94–96. doi:10.4103/0253-7176.96171 PMID:22661819

Harley, D. A., & Dillard, J. M. (Eds.). (2005). *Contemporary mental health issues among African Americans*. Amer Counseling Assn.

Harper, F. D., & Dawkins, M. P. (1977). Alcohol abuse in the Black community. *The Black Scholar*, *8*(6), 23–31. doi:10.1080/00064246.1977.11658635

Harper, J. I., & Copeman, P. W. (1983). Dermatitis artefacta presenting as a "vasculitis". *Journal of the Royal Society of Medicine*, *76*(11), 970–971. doi:10.1177/014107688307601118 PMID:6631880

Harris, Y. R., & Graham, J. A. (2014). In the African American child: Development and challenges (pp. 65–80). Springer Publishing Company.

Harris, J. R. A., McKinney, J. L. G., & Fripp, J. (2019). "God Is a Keeper": A Phenomenological Investigation of Christian African American Women's Experiences With Religious Coping. *The Professional Counselor*, *9*(3), 171–184. doi:10.15241/jrah.9.3.171

Harris, J. R., Crowe, A., & McKinney, J. G. (2020). African Americans' perceptions of mental illness and preferences for treatment. *Journal of Counselor Practice*, *11*(1), 1–33. doi:10.22229/afa1112020

Harris, S. M. (1995). Psychosocial development and Black male masculinity: Implications for counseling economically disadvantaged African American male adolescents. *Journal of Counseling and Development*, *73*(3), 279–287. doi:10.1002/j.1556-6676.1995.tb01749.x

Harris, S. M. (2015). Black American female eating dysfunctions and body image: A bioecological perspective. *Negro Educational Review*, *66*(1-4), 27–54. doi:10.13140/RG.2.1.4962.6640

Haughwout, S. P., Harford, T. C., Castle, I.-J. P., & Grant, B. F. (2016). Treatment Utilization Among Adolescent Substance Users: Findings from the 2002 to 2013 National Survey on Drug Use and Health. *Alcoholism, Clinical and Experimental Research*, *40*(8), 1717–1727. https://doi-org.proxy.tamuc.edu/10.1111/acer.13137. doi:10.1111/acer.13137 PMID:27427179

Haw, C., Hawton, K., Houston, K., & Townsend, E. (2001). Psychiatric and personality disorders in deliberate self-harm patients. *The British Journal of Psychiatry*, *178*(1), 48–54. doi:10.1192/bjp.178.1.48 PMID:11136210

Hays, K. (2015). Black churches' capacity to respond to the mental health needs of African Americans. *Social Work & Christianity*, *42*(3), 293–312.

Hazlett-Stevens, H., & Craske, M. (2002). *Brief Cognitive-Behavioral Therapy: Definition and Scientific Foundations*. John Wiley & Sons Ltd.

HeadUpGuys. (n.d.). *Manage & Prevent Depression in Men. Vancouver (BC)*. HeadsUpGuys. https://headsupguys.org

Henry, T. L., Jetty, A., Petterson, S., Jaffree, H., Ramsay, A., Heiman, E., & Bazemore, A. (2020). Taking a closer look at mental health treatment differences: Effectiveness of mental health treatment by provider type in racial and ethnic minorities. *Journal of Primary Care & Community Health*, *11*, 2150132720966403. doi:10.1177/2150132720966403 PMID:33089752

Heron M. (2018). Deaths: leading causes for 2016 [PDF-2.3M]. *National Vital Statistics Report*, *67*(6), 1–77.

Hertz, R. P., Unger, A. N., Cornell, J. A., & Saunders, E. (2005). Racial disparities in hypertension prevalence, awareness, and management. *Archives of Internal Medicine*, *165*(18), 2098–2104. doi:10.1001/archinte.165.18.2098 PMID:16216999

Hewitt, C. M. (2004). African-American concentration in jobs the political economy of job segregation and contestation in Atlanta. *Urban Affairs Review, 39*(3), 318–341. doi:10.1177/1078087403253416

Highland, K. B., & Flume, P. A. (2002). A "story" of a woman with cystic fibrosis. *Chest, 121*(5), 1704–1707. doi:10.1378/chest.121.5.1704 PMID:12006467

Hirayama, Y., Sakamaki, S., Tsuji, Y., Sagawa, T., Takayanagi, N., Chiba, H., Matsunaga, T., Kato, J., & Niitsu, Y. (2003). Fatality caused by self-bloodletting in a patient with factitious anemia. *International Journal of Hematology, 78*(2), 146–148. doi:10.1007/BF02983383 PMID:12953809

Holden, K. B., McGregor, B. S., Blanks, S. H., & Mahaffey, C. (2012). Psychosocial, socio-cultural, and environmental influences on mental health help-seeking among African-American men. *The Journal of Men's Health, 9*(2), 63–69. doi:10.1016/j.jomh.2012.03.002 PMID:22905076

Hooley, J. M. (2007). *Expressed emotion and relapse of psychopathology*. Annual Review of Clinical Psychology. doi:10.1146/annurev.clinpsy.2.022305.095236

Hooley, J. M., & Gotlib, I. H. (2000). A diathesis-stress conceptualization of expressed emotion and clinical outcome. *Applied & Preventive Psychology, 9*(3), 135–151. doi:10.1016/S0962-1849(05)80001-0

Horsman, E. N. (2018). Underage drinking as a predictor of alcohol use disorder among African Americans. *Journal of Psychology in Africa, 28*(4), 323–329. doi:10.1080/14330237.2018.1507097

Howard, L. M., Haislip, B. N., Heron, K. E., & Xiao, X. H. (2019). Associations among social connections, body dissatisfaction, and disordered eating in African American and European American college women. *Psi Chi Journal of Psychological Research, 24*(1), 33–42. doi:10.24839/2325-7342.JN24.1.33

Hudson, D. L., Neighbors, H. W., Geronimus, A. T., & Jackson, J. S. (2016). Racial discrimination, john henryism, and depression among African Americans. *The Journal of Black Psychology, 42*(3), 221–243. doi:10.1177/0095798414567757 PMID:27529626

Hudson, D., Collins-Anderson, A., & Hutson, W. (2023). Understanding the Impact of Contemporary Racism on the Mental Health of Middle Class Black Americans. *International Journal of Environmental Research and Public Health, 20*(3), 1660. doi:10.3390/ijerph20031660 PMID:36767028

Hunter, A. G., & Davis, J. E. (1992). Constructing gender: An exploration of Afro-American men's conceptualization of manhood. *Gender & Society, 6*(3), 464–479. doi:10.1177/089124392006003007

Hunter, A. G., & Davis, J. E. (1994). Hidden voices of Black men: Meaning, structure, and complexity of manhood. *Journal of Black Studies, 25*(1), 20–40. doi:10.1177/002193479402500102

Hyde, J. S., & DeLamater, J. D. (2017). Understanding Human Sexuality (13ed.). New York: McGraw-Hill.

Ingoldsby, B. (1991). The Latin American family: Familism vs. machismo. *Journal of Comparative Family Studies*, *1*(1), 57–64. doi:10.3138/jcfs.22.1.57

International O. C. D. Foundation. (2010). Obsessive Compulsive Personality Disorder (OCPD). IOCD. https://iocdf.org/wp-content/uploads/2014/10/OCPD-Fact-Sheet.pdf

Ivezić, S. Š., Sesar, M. A., & Mužinić, L. (2017) Effects of a group psychoeducation program on self-stigma, empowerment and perceived discrimination of persons with schizophrenia. Psychiatria Danubina, 29(1), pp 66-73.

Iwamoto, D. K., Liao, L., & Liu, W. M. (2010). Masculine norms, avoidant coping, Asian values, and depression among Asian American men. *Psychology of Men & Masculinity*, *11*(1), 15–24. doi:10.1037/a0017874 PMID:20657794

Jackson, B. K. (2015). Licensed professional counselors' perceptions of pastoral counseling in the African American community. *The Journal of Pastoral Care & Counseling*, *69*(2), 85–101. doi:10.1177/1542305015586773 PMID:26227938

Jackson, J. S., Campbell, L., & Williams, D. (1989). The influence of racial factors on psychiatric diagnosis: A review and suggestions for research. *Community Mental Health Journal*, *25*(4), 301–311. doi:10.1007/BF00755677 PMID:2697490

Jackson, J. S., Neighbors, H. W., Torres, M., Martin, L. A., Williams, D. R., & Baser, R. (2007). Use of mental health services and subjective satisfaction with treatment among Black Caribbean immigrants: Results from the National Survey of American Life. *American Journal of Public Health*, *97*(1), 60–67. doi:10.2105/AJPH.2006.088500 PMID:17138907

Jacobs, M. D., Rolle, I., Ferrans, C. E., Whitaker, E. E., & Warnecke, R. B. (2006). Understanding African Americans' View of the Trushworthiness of Physicians. *Journal of General Internal Medicine*, *21*(6), 642–647. doi:10.1111/j.1525-1497.2006.00485.x PMID:16808750

Jacobson, J. O., Robinson, P., & Bluthenthal, R. N. (2007). A multilevel decomposition approach to estimate the role of program location and neighborhood disadvantage in racial disparities in alcohol treatment completion. *Social Science & Medicine*, *64*(2), 462–476. doi:10.1016/j.socscimed.2006.08.032 PMID:17055634

Jafferany, M. D., & Mohammad, F. A. P. A. (2018). The Primary Care Companion for CNS Disorders.

Jaghab, K. (2006). Munchausen's Syndrome and Other Factitous Disorder in Children. *Psychiatry (Edgmont, Pa.)*, *3*(3), 46–55.

Jahraus, J. (2018). Medical complications of eating disorders. *Psychiatric Annals*, *48*(10), 463–467. doi:10.3928/00485713-20180912-04

Jauk, E., Ulbrich, L., Jorschick, P., Höfler, M., Kaufman, S. B., & Kanske, P. (2022). The nonlinear association between grandiose and vulnerable narcissism: An individual data meta-analysis. *Journal of Personality*, *90*(5), 703–726. doi:10.1111/jopy.12692 PMID:34860434

Javaras, K. N., Runfola, C. D., Thornton, L. M., Agerbo, E., Birgegård, A., Norring, C., Yao, S., Råstam, M., Larsson, H., Lichtenstein, P., & Bulik, C. M. (2015). Sex- and age-specific incidence of healthcare- register-recorded eating disorders in the complete Swedish 1979–2001 birth cohort. *International Journal of Eating Disorders, 48*(8), 1070–1081. doi:10.1002/eat.22467 PMID:26769444

Jegede, O., Muvvala, S., Katehis, E., Paul, S., Soipe, A., & Jolayemi, A. (2021). Perceived barriers to access care, anticipated discrimination and structural vulnerability among African Americans with substance use disorders. *The International Journal of Social Psychiatry, 67*(2), 136–143. https://doi-org.proxy.tamuc.edu/10.1177/0020764020934512. doi:10.1177/0020764020934512 PMID:32666877

Jerome, R., Halkitis, P., & Coley, M.The Hope Team. (2009). Methamphetamine use patterns among urban Black men who have sex with men. *Culture, Health & Sexuality, 11*(4), 399–413. https://doi-org.proxy.tamuc.edu/10.1080/13691050902780768. doi:10.1080/13691050902780768 PMID:19301167

Jin, W. K., Morgan, E., & Nyhan, B. (2020). Treatment versus Punishment: Undersdanding Racial Inequalities in Drug Policy. *Journal of Health Politics, Policy & Law, 45*(2), 177–209. https://doi-org.proxy.tamuc.edu/10.1215/03616878-8004850

Johnson, B. L., McShane, T. O., & Salgado, D. M. (2015, May). *Effects of masculine norms on health behaviors in men.* Poster presented at the Western Psychological Association Convention, Las Vegas, NV.

Johnson, T. (2022, January 1). *5 meaningful ways to embrace black mental health this February.* Anxiety and Depression Association of America, ADAA. Retrieved February 28, 2023, from https://adaa.org/living-with-anxiety/personal-stories/5-meaningful-ways-embrace-black-mental-health-february

Johnson, B. R., & Harrison, J. A. (2000). Suspected Munchausen's syndrome and civil commitment. *The Journal of the American Academy of Psychiatry and the Law, 28*(1), 74–76. PMID:10774844

Jones, B. L., Vyhlidal, C. A., Bradley-Ewing, A., Sherman, A., & Goggin, K. (2017). If we would only ask: How Henrietta Lacks continues to teach us about perceptions of research and genetic research among African Americans today. *Journal of Racial and Ethnic Health Disparities, 4*(4), 735–745. doi:10.100740615-016-0277-1 PMID:27664025

Jones, W. (2020). The lives of Douglass, Du Bois, and Washington: Self-actualization among African American males. *Journal of Humanistic Psychology, 60*(3), 303–329. https://doi-org.proxy.tamuc.edu/10.1177/0022167817739761. doi:10.1177/0022167817739761

Jordan, S. (2021). Neurodiversity in children and the struggles of being misdiagnosed. *Black Wall Street Media.* https://blackwallst.media/neurodiversity-in-children-and-the-struggles-of-being-misdiagnosed

Kahn, A., Boroff, E. S., Martin, K. A., Northfelt, D. W., & Heigh, R. I. (2015). Factitious disorder in Crohn's disease: Recurrent pancytopenia caused by surreptitious ingestion of 6-Mercaptopurine. *Case Reports in Gastroenterology*, *9*(2), 137–141. doi:10.1159/000382073 PMID:26078732

Kanaan, R. A., & Wessely, S. C. (2010). Factitious disorders in neurology: An analysis of reported cases. *Psychosomatics*, *51*(1), 47–54. doi:10.1016/S0033-3182(10)70658-7 PMID:20118440

Kane, C. M. (2000). African American family dynamics as perceived by family members. *Journal of Black Studies*, *30*(5), 691–702. doi:10.1177/002193470003000504

Kang, E., Wen, Z., Song, H., Christian, K. M., & Ming, G. (2016). Adult neurogenesis and psychiatric disorders. *Cold Spring Harbor Perspectives in Biology*, *8*(9), a019026. doi:10.1101/cshperspect.a019026 PMID:26801682

Kanny, D., Liu, Y., & Drewer, R. D. (2009). Binge drinking—United States, 2009. Morbidity and Mortality Weekly Report. National Center for Chronic Disease Prevention and Health Promotion.

Kapfhammer, H. P., Rothenhäusler, H. B., Dietrich, E., Dobmeier, P., & Mayer, C. (1998). Artifactual disorders–between deception and self-mutilation. Experiences in consultation psychiatry at a university clinic. *Der Nervenarzt*, *69*(5), 401–409. doi:10.1007001150050289 PMID:9629556

Karlstad, J., Moe, C. F., Stokland, R. A., & Brinchmann, B. S. (2022). "Balancing within a closed family system": A grounded theory study of how family life is affected by having a family member with an eating disorder. *Journal of Eating Disorders*, *10*(1), 1–10. doi:10.118640337-022-00669-9 PMID:36217195

Kashyap, N. (2022, September 21). *Transference-focused psychotherapy: Using the therapist-individual relationship to heal.* Verywell Health. https://www.verywellhealth.com/transference-focused-psychotherapy-5323806

Kawaii-Bogue, B., Williams, N. J., & MacNear, K. (2017). Mental health care access and treatment utilization in African American communities: An integrative care framework. *Best Practices in Mental Health*, *13*(2), 11–29.

Kazdin, A. E., Fitzsimmons-Craft, E. E., & Wilfley, D. E. (2017). Addressing critical gaps in the treatment of eating disorders. *International Journal of Eating Disorders*, *50*(3), 170–189. doi:10.1002/eat.22670 PMID:28102908

Kelly, N. R., Cotter, E. W., Guidinger, C., & Williamson, G. (2020). Perceived discrimination, emotion dysregulation and loss of control eating in young men. *Eating Behaviors*, *37*, 101387. doi:10.1016/j.eatbeh.2020.101387 PMID:32353703

Kelly, N. R., Smith, T. M., Hall, G. C., Guidinger, C., Williamson, G., Budd, E. L., & Giuliani, N. R. (2018). Perceptions of general and postpresidential election discrimination are associated with loss of control eating among racially/ethnically diverse young men. *International Journal of Eating Disorders*, *51*(1), 28–38. doi:10.1002/eat.22803 PMID:29149497

Kendler, K. S., Thornton, L. M., & Gardner, C. O. (2000). Stressful life events and previous episodes in the etiology of major depression in women: An evaluation of the "kindling" hypothesis. *The American Journal of Psychiatry*, *157*(8), 1. doi:10.1176/appi.ajp.157.8.1243 PMID:10910786

Kenedi, C. A., Shirey, K. G., Hoffa, M., Zanga, J., Lee, J. C., & Harrison, J. D. (2011). Laboratory diagnosis of factitious disorder: A systematic review of tools useful in the diagnosis of Munchausen's syndrome. *The New Zealand Medical Journal*, *124*(1342), 66–81. PMID:21963927

Keshavarzpir, Z., Seyedfatemi, N., Mardani-Hamooleh, M., Esmaeeli, N., & Boyd, J. E. (2020). The Effect of Psychoeducation on Internalized Stigma of the Hospitalized Patients with Bipolar Disorder: A Quasi-Experimental Study. *Issues in Mental Health Nursing*, 1–8. doi:10.1080/01612840.2020.1779881 PMID:32881602

Kessler, R. C., Berglund, P. A., Chiu, W. T., Deitz, A. C., Hudson, J. I., Shahly, V., Aguilar-Gaxiola, S., Alonso, J., Angermeyer, M. C., Benjet, C., Bruffaerts, R., de Girolamo, G., de Graaf, R., Maria Haro, J., Kovess-Masfety, V., O'Neill, S., Posada-Villa, J., Sasu, C., Scott, K, & Xavier, M. (2013). The prevalence and correlates of binge eating disorder in the World Health Organization world mental health surveys. *Biological Psychiatry*, *73*(9), 904–914. doi:10.1016/j.biopsych.2012.11.020 PMID:23290497

Kim, M. (2016). Understanding the etiology and treatment approaches of schizophrenia: Theoretical perspectives and their critique. *Journal of Psychiatry*, *6*, 1–9.

King, L. M., Moody, S., Thompson, O., & Bennett, M. (1983). Black psychology reconsidered: Notes toward curriculum development. In J. C. Chunn II, P. J. Dunston, & F. Ross-Sheriff (Eds.), *Mental health & people of color: Curriculum development and change* (pp. 3–22). Howard University Press.

King, R. M., Grenyer, B. F., Gurtman, C. G., & Younan, R. (2020). A clinician's quick guide to evidence-based approaches: Narcissistic personality disorder. *Clinical Psychologist*, *24*(1), 91–95. doi:10.1111/cp.12214

King, T. F., Shea, P. O., Sullivan, E. P., Srinivasan, R., Griffin, A., Fitzgerald, R., Tormey, W., & Smith, D. (2008). An apparent phaeochromocytoma and abnormal thyroid function tests. *Annals of Clinical Biochemistry*, *45*(2), 215–217. doi:10.1258/acb.2007.007106 PMID:18325190

Kinns, H., Housley, D., & Freedman, D. B. (2013). Munchausen syndrome and factitious disorder: The role of the laboratory in its detection and diagnosis. *Annals of Clinical Biochemistry*, *50*(3), 194–203. doi:10.1177/0004563212473280 PMID:23592802

Kiselica, M. S. (2011). Promoting positive masculinity while addressing gender role conflict: A balanced theoretical approach to clinical work with boys and men. In C. Blazina & D. S. Shen-Miller (Eds.), An international psychology of men: Theoretical advances, case studies, and clinical innovations (pp. 127–156). Routledge/Taylor & Francis Group.

Kiselica, M. S., Englar-Carlson, M., Horne, A. M., & Fisher, M. (2008). A positive psychology perspective on helping boys. *Counseling troubled boys: A guidebook for professionals*, 31-48.

Kiselica, M. S., & Englar-Carlson, M. (2010). Identifying, affirming, and building upon male strengths: The positive psychology/positive masculinity model of psychotherapy with boys and men. *Psychotherapy (Chicago, Ill.)*, *47*(3), 276–287. doi:10.1037/a0021159 PMID:22402085

Klaus, L., Zararini, M., Schmahl, C., Linehan, M., & Bohus, M. (2004, July 31). *Borderline personality disorder - the lancet*. The Lancet. https://www.thelancet.com/journals/lancet/article/PIIS0140-6736(04)16770-6/fulltext

Klonsky, E. D., Oltmanns, T. F., & Turkheimer, E. (2014). Deliberate self-harm in a nonclinical population: Prevalence and psychological correlates. *The American Journal of Psychiatry*, 9. PMID:12900314

Kolvenbach, S., Fernández de la Cruz, L., Mataix, C. D., Patel, N., & Jassi, A. (2018). Perceived treatment barriers and experiences in the use of services for obsessive–compulsive disorder across different ethnic groups: A thematic analysis. *Child and Adolescent Mental Health*, *23*(2), 99–106. doi:10.1111/camh.12197 PMID:32677337

Kopelowicz, A., Zarate, R., Gonzalez, V., Lopez, S. R., Ortega, P., Obregon, N., & Mintz, J. (2002). Evaluation of expressed emotion in schizophrenia: A comparison of Caucasians and Mexican-Americans. *Schizophrenia Research*, *55*(1-2), 179–186. doi:10.1016/S0920-9964(01)00193-1 PMID:11955977

Koufagued, K., Chafry, B., Benyass, Y., Abissegue, Y., Benchebba, D., Bouabid, S., & Belkacem, C. (2015). Munchausen syndrome revealed by subcutaneous limb emphysema: A case report. *Journal of Medical Case Reports*, *9*(1), 1–4. doi:10.118613256-015-0649-x PMID:26282124

Kraepelin, E. (1921). Manic Depressive Insanity and Paranoia. Arno Press. doi:10.1097/00005053-192104000-00057

Krahn, L., Li, H., & O'Connor, M.K. (2014). Patients who strive to be ill: factitious disorder with physical symptoms. *Am J Psychiatry, 9.*

Kranke, D., Guada, J., Kranke, B., & Floersch, J. (2012). What do African American youth with a mental illness think about help-seeking and psychiatric medication?: Origins of stigmatizing attitudes. *Social Work in Mental Health*, *10*(1), 53–71. doi:10.1080/15332985.2011.618076

Krochmalik, A., & Menzies, R. G. (2003). The classification and diagnosis of obsessive- compulsive disorder. In R. G. Menzies & P. de Silva (Eds.), *Obsessive-compulsive disorder: Theory, research and treatment* (pp. 3–20). Wiley & Sons.

Kroon Van Diest, A. M., Tartakovsky, M., Stachon, C., Pettit, J. W., & Perez, M. (2014). The relationship between acculturative stress and eating disorder symptoms: Is it unique from general life stress? *Journal of Behavioral Medicine*, *37*(3), 445–457. doi:10.100710865-013-9498-5 PMID:23456250

Kyle, M., Miller, C. B., Rogers, Z., Siriwardena, A. N., MacMahon, K. M., & Espie, C. A. (2014). Sleep restriction therapy for insomnia is associated with reduced objective total sleep time, increased daytime somnolence, and objectively impaired vigilance: Implications for the clinical management of insomnia disorder. *Sleep*, *37*(2), 229–237. doi:10.5665leep.3386 PMID:24497651

Kymalainen, J. A., & Weisman de Mamani, A. G. (2008). Expressed emotion, communication deviance, and culture in families of patients with schizophrenia: A review of the literature. *Cultural Diversity & Ethnic Minority Psychology*, *14*(2), 85–91. doi:10.1037/1099-9809.14.2.85 PMID:18426280

Kymalainen, J. A., Weisman, A. G., Rosales, G. A., & Armesto, J. C. (2006). Ethnicity expressed emotion and communication deviance in family members of patients with schizophrenia. *The Journal of Nervous and Mental Disease*, *194*(6), 391–396. doi:10.1097/01.nmd.0000221171.42027.5a PMID:16772854

Lacey, K. K., Mouzon, D. M., Govia, I. O., Matusko, N., Forsythe-Brown, I., Abelson, J. M., & Jackson, J. S. (2016). Substance Abuse Among Blacks Across the Diaspora. *Substance Use & Misuse*, *51*(9), 1147–1158. https://doi-org.proxy.tamuc.edu/10.3109/10826084.2016.1160124. doi:10.3109/10826084.2016.1160124 PMID:27191862

Lader. (1999). Limitations on the use of benzodiazepines in anxiety and insomnia: are they justified? *European Neuropsychopharmacology*, *9*, S399–S405. doi:10.1016/S0924-977X(99)00051-6

Lai, Y., Wang, T., Zhang, C., Lin, G., Voon, V., Chang, J., & Sun, B. (2020). Effectiveness of and safety of neuroablation for severe and treatment-resistant obsessive-compulsive disorder: A systematic review and meta-analysis. *Journal of Psychiatry & Neuroscience*, *45*(5), 356–368. doi:10.1503/jpn.190079 PMID:32549057

Lancaster, V. (2022, August 3). Borderline personality disorder and the danger of self-destruction. *Psychology Today*. https://www.psychologytoday.com/us/blog/the-complex-diagnosis/202208/borderline-personality-disorder-and-the-danger-self-destruction

Lande, R. Gregory, Williams, MC USA (Ret), Lisa Banks, MSN, APRN-BC. (2013). Prevalence and Characteristics of Military Malingering. *Oxford Academic Journal Article*, *178*(1), 50–54. PMID:23356119

Latendresse, S. J., Ye, F., Chung, T., Hipwell, A., & Sartor, C. E. (2017). Parental monitoring and alcohol use across adolescence in Black and White girls: A cross-lagged panel mixture model. *Alcoholism, Clinical and Experimental Research*, *41*(6), 1144–1153 https://doi-org/10 1111/acer 13386 PMID:28391598

Latzman, R. D., Naifeh, J. A., Watson, D., Vaidya, J. G., Heiden, L. J., Damon, J. D., Hight, T. L., & Young, J. (2011). Racial differences in symptoms of anxiety and depression among three cohorts of students in the southern United States. *Psychiatry*, *74*(4), 332–348. doi:10.1521/psyc.2011.74.4.332 PMID:22168294

Laurencin, C. T., & Walker, J. M. (2020). A pandemic on a pandemic: Racism and COVID-19 in Blacks. *Cell Systems*, *11*(1), 9–10. doi:10.1016/j.cels.2020.07.002 PMID:32702320

Lawlor, A., & Kirakowski, J. (2014). When the lie is the truth: Grounded theory analysis of an online support group for factitious disorder. *Psychiatry Research, 218*(1), 209–218. doi:10.1016/j.psychres.2014.03.034 PMID:24745468

Laws, T. (2018). Tuskegee as sacred rhetoric: Focal point for the emergent field of African American religion and health. *Journal of Religion and Health, 57*(1), 408–419. doi:10.100710943-017-0505-y PMID:29064071

Leaper, C., & Van, S. R. (2008). Masculinity ideology, covert sexism, and perceived gender typicality in relation to young men's academic motivation and choices in college. *Psychology of Men & Masculinity, 9*(3), 139–153. doi:10.1037/1524-9220.9.3.139

Lease, S. H., Shuman, W. A., & Gage, A. N. (2019). Incorporating traditional masculinity ideology into health promotion models: Differences for African American/Black and White men. *Psychology of Men & Masculinity, 20*(1), 128–141. doi:10.1037/men0000151

LeBlanc, M., Mérette, C., Savard, J., Ivers, H., Baillargeon, L., & Morin, C. M.LEBLANC. (2009). Incidence and Risk Factors of Insomnia in a Population-Based Sample. *Sleep, 32*(8), 1027–1037. doi:10.1093leep/32.8.1027 PMID:19725254

Lee, S. (2020, August 6). Racial disparities lead to poor mental health care for Black Americans. *Verywell Mind.* https://www.verywellmind.com/racial-disparities-mental-health-5072490

Leedy, M. J., Jackson, M., & Callahan, J. L. (2007). Treating depression and compensatory narcissistic personality style in a man with chronic Lyme disease. *Clinical Case Studies, 6*(5), 430–442. doi:10.1177/1534650106295847

Lee, K., Kwon, Y.-J., Lee, K., Lim, E., Jang, S.-H., & Sohn, I.-K. (2022). Psychological Characteristics of Community People with Insomnia Focused on : Attention deficit hyperactivity symptoms, Depression, Anxiety and Mood Disorder. *Sleep Medicine, 100*, S134–S135. doi:10.1016/j.sleep.2022.05.368

Lee, R. J. (2017). Mistrustful and misunderstood: A review of paranoid personality disorder. *Current Behavioral Neuroscience Reports, 4*(2), 151–165. doi:10.100740473-017-0116-7 PMID:29399432

Lenzenweger, M. F., Lane, M. C., Loranger, A. W., & Kessler, R. C. (2007, January 11). DSM-IV personality disorders in the National Comorbidity Survey Replication. *Biological Psychiatry, 62*(6), 553–564. doi:10.1016/j.biopsych.2006.09.019 PMID:17217923

Levant, R. F. (2006). Forward. In M. Englar-Carlson & M. A. Stevens (Eds.), *In the room with men: A casebook of therapeutic change* (pp. xv–xx). American Psychological Association.

Levant, R. F. (2011). Research in the psychology of men and masculinity using the gender role strain paradigm as a framework. *The American Psychologist, 66*(8), 765–776. doi:10.1037/a0025034 PMID:22082409

Levant, R. F., Rankin, T. J., Williams, C. M., Hasan, N. T., & Smalley, K. B. (2010). Evaluation of the factor structure and construct validity of scores on the Male Role Norms Inventory—Revised (MRNI-R). *Psychology of Men & Masculinity, 11*(1), 25–37. doi:10.1037/a0017637

Levant, R. F., Wimer, D. J., Williams, C. M., Smalley, K. B., & Noronha, D. (2009). The relationships between masculinity variables, health risk behaviors and attitudes toward seeking psychological help. *International Journal of Men's Health*, *8*(1), 3–21. Advance online publication. doi:10.3149/jmh.0801.3

Levenson, J. L., Chafe, W., & Flanagan, P. (2007, January). (207). Factitious ovarian cancer: Feigning via resources on the internet. *Psychosomatics*, *48*(1), 71–73. doi:10.1176/appi.psy.48.1.71 PMID:17209154

Levin, J. S. (1984). The Role of the black church in community medicine. *Journal of the National Medical Association*, *76*, 477–483. PMID:6737505

Lewis, J. A., Mendenhall, R., Harwood, S. A., & Browne Huntt, M. (2013). Coping with gendered racial microaggressions among Black women college students. *Journal of African American Studies*, *17*(1), 51–73. doi:10.100712111-012-9219-0

Liao, Z., Zhu, S., & Li, X. (2018). Anxiety and depression in paradoxical insomnia: A case-control study. *Neuropsychiatric Disease and Treatment*, *14*, 231–238. doi:10.2147/NDT.S156058 PMID:29386896

Libow, J. A. (2000). Child and adolescent illness falsification. *Pediatrics*, *105*(2), 336–342. doi:10.1542/peds.105.2.336 PMID:10654952

Liddon, L., Kingerlee, R., & Barry, J. A. (2017). Gender differences in preferences for psychological treatment, coping strategies, and triggers to help-seeking. *British Journal of Clinical Psychology*, *57*(1), 42–58. doi:10.1111/bjc.12147 PMID:28691375

Linardon, J., Wade, T. D., de la Piedad Garcia, X., & Brennan, L. (2017). The efficacy of cognitive- behavioral therapy for eating disorders: A systematic review and meta-analysis. *Journal of Consulting and Clinical Psychology*, *85*(11), 1080–1094. doi:10.1037/ccp0000245 PMID:29083223

Lincoln, T. M., Lullman, E., & Rief, W. (2007). Correlates and long-term consequences of poor insight in patients with schizophrenia: A systematic review. *Schizophrenia Bulletin*, *33*(6), 1324–1342. doi:10.1093chbulbm002 PMID:17289653

Lindsey, K. P., & Paul, G. L. (1989). Involuntary commitment to public mental institutions: Issues involving the overrepresentation of Blacks and assessment of relevant functioning. *Psychological Bulletin*, *106*(2), 171–183. doi:10.1037/0033-2909.106.2.171 PMID:2678200

Linehan, M. M. (1993, May 14). *Cognitive-behavioral treatment of borderline personality disorder* (2nd ed.). Guildford Press.

Lin, J. L., Servat, J. J., Bernardino, C. R., Goldberg, R. A., & Levin, F. (2012). Bilateral corneal perforations and autoproptosis as self-induced manifestations of ocular Munchausen's syndrome. *Orbit (Amsterdam, Netherlands)*, *31*(4), 252–255. doi:10.3109/01676830.2012.669013 PMID:22571651

Linszen, D. H., Dingemans, P. M., Nugter, M. A., Van der Does, J. W., Scholte, W. F., & Lenior, M. A. (1997). Patient attributes and expressed emotion as risk factors for psychotic relapse. *Schizophrenia Bulletin, 23*(1), 119–130. doi:10.1093chbul/23.1.119 PMID:9050118

Linton, S. L., Cooper, H. L. F., Luo, R., Karnes, C., Renneker, K., Haley, D. F., Hunter-Jones, J., Ross, Z., Bonney, L., & Rothenberg, R. (2016). People and places: Relocating to neighborhoods with better economic and social conditions is associated with less risky drug/alcohol network characteristics among African American adults in Atlanta, GA. *Drug and Alcohol Dependence, 160*, 30–41. https://doi-org.proxy.tamuc.edu/10.1016/j.drugalcdep.2015.11.036. doi:10.1016/j.drugalcdep.2015.11.036 PMID:26781062

Lipson, S. K., Kern, A., Eisenberg, D., & Breland-Noble, A. M. (2018). Mental Health Disparities Among College Students of Color. *The Journal of Adolescent Health, 63*(3), 348–356. doi:10.1016/j.jadohealth.2018.04.014 PMID:30237000

Livaoğlu, M., Kerimoğlu, S., Hocaoğlu, C., Arvas, L., & Karacal, N. (2008). Munchausen's syndrome: A rare self-mutilation syndrome. *Dermatologic Surgery, 34*(9), 1288–1291. doi:10.1097/00042728-200809000-00024 PMID:18616542

Lo, C. C., Howell, R. J., & Cheng, T. C. (2012). Problem drinking by race and nativity: What is learned from social structural and mental health-related data of US-born and immigrant respondents? *The American Journal on Addictions, 21*, S77–S87. https://doi-org.proxy.tamuc.edu/10.1111/j.1521-0391.2012.00292.x. doi:10.1111/j.1521-0391.2012.00292.x PMID:23786515

Lorber, J. (1997). *The Variety of Feminisms and Their Contributions to Gender Equality*. Germany: Bis.

Lucksted, A., Drapalski, A. L., Brown, C. H., Wilson, C., Charlotte, M., Mullane, A., & Fang, L. J. (2017). Outcomes of a Psychoeducational Intervention to Reduce Internalized Stigma Among Psychosocial Rehabilitation Clients. *Psychiatric Services (Washington, D.C.), 68*(4), 360–367. doi:10.1176/appi.ps.201600037 PMID:27903136

Lu, W., Silverstein, S. M., Mueser, K. T., Minsky, S., Bullock, D., Buchbinder, S., Chen, Q., Eubanks, R., & Guillaume-Salvant, A. (2022). Undocumented PTSD among African American clients with serious mental illness in a statewide mental health system. *Psychological Trauma: Theory, Research, Practice, and Policy*, 1–10. doi:10.1037/tra0001243 PMID:35797171

Lydecker, J. A., & Grilo, C. M. (2019). Food insecurity and bulimia nervosa in the United States. *International Journal of Eating Disorders*. https://doi. doi:org/10.1002/eat.23074

Lydecker, J. A., & Grilo, C. M. (2016). Different yet similar: Examining race and ethnicity in treatment-seeking adults with binge eating disorder. *Journal of Consulting and Clinical Psychology, 84*(1), 88–94. [REMOVED HYPERLINK FIELD] doi:10.1037/ccp0000048 PMID:26348841

MacIntyre, M. M., Zare, M., & Williams, M. (2023). Anxiety-Related Disorders in the Context of Racism. *Current Psychiatry Reports, 25*(2), 31–43. doi:10.100711920-022-01408-2 PMID:36645562

Mahalik, J. R., Burns, S. M., & Syzdek, M. (2007). Masculinity and perceived normative health behaviors as predictors of men's health behaviors. *Social Science & Medicine*, *64*(11), 2201–2209. doi:10.1016/j.socscimed.2007.02.035 PMID:17383784

Mahalik, J. R., Good, G. E., Tager, D., Levant, R. F., & Mackowiak, C. (2012). Developing a taxonomy of helpful and harmful practices for clinical work with boys and men. *Journal of Counseling Psychology*, *59*(4), 591–603. doi:10.1037/a0030130 PMID:23088685

Mailis-Gagnon, A., Nicholson, K., Blumberger, D., & Zurowski, M. (2008). Characteristics and period prevalence of self-induced disorder in patients referred to a pain clinic with the diagnosis of complex regional pain syndrome. *The Clinical Journal of Pain*, *24*(2), 176–185. doi:10.1097/AJP.0b013e31815ca278 PMID:18209524

Majors, R., & Billson, J. (1992). *Cool pose: The dilemmas of Black manhood in America*. Touchstone.

Males, M. (2018). Racial implications of the narcissistic personality inventory reinterpreting popular depictions of narcissism trends. *Journal of Psychology and Psychiatry*, *2*(1), 1–4. doi:10.15761/JPP.1000106

Malhi, & Mann, J. J. (2018). Depression. *The Lancet (British Edition)*, *392*(10161), 2299–. https://doi.org/ doi:10.1016/S0140-6736(18)31948

Mallinger, J., Fisher, S., Brown, T., & Lamberti, J. A. (2006). Racial disparities in the use of second-generation antipsychotics for the treatment of schizophrenia. *Psychiatric Services (Washington, D.C.)*, *57*(1), 133–136. https://www.researchgate.net/profile/J-Lamberti/publication/7371795_Racial_Disparities_in_the_Use_of_Second-Generation_Antipsychotics_for_the_Treatment_of_Schizophrenia/links/56c39c0f08ae60234250a2d0/Racial-Disparities-in-the-Use-of-Second-Generation-Antipsychotics-for-the-Treatment-of-Schizophrenia.pdf. doi:10.1176/appi.ps.57.1.133 PMID:16399976

Mannes, Z. L., Burrell, L. E., Bryant, V. E., Dunne, E. M., Hearn, L. E., & Whitehead, N. E. (2016). Loneliness and substance use: The influence of gender among HIV+ Black/African American adults 50+. *AIDS Care*, *28*(5), 598–602. https://doi-org.proxy.tamuc.edu/10.1080/09540121.2015.1120269. doi:10.1080/09540121.2015.1120269 PMID:26654243

Mao, J., Ji, Y., Xu, Y., Tang, G., Yu, Z., Xu, L., Shen, C., & Wang, W. (2017). Group cognitive-behavioral therapy in insomnia: A cross-sectional case-controlled study. *Neuropsychiatric Disease and Treatment*, *13*, 2841–2848. doi:10.2147/NDT.S149610 PMID:29200858

Margolis, S. (2002). *The Johns Hopkins medical guide to health after 50*. Medlette Associates, Inc.

Marker, C. D., & Aylward, A. G. (2012). Description. In D. Wedding, L. Beutler, K. E. Freedland, L. C. Sobell, & D. A. Wolfe (Eds.), *Generalized Anxiety Disorder* (pp. 6–7). Hogrefe.

Marquez-Velarde, G., Miller, G. H., Ma, G., & Keith, V. M. (2022). Psychological Distress among Black Immigrants by Region of Birth. *Journal of Immigrant and Minority Health*, *24*(2), 368–375. https://doi-org.proxy.tamuc.edu/10.1007/s10903-021-01203-w. doi:10.100710903-021-01203-w PMID:33905047

Martin, L. A., Neighbors, H. W., & Griffith, D. M. (2013). The experience of symptoms of depression in men vs women: Analysis of the National Comorbidity Survey Replication. *JAMA Psychiatry*, *70*(10), 1100–1106. doi:10.1001/jamapsychiatry.2013.1985 PMID:23986338

Mason, T. B., Lewis, R. J., & Heron, K. E. (2017). Indirect pathways connecting sexual orientation and weight discrimination to disordered eating among young adult lesbians. *Psychology of Sexual Orientation and Gender Diversity*, *4*(2), 193–204. doi:10.1037gd0000220

Mathews, A., Corrigan, P., Smith, B., & Aranda, F. (2006). A qualitative exploration of African Americans' attitudes toward mental illness and mental illness treatment seeking. *Rehabilitation Education*, *20*(4), 253–268. doi:10.1891/088970106805065331

Mathis, J. E. (2018). *Comparing Treatment Outcomes of Young Adult Males and Females in Wilderness Therapy Programs through a Gender Schema Lens* [Doctoral dissertation, Northcentral University].

Matthews, L. R., Gerald, J., & Jessup, G. M. (2021). Exploring men's use of mental health support offered by an Australian Employee Assistance Program (EAP): Perspectives from a focus-group study with males working in blue-and white-collar industries. *International Journal of Mental Health Systems*, *15*(1), 1–17. doi:10.118613033-021-00489-5 PMID:34348756

Maura, J., & Weisman de Mamani, A. (2017). Mental health disparities, treatment engagement, and attrition among racial/ethnic minorities with severe mental illness: A review. *Journal of Clinical Psychology in Medical Settings*, *24*(3-4), 187–210. doi:10.100710880-017-9510-2 PMID:28900779

Maur, K. V., Wasson, K. R., DeFord, J. W., & Caranasos, G. J. (1973). Munchausen's syndrome: A thirty-year history of peregrination par excellence. *Southern Medical Journal*, *66*(6), 629. doi:10.1097/00007611-197306000-00001 PMID:4733204

Mayer, L., Corrigan, P. W., Eisheuer, D., Oexle, N., & Rüsch, N. (2021). Attitudes towards Disclosing a Mental Illness: Impact on Quality of Life and Recovery. *Social Psychiatry and Psychiatric Epidemiology*, *57*(2), 363–374. doi:10.100700127-021-02081-1 PMID:33895868

Mayes, S. D., Fernandez-Mendoza, J., Baweja, R., Calhoun, S., Mahr, F., Aggarwal, R., & Arnold, M. (2014). Correlates of suicide ideation and attempts in children and adolescents with eating disorders. *Eating Disorders*, *22*(4), 352–366. doi:10.1080/10640266.2014.915694 PMID:24842006

Mayo Clinic. (2019). *Factitious Discorder*. Middlesex Heatlth.

Mayo Clinic. (2022, October 14) *Depression (major depressive disorder)*. Mayo Clinic. https://www.mayoclinic.org/diseases-conditions/depression/diagnosis-treatment/drc-20356013

May, R. A. B. (2018). Velvet rope racism, racial paranoia, and cultural scripts: Alleged dress code discrimination in urban nightlife, 2000–2014. *City & Community*, *17*(1), 44–64. doi:10.1111/cico.12286

Mays, V. M., Cochran, S. D., & Barnes, N. W. (2007). Race, race-based discrimination, and health outcomes among African Americans. *Annual Review of Psychology*, *58*(1), 201–225. doi:10.1146/annurev.psych.57.102904.190212 PMID:16953796

Mays, V. M., Jones, A. L., Delany-Brumsey, A., Coles, C., & Cochran, S. D. (2017). Perceived Discrimination in Health Care and Mental Health/Substance Abuse Treatment Among Blacks, Latinos, and Whites. *Medical Care*, *55*(2), 173–181. https://doi-org.proxy.tamuc.edu/10.1097/MLR.0000000000000638. doi:10.1097/MLR.0000000000000638 PMID:27753743

Mazza, C., Formica, F., Ferracuti, S., Ricci, E., Colasanti, M., Biondi, S., Di Domenico, A., & Roma, P. (2022). High expressed emotion (HEE), assessed using the Five-Minute Speech Sample (FMSS), as a predictor of psychiatric relapse in patients with schizophrenia and major depressive disorder: A meta-analysis and meta-regression. *Journal of Clinical Medicine*, *11*(21), 6533. doi:10.3390/jcm11216533 PMID:36362760

McCarthy, J., & Holliday, E. L. (2004). Help-seeking and counseling within a traditional male gender role: An examination from a multicultural perspective. *Journal of Counseling and Development*, *82*(1), 25–30. doi:10.1002/j.1556-6678.2004.tb00282.x

McCleary-Gaddy, A. T. & James, D. (2020). Skin tone, life satisfaction, and psychological distress among African Americans: The mediating effect of stigma consciousness. *Journal of Health Psychology*. doi:10.1177/1359105320954251

McCloud, M. (2013, February 26). Borderline personality afflicts all races and both genders. *Psychology Today*. https://www.psychologytoday.com/us/blog/black-womens-health-and-happiness/201302/borderline-personality-afflicts-all-races-and-both

McCreary, D. R. (2012). Muscularity and body image. Encyclopedia of Body Image and Human Appearance, 2, 561–567. doi:10.1016/B978-0-12-384925-0.00088-2

McCutcheon, R., Marques, T., & Howes, O. (2020). Schizophrenia-an overview. *JAMA Psychiatry*. https://jamanetwork.com/journals/jamapsychiatry/article-abstract/2753514

McEwen, D. R. (1998). Recognizing Munchausen's syndrome. *J Assoc Perioper Regist Nurs*, *67*(2), 440–442. PMID:9505125

McGilloway, A., Hall, R. E., Lee, T., & Bhui, K. S. (2010). A systematic review of personality disorder, race and ethnicity: Prevalence, aetiology, and treatment. *BMC Psychiatry*, *10*(1), 1–14. doi:10.1186/1471-244X-10-33 PMID:20459788

McGrew, S. J., Raines, A. M., Walker, R. L., Leonard, S. J., & Vujanovic, A. A. (2023). Posttraumatic Stress, Alcohol Use, and Alcohol Use Motives among Non-Hispanic Black/African American College Students: The Role of Emotion Regulation. *Journal of Dual Diagnosis*, *19*(1), 3–15. https://doi-org.proxy.tamuc.edu/10.1080/15504263.2022.2160037. doi:10.1080/15504263.2022.2160037 PMID:36583682

McLean, S. A., Caldwell, B., & Roberton, M. (2019). Reach out and recover: Intentions to seek treatment in individuals using online support for eating disorders. *International Journal of Eating Disorders*, *52*(10), 1137–1149. doi:10.1002/eat.23133 PMID:31298791

McNeil Smith, S., & Taylor, J. (2015). The Relationship Between Social Stress and Substance Use Among Black Youths Residing in South Florida. *Journal of Child & Adolescent Substance Abuse*, *24*(6), 372–378. https://doi-org.proxy.tamuc.edu/10.1080/1067828X.2013.872062. doi:10.1080/1067828X.2013.872062

Meds Safety. (2023, March 14). *Borderline personality disorder*. Meds Safety. https://medssafety.com/borderline-personality-disorder/

Mehta, N. J., & Khan, I. A. (2002). Cardiac Munchausen syndrome. *Chest*, *122*(5), 1649–1653. doi:10.1378/chest.122.5.1649 PMID:12426266

Mendez-Miller, M., Naccarato, J., & Radico, J. A. (2022, February 1). Borderline Personality Disorder. *American Family Physician*, *105*(2), 156–161. PMID:35166488

Mental Health America. (n.d.). *Black and African American Communities and Mental Health*. MHA. https://www.mhanational.org/issues/black-and-african-american-communities-and-mental-health

Menzies, R. G., & de Silva, P. (Eds.). (2003). Obsessive-compulsive disorder: Theory, research and treatment. Hoboken, NJ: Wiley & Sons. –175. https://doi.org/. 2020.1817554 doi:10.1080/08039488

Metzl, J. M. (2009). *The protest psychosis: How schizophrenia became a Black disease*. Beacon Press.

Micali, N., Hagberg, K. W., Petersen, I., & Treasure, J. L. (2013). The incidence of eating disorders in the UK in 2000–2009: Findings from the General Practice Research Database. *BMJ Open*, *3*(5), e002646. doi:10.1136/bmjopen-2013-002646 PMID:23793681

Michalopoulou, G., Falzarano, P., & Rosenberg, D. (2009). Recruitment of African Americans for obsessive compulsive disorder treatment research. *Journal of Health Disparities Research and Practice*, *3*(1), 71–82.

Miller, J. D., Back, M. D., Lynam, D. R., & Wright, A. G. (2021). Narcissism today: What we know and what we need to learn. *Current Directions in Psychological Science*, *30*(6), 519–525. doi:10.1177/09637214211044109

Miller, J. D., Maples, J. L., Cai, H., Kisbu-Sakarya, Y., LoPilato, A., Sedikides, C., Buffardi, L., Gentile, B., Kwan, V. S., Pendry, L. F., Siedor, L., & Campbell, W. K. (2015). Narcissism and United States' culture: The view from home and around the world. *Journal of Personality and Social Psychology*, *109*(6), 1068–1089. doi:10.1037/a0039543 PMID:26389797

Miller, W. R., Sorensen, J. L., Selzer, J. A., & Brigham, G. S. (2006). Disseminating evidence-based practices in substance abuse treatment: A review with suggestions. *Journal of Substance Abuse Treatment*, *31*(1), 25–39. doi:10.1016/j.jsat.2006.03.005 PMID:16814008

Mincey, K., Alfonso, M., Hackney, A., & Luque, J. (2014). Understanding masculinity in undergraduate African American men: A qualitative study. *American Journal of Men's Health*, *8*(5), 387–398. doi:10.1177/1557988313515900 PMID:24356494

Miranda, J., & Cooper, L. A. (2004). Disparities in care for depression among primary care patients. *Journal of General Internal Medicine*, *19*(2), 120–126. doi:10.1111/j.1525-1497.2004.30272.x PMID:15009791

Mirande´, A. (1988). Chicano fathers: Traditional perceptions and current realities. In P. Bronstein & C. P. Cowan (Eds.), *Fatherhood today: Men's changing role in the family* (pp. 93–106). Wiley.

Mirande´, A. (1997). *Hombres y machos: Masculinity and Latino culture*. Westview Press.

Misra, S., Jackson, V. W., Chong, J., Choe, K., Tay, C., Wong, J., & Yang, L. H. (2021). Systematic review of cultural aspects of stigma and mental illness among racial and ethnic minority groups in the United States: Implications for interventions. *American Journal of Community Psychology*, *68*(3-4), 486–512. doi:10.1002/ajcp.12516 PMID:33811676

Montgomery, L., Burlew, A. K., & Korte, J. E. (2017). Does change in readiness influence retention among African American women and men in substance abuse treatment? *Journal of Ethnicity in Substance Abuse*, *16*(4), 420–431. https://doi-. doi:10.1080/15332640.2017.1300553 PMID:28368681

Mooney, L. A., Knox, D., & Schacht, C. (2015). Understanding Social Problems (9thed.). Standford, CT: Cengage Learning.

Morin, A. (2020, October 26). Exploring the mental health stigma in black communities. *Verywell Mind.* https://www.verywellmind.com/exploring-the-mental-health-stigma-in-black-communities-5078964

Morison, L., Trigeorgis, C., & John, M. (2014). Are mental health services inherently feminised? *The Psychologist*, *27*(6), 414–416.

Mosher, D., & Tompkins, S. (1988). Scripting the macho man: Hypermasculine socialization and enculturation. *Journal of Sex Research*, *25*(1), 60–84. doi:10.1080/00224498809551445

Mosley, B., Atkins, B. J., & Klein, M. (1988). Alcoholism and Blacks. *Journal of Alcohol and Drug Education*, *33*(4), 51–58.

Motlova, L. B., Balon, R., Beresin, E. V., Brenner, A. M., Coverdale, J. H., Guerrero, A. P. S., Louie, A. K., & Roberts, L. W. (2017). Psychoeducation as an Opportunity for Patients, Psychiatrists, and Psychiatric Educators: Why Do We Ignore It? *Academic Psychiatry*, *41*(4), 447–451. doi:10.100740596-017-0728-y PMID:28536990

Mount, D. L., Johnson, D. M., Rego, M. I., Schofield, K., Amponsah, A., & Graham, L. F. (2012). Preliminary findings exploring the social determinants of Black males' lay health perspectives. *American Journal of Men's Health*, *6*(1), 71–79. doi:10.1177/1557988311420993 PMID:22105065

Mouzon, D. M., Watkins, D. C., Perry, R., Simpson, T. M., & Mitchell, J. A. (2019). Intergenerational Mobility and Goal-Striving Stress Among Black Americans: The Roles of Ethnicity and Nativity Status. *Journal of Immigrant and Minority Health*, *21*(2), 393–400. https://doi-org.proxy.tamuc.edu/10.1007/s10903-018-0735-4. doi:10.100710903-018-0735-4 PMID:29611019

Mowatt, R. A., French, B. H., & Malebranche, D. A. (2013). Black/female/body hypervisibility and invisibility: A Black feminist augmentation of feminist leisure research. *Journal of Leisure Research*, *45*(5), 644–660. doi:10.18666/jlr-2013-v45-i5-4367

Moynihan, D. P. (1965). *The Negro family: The case for national action*. Washington, DC: U. S. Government Printing Office.

Muacevic, A., Adler, J. R., Sinha, A., & Smolik, T. (2021). Striving to Die: Medical, Legal, and Ethical Dilemmas Behind Factitous Disorder. *Cureus Publishing Beyond Open Access*, *13*(2), e13243.

Mukai, K., Matsuura, N., Miyauchi, M., Hashimoto, T., Yamanishi, K., Maebayashi, K., Hayashida, K., & Matsunaga, H. (2021). Evaluation of hemodynamic changes using near-infrared spectroscopy in patients with tic-related obsessive–compulsive disorder. *Psychiatry and Clinical Neurosciences*, *75*(6), 191–199. doi:10.1111/pcn.13207 PMID:33543818

Mulia, N., Witbrodt, J., Karriker, J. K. J., Li, L., Lui, C. K., & Zapolski, T. (2022). Education matters: Longitudinal pathways to mid-life heavy drinking in a national cohort of black Americans. *Addiction (Abingdon, England)*, *117*(8), 2225–2234. https://doi-org.proxy.tamuc.edu/10.1111/add.15882. doi:10.1111/add.15882 PMID:35320593

Mulia, N., Ye, Y., Zemore, S. E., & Greenfield, T. K. (2008). Social Disadvantage, Stress, and Alcohol Use Among Black, Hispanic, and White Americans: Findings From the 2005 U.S. National Alcohol Survey. *Journal of Studies on Alcohol and Drugs*, *69*(6), 824–833. https://doi-org.proxy.tamuc.edu/10.15288/jsad.2008.69.824. doi:10.15288/jsad.2008.69.824 PMID:18925340

Munn-Chernoff, M. A., Grant, J. D., Agrawal, A., Koren, R., Glowinski, A. L., Bucholz, K. K., Madden, P. A. F., Heath, A. C., & Duncan, A. E. (2015). Are there common familial influences for major depressive disorder and an overeating–binge eating dimension in both European American and African American female twins? *International Journal of Eating Disorders*, *48*(4), 375–382. doi:10.1002/eat.22280 PMID:24659561

Murphy, S. L., Kochanek, K. D., Xu, J. Q., & Arias, E. (2021). *Mortality in the United States, 2020. NCHS Data Brief, no 427*. National Center for Health Statistics., doi:10.15620/cdc:112079

Nagendra, A., Black, C., & Penn, D. (2022). Black Americans and schizophrenia: Racism as a driver of inequities in psychosis diagnosis, assessment, and treatment. *Schizophrenia Research*. doi:10.1016/j.schres.2022.10.007 PMID:36396493

Nagendra, A., Weiss, D., Merritt, C., Cather, C., Sosoo, E., Mueser, K., & Penn, D. (2023). Clinical and psychosocial outcomes of Black Americans in the Recovery After an Initial Schizophrenia Episode Early Treatment Program (RAISE-ETP) study. *Social Psychiatry and Psychiatric Epidemiology*, *58*(1), 77–89. doi:10.100700127-022-02297-9 PMID:35932309

Narkhede, A. (2020, August 14). *Barriers to Mental Health Treatment in the Black Community.* Cleveland Clinic.

National Alliance of Mental Health. (2022, March 23). *Black/African Americans-Mental Health.* National Alliance of Mental Health. https://nami.org/Your-Journey/Identity-and-Cultural-Dimensions/Black-African-American

National Alliance of Mental Illness. (n.d.). *Black/African American.* NAMI. https://www.nami.org/Your-Journey/Identity-and-Cultural-Dimensions/Black-African-American

National Alliance on Mental Illness. (2019). *African American Mental Health.* NAMI. https://www.nami.org/Your-Journey/Identity-and-Cultural-Dimensions/Black-African- American

National Alliance on Mental Illness. (2020a). *Mental health in Black communities: Challenges, resources, community voices.* NAMICA. https://namica.org/mental-health-challenges-in-african-american-communities/

National Alliance on Mental Illness. (2020b). *The annual state of the communities' reports with diverse communities.* NAMICA. https://namica.org/wp-content/uploads/2019/12/nca_Diverse-Communities-ASoCR-Summary-18-19_Final.test_.pdf

National Alliance on Mental Illness. (2022). *Black/African American.* NAMI. https://www.nami.org/Your-Journey/Identity-and-Cultural-Dimensions/Black-African-American

National Alliance on Mental Illness. (n.d). Black/African American. *National Alliance on Mental Illness.* NAMI. https://www.nami.org/Your-Journey/Identity-and-Cultural-Dimensions/Black-African-American

National Association of Social Workers (NASW). (2015). *Standards and indicators for cultural competence in social work practice.* NASW. https://www.socialworkers.org/Practice/Practice-Standards-Guidelines

National Center for Health Statistics (US). (2018). *Health, United States, 2017: With Special Feature on Mortality.* National Center for Health Statistics.

National Collaborating Centre for Mental Health. U. K. (2009). Borderline personality disorder: Treatment and management. British Psychological Society.

National Institute of Mental Health. (2019). *Mental health information, statistics. Major Depression.* NIH. https://www.nimh.nih.gov/health/statistics/major-depression.shtml

National Institute of Mental Health. (2021). *Schizophrenia.* NIMH. https://www.nimh.nih.gov/health/publications/schizophrenia

National Institute of Mental Health. (2022, January). *Mental Health Information*. NAMI. https://www.nimh.nih.gov/health/statistics/major-depression

National Institute on Alcohol Abuse and Alcoholism. (1990). *Seventh special report to the U.S. congress on alcohol and health Rockville*. U. S. Department of Health and Human Services.

National Urban League. (2007). *State of Black America: Portrait of the Black Male*. Beckham Publications Group.

Neal-Barnett, A., Statom, D., & Stadulis, R. (2011). Trichotillomania symptoms in African American women: Are they related to anxiety and culture? *CNS Neuroscience & Therapeutics*, *17*(4), 207–213. doi:10.1111/j.1755-5949.2010.00138.x PMID:20406247

Neely-Fairbanks, S. Y., Rojas-Guyler, L., Nabors, L., & Banjo, O. (2018). Mental illness knowledge, stigma, help-seeking behaviors, spirituality and the African American church. *American Journal of Health Studies*, *33*(4), 162–174. doi:10.47779/ajhs.2018.69

Nellis, A. 2021. *The Color of Justice: Racial and Ethnic Disparity in State Prisons*, The Sentencing Project. https://policycommons.net/artifacts/3351700/the-color-of-justice-racial-and-ethnic-disparity-in-state-prisons/.

Nelson, K., Norris, K., & Mangione, C. M. (2002). Disparities in the diagnosis and pharmacologic treatment of high serum cholesterol by race and ethnicity: Data from the Third National Health and Nutrition Examination Survey. *Archives of Internal Medicine*, *162*(8), 929–935. doi:10.1001/archinte.162.8.929 PMID:11966345

Nelson, S. M., Griffin, C. A., Hein, T. C., Bowersox, N., & McCarthy, J. F. (2022). Personality disorder and suicide risk among patients in the veterans affairs health system. *Personality Disorders*, *13*(6), 563–571. doi:10.1037/per0000521 PMID:34726449

Neukrug, E., Britton, B. S., & Crews, R. C. (2013). Common health-related concerns of men: Implications for counselors. *Journal of Counseling and Development*, *91*(4), 390–397. doi:10.1002/j.1556-6676.2013.00109.x

Newhill, C. E., Eack, S. M., & Conner, K. O. (2009, April 21). *Racial differences between African and White Americans in the presentation of borderline personality disorder - race and Social Problems*. Springer. https://link.springer.com/article/10.1007/s12552-009-9006-2

Newhill, C., & Harris, D. (2007). African American consumers' perceptions of racial disparities in mental health services. *Social Work in Public Health*, *23*(2/3), 107–124. doi:10.1080/19371910802151861 PMID:19306590

Nichols, G. R. II, Davis, G. J., & Corey, T. S. (1990). In the shadow of the baron: Sudden death due to Munchausen syndrome. *The American Journal of Emergency Medicine*, *8*(3), 216–219. doi:10.1016/0735-6757(90)90326-U PMID:2184806

NIDCR. (2009). *Oral Cancer: What African American Men Need to Know*. Bethesda, MD: National Institute of Dental and Craniofacial Research. http://www.nidcr.nih.gov/Oral Health/Topics/OralCancer/AfricanAmericanMen.htm

Nishimura, K., Kobayashi, S., Sugawara, H., Nakajima, I., Ishida, H., Fuchinoue, S., Tanabe, K., & Ishigooka, J. (2012). Psychiatric consultation after kidney transplantation: A 10-year single-center study including outpatients in Japan. *International Journal of Psychiatry in Medicine, 43*(3), 197–209. doi:10.2190/PM.43.3.a PMID:22978079

Nock, M. K., Borges, G., Bromet, E. J., Alonso, J., Angermeyer, M., Beautrais, A., Bruffaerts, R., Chiu, W. T., de Girolamo, G., Gluzman, S., de Graaf, R., Gureje, O., Haro, J. M., Huang, Y., Karam, E., Kessler, R. C., Lepine, J. P., Levinson, D., Medina-Mora, M. E., & Williams, D. (2008). Cross-national prevalence and risk factors for suicidal ideation, plans and attempts. *The British Journal of Psychiatry, 192*(2), 98–105. doi:10.1192/bjp.bp.107.040113 PMID:18245022

Noone, J. H., & Stephens, C. (2008). Men, masculine identities, and health care utilisation. *Sociology of Health & Illness, 30*(5), 711–725. doi:10.1111/j.1467-9566.2008.01095.x PMID:18564976

Norcliffe-Kaufmann, L., Gonzalez-Duarte, A., Martinez, J., & Kaufmann, H. (2010). Tachyarrythmias with elevated cardiac enzymes in Münchausen syndrome. *Clinical Autonomic Research, 20*(4), 259–261. doi:10.100710286-010-0066-6 PMID:20424883

Norman, R.E., Byambaa, M., Butchart, J., Scott, T., & Vos. (2012). *The long-term health consequences of child physical abuse, emotional abuse, and neglect.* NIH.

O'Reilly, R. A., & Aggeler, P. M. (1976). Covert anticoagulant ingestion: Study of 25 patients and review of world literature. *Medicine, 55*(5), 389–399. doi:10.1097/00005792-197609000-00003 PMID:957998

Office of Minority Health. (2023, February 17). *Mental and behavioral health- African Americans.* Office of Minority Health. https://www.minorityhealth.hhs.gov/omh/browse.aspx?lvl=4&lvlid=24

Office of Minority Mental Health, U.S. Department of Health and Human Services. (2017). Mental health and African Americans. *Minority Health.* https://minorityhealth.hhs.gov/omh/browse.aspx?lvl=4&lvlid=24

Ogbonmwan, S. E., & Abidogun, K. (2008). A variant of Munchausen syndrome presenting as a gynaecological emergency. *British Journal of Hospital Medicine (London, England), 69*(7), 414–415. doi:10.12968/hmed.2008.69.7.30421 PMID:18833980

Ogborne, A. C., Wild, T. C., Braun, K., & Newton-Taylor, B. (1998). Measuring treatment process beliefs among staff of specialized addiction treatment services. *Journal of Substance Abuse Treatment, 15*(4), 301–312. doi:10.1016/S0740-5472(97)00196-7 PMID:9650138

Okoro, O., Vosen, E. C., Allen, K., Kennedy, J., Roberts, R., & Aremu, T. (2022). COVID-19 impact on mental health, healthcare access and social wellbeing–a Black community needs assessment. *International Journal for Equity in Health, 21*(1), 1–11. doi:10.118612939-022-01743-z PMID:36138403

Olbert, C. M., Nagendra, A., & Buck, B. (2018). Meta-analysis of Black vs. White racial disparity in schizophrenia diagnosis in the United States: Do structured assessments attenuate racial disparities? *Journal of Abnormal Psychology, 127*(1), 104–115. doi:10.1037/abn0000309 PMID:29094963

Olfson, M., Zuvekas, S. H., McClellan, C., Wall, M. M., Hankerson, S. H., & Blanco, C. (2023). Racial-ethnic disparities in outpatient mental health care in the United States. *Psychiatric services*.

Oner, E., Unlu, M., Solgun, B., Kocyigit, H., & Cimen, P. (2015). Munchausen's syndrome: Hemoptysis, hematochezia, hematuria. *Journal of Evolution of Medical and Dental Sciences*, 8091.

Ong, & Sholtes, D. (2010). A mindfulness-based approach to the treatment of insomnia. *Journal of Clinical Psychology, 66*(11), 1175–1184. doi:10.1002/jclp.20736

Onnela, A., Hurtig, T., & Ebeling, H. (2021). A psychoeducational mental health promotion intervention in comprehensive schools: Recognising problems and reducing stigma. *Health Education Journal, 80*(5), 554–566. doi:10.1177/0017896921994134

Operario, D., & Fiske, S. (2008). Stereotypes: Content, structures, processes, and context. In Social Cognition (pp. 22–44). doi:10.1002/9780470693421.ch2

Orem, S. (2017). (Un)necessary procedures: Black women, disability, and work in Grey's Anatomy. *African American Review, 50*(2), 169–183. doi:10.1353/afa.2017.0020

Ormond, A., Barbour, R., Lewis, R. K., Montgomery, A., & Ponds, A. (2021). Results from a community mental health assessment in a historically Black church: A call for action. *Journal of Prevention & Intervention in the Community, 49*(3), 235–250. doi:10.1080/10852352.2019.1654257 PMID:31460840

Osa, M. L., & Kelly, N. R. (2021, March 4). Experiences of Discrimination Are Associated With Drive for Muscularity Among African American Men. *Psychology of Men & Masculinity, 22*(2), 365–374. doi:10.1037/men0000287

Otowa, T., Gardner, C. O., Kendler, K. S., & Hettema, J. M. (2013). Parenting and risk for mood, anxiety and substance use disorders: A study in population-based male twins. *Social Psychiatry and Psychiatric Epidemiology, 48*(11), 1841–1849. doi:10.100700127-013-0656-4 PMID:23344783

Parcesepe, A. M., & Cabassa, L. J. (2013). Public stigma of mental illness in the United States: A systematic literature review. *Administration and Policy in Mental Health, 40*(5), 384–399. doi:10.100710488-012-0430-z PMID:22833051

Parent, D. J., Krafft, T., Noel, J. C., Askenasi, R., Goldschmidt, D., Heenen, M., & Linkowski, P. (1994). Cutaneous Münchausen syndrome with presentation simulating pyoderma gangrenosum. *Journal of the American Academy of Dermatology, 31*(6), 1072–1074. doi:10.1016/S0190-9622(09)80093-5 PMID:7962767

Parent, M. C., Hammer, J. H., Bradstreet, T. C., Schwartz, E. N., & Jobe, T. (2018). Men's mental health help-seeking behaviors: An intersectional analysis. *American Journal of Men's Health, 12*(1), 64–73. doi:10.1177/1557988315625776 PMID:29226771

Paris, J. (2005, June 7). *Borderline personality disorder*. CMAJ. https://www.cmaj.ca/content/172/12/1579

Pascual, A., Miguélez, A., Vanaclocha, F., Rubio, G., & Iglesias, L. (2001). Periocular and perioral artefactual dermatitis: Dermatological and psychiatric management in a hospital setting. *Dermatol Psychosom*, *2*(4), 200–202. doi:10.1159/000049672

Pate, K., Cherian, J., Gohil, K., & Atkinson, D. (2014). Schizophrenia: Overview and treatment options. *Journal of Pharmacy and Therapeutics*, *39*(9), 638–645. PMID:25210417

Patenaude, B., Zitsch, R. III, & Hirschi, S. D. (2006). Blood — but not bleeding — at a tracheotomy site: A case of Munchausen's syndrome. *Ear, Nose, and Throat Journal*, *85*(10), 677–679. doi:10.1177/014556130608501020 PMID:17124944

Patterson, D. A., Dulmus, C. N., & Maguin, E. (2013). Is openness to using empirically supported treatments related to organizational culture and climate? *Journal of Social Service Research*, *39*(4), 562–571. doi:10.1080/01488376.2013.804023 PMID:24159247

Patterson, D. A., Ramsey, A. T., & van den Berk-Clark, C. (2015). Implementing outside the box: Community-based social service provider experiences with using an alcohol screening and intervention. *Journal of Social Service Research*, *41*, 233–245. doi:10.1080/01488376.2014.980963 PMID:25798019

Pederson, A., Tsai, A. C., Hawkins, D., Moskowitz, J., & Dixon, L. (2023). Understanding the association between mental health knowledge and mental health service utilization among black adults. *Community Mental Health Journal*, *59*(1), 57–67. doi:10.100710597-022-00988-w PMID:35794413

Pederson, S. D., Curley, E. J., & Collins, C. J. (2021). A Systematic Review of Motivational Interviewing to Address Substance Use with Justice-Involved Adults. *Substance Use & Misuse*, *56*(5), 639–649. https://doi-org.proxy.tamuc.edu/10.1080/10826084.2021.1887247. doi:10.1080/10826084.2021.1887247 PMID:33726607

Peoples, J. E., Butler-Barnes, S. T., Stafford, J. D., Williams, S.-L., & Smith, I. (2023). Exploring the association between mental health climate and depression: the protective role of positive mental health and sense of belonging among Black college students. *Journal of American College Health*, 1–11. https://doi-org.proxy.tamuc.edu/10.1080/07448481.2022.2155466

Perlis, P. D., Riemann, D., Bastien, C. H., Teel, J., & Thase, M. (2022). Insomnia. The Lancet (British Edition), 400(10357), 1047–1060. doi:10.1016/S0140-6736(22)00879-0

Pescosolido, B., Halpern-Manners, A., & Luo, L. (2021). Trends in public stigma of mental illness in the US, 1996-2018. *JAMA Netw Open.* doi:10.1001/jamanetworkopen.2021.40202 PMID:34932103

Peteet, B., Watts, V., Tucker, E., Brown, P., Hanna, M., Saddlemire, A., Rizk, M., Belliard, J. C., Abdul-Mutakabbir, J. C., Casey, S., & Simmons, K. (2022). Faith, fear, and facts: A covid-19 vaccination hesitancy intervention for black church congregations. *Vaccines*, *10*(7), 1–11. doi:10.3390/vaccines10071039 PMID:35891203

Petersdorf, R. G., & Beeson, P. B. (1961). Fever of unexplained origin: Report on 100 cases. *Medicine*, *40*(1), 1–30. doi:10.1097/00005792-196102000-00001 PMID:13734791

Peters, Z. J., Santo, L., Davis, D., & DeFrances, C. J. (2023). *Emergency department visits related to mental health disorders among adults, by race and Hispanic ethnicity: United States, 2018–2020. National Health Statistics Reports; no 181*. National Center for Health Statistics. doi:10.15620/cdc:123507

Pickard, J. G., Williams Woodson, S.-L., & Johnson, S. D. (2021). The relationship of public and private religiosity to African American women caregivers' use of alcohol for coping with caregiving burden. *Aging & Mental Health*, *25*(3), 551–558. https://doi-org.proxy.tamuc.edu/10.1080/13607863.2019.1699020. doi:10.1080/13607863.2019.1699020 PMID:31809587

Pike, K. M., Hoek, H. W., & Dunne, P. E. (2014). Cultural trends and eating disorders. *Current Opinion in Psychiatry*, *27*(6), 436–442. doi:10.1097/YCO.0000000000000100 PMID:25211499

Pinedo, M. (2019). A current re-examination of racial/ethnic disparities in the use of substance abuse treatment: Do disparities persist? *Drug and Alcohol Dependence*, *202*, 162–167. https://doi-org.proxy.tamuc.edu/10.1016/j.drugalcdep.2019.05.017. doi:10.1016/j.drugalcdep.2019.05.017 PMID:31352305

Pinedo, M., Zemore, S., & Mulia, N. (2022). Black-White differences in barriers to specialty alcohol and drug treatment: Findings from a qualitative study. *Journal of Ethnicity in Substance Abuse*, *21*(1), 112–126. https://doi-org.proxy.tamuc.edu/10.1080/15332640.2020.1713954. doi:10.1080/15332640.2020.1713954 PMID:31961283

Piowowarczyk, L., Bishop, H., Yusuf, A., Mudymba, F., & Raj, A. (2014). Congolese and Somali beliefs about mental health services. *The Journal of Nervous and Mental Disease*, *202*(3), 209–216. doi:10.1097/NMD.0000000000000087 PMID:24566506

Pittman, D. M., & Kaur, P. (2018). Examining the role of racism in the risky alcohol use behaviors of black female college students. *Journal of American College Health*, *66*(4), 310–316. https://doi-org.proxy.tamuc.edu/10.1080/07448481.2018.1440581. doi:10.1080/07448481.2018.1440581 PMID:29448892

Plassmann, R. (1994). Münchhausen syndromes and factitious diseases. *Psychotherapy and Psychosomatics*, *62*(1–2), 7–26. doi:10.1159/000288899 PMID:7984770

Pleck, J. H., Sonenstein, F. L., & Ku, L. C. (1993). Masculinity ideology: Its impact on adolescent males' heterosexual relationships. *The Journal of Social Issues*, *49*(3), 11–29. doi:10.1111/j.1540-4560.1993.tb01166.x

Plowden, K. O., Thompson Adams, L., & Wiley, D. (2016). Black and blue: Depression and African American men. *Archives of Psychiatric Nursing*, *30*(5), 630–635. doi:10.1016/j.apnu.2016.04.007 PMID:27654249

Plunkett, D. (2014). The black church, values, and secular counseling: Implications for counselor education and practice. *Counseling and Values*, *59*(2), 208–221. doi:10.1002/j.2161-007X.2014.00052.x

Pugle, M. (2022, September 2). What are the types of borderline personality disorders? *Verywell Health*. https://www.verywellhealth.com/types-of-bpd-5193843

Ralph, A. F., Brennan, L., Bryne, S., Caldwell, B., Farmer, J., Hart, L. M., & Hay, P. (2022). Management of eating disorders for people with higher weight: Clinical practice guideline. *Journal of Eating Disorders*, *10*(121), 1–42. doi:10.118640337-022-00622-w PMID:35978344

Randall, J., Cunningham, P. B., & Henggeler, S. W. (2018). The Development and Transportability of Multisystemic Therapy-Substance Abuse: A Treatment for Adolescents with Substance Use Disorders. *Journal of Child & Adolescent Substance Abuse*, *27*(2), 59–66. https://doi-org.proxy.tamuc.edu/10.1080/1067828X.2017.1411301. doi:10.1080/1067828X.2017.1411301

Ransome, Y., & Gilman, S. E. (2016). The role of religious involvement in black-white differences in alcohol use severity. *Journal of Studies on Alcohol and Drugs*, *77*(5), 792–801. doi:10.15288/jsad.2016.77.792 PMID:27588538

Raz, M. (2020, April 21). Psychiatry under the shadow of White Supremacy. *Nature News*. https://www.nature.com/articles/d41586-020-01126-w

Redmond, M. L., Smith, S., & Collins, T. C. (2020). Exploring African-American womens' experiences with substance use treatment: A review of the literature. *Journal of Community Psychology*, *48*(2), 337–350. https://doi-org.proxy.tamuc.edu/10.1002/jcop.22241. doi:10.1002/jcop.22241 PMID:31609461

Reed-Knight, B., & Fischer, S. (2011). Treatment of narcissistic personality disorder symptoms in a dialectical behavior therapy framework: A discussion and case example. In W. K. Campbell & J. D. Miller (Eds.), *The handbook of narcissism and narcissistic personality disorder: Theoretical approaches, empirical findings, and treatments* (pp. 466–475). doi:10.1002/9781118093108.ch42

Reich, P., & Gottfried, L. A. (1983). Factitious Disorder in a Teaching Hospital. *Clinical Review*.

Reich, J. D. &, Hanno, P. (1997). Factitious Renal Colic. *Science Direct*, *50*(6), 858–862. PMID:9426714

Reich, P., & Gottfried, L. A. (1983). Factitious disorders in a teaching hospital. *Annals of Internal Medicine*, *99*(2), 240–247. doi:10.7326/0003-4819-99-2-240 PMID:6881779

Reinert, M., Fritze, D., & Nguyen, T. (2021). *The State of Mental Health in America 2022*. Mental Health America, Alexandria VA.

Released, S. I. (2015). *SPSS statistics for windows, version 23.0*. SPSS Inc.

Rezaie, Vakili-Amini, Y. Y., Paschall, E. E., & Khazaie, H. H. (2020). Personality profiles in paradoxical insomnia: a case-control study. *Sleep Science (São Paulo, SP)*, *13*(4), 242–248. https://doi.org/ doi:10.5935/1984-0063.20190148

Rice, S. M., Fallon, B. J., Aucote, H. M., & Möller-Leimkühler, A. M. (2013). Development and preliminary validation of the male depression risk scale: Furthering the assessment of depression in men. *Journal of Affective Disorders*, *151*(3), 950–958. doi:10.1016/j.jad.2013.08.013 PMID:24051100

Ridley, C. R. (1984). Clinical treatment of the nondisclosing Black client: A therapeutic paradox. *The American Psychologist*, *39*(11), 1234–1244. doi:10.1037/0003-066X.39.11.1234 PMID:6507987

Riedel, B. W. (2000). Sleep hygiene. In K. L. Lichstein & C. M. Morin (Eds.), *Treatment of Late-life Insomnia* (pp. 125–146). Sage. doi:10.4135/9781452225555.n5

Rigg, K. K. (2017). Motivations for Using MDMA (Ecstasy/Molly) among African Americans: Implications for Prevention and Harm-Reduction Programs. *Journal of Psychoactive Drugs*, *49*(3), 192–200. https://doi-org.proxy.tamuc.edu/10.1080/02791072.2017.1305518. doi:10.1080/02791072.2017.1305518 PMID:28406348

Rivas-Vazquez, R. A., & Blais, M. A. (2002). Pharmacologic treatment of personality disorders. *Professional Psychology, Research and Practice*, *33*(1), 104–107. doi:10.1037/0735-7028.33.1.104

Roberts-Douglass, K., & Curtis-Boles, H. (2013). Exploring positive masculinity development in African American men: A retrospective study. *Psychology of Men & Masculinity*, *14*(1), 7–15. doi:10.1037/a0029662

Robertson, M. M., & Hossain, G. (1997). Munchausen's syndrome coexisting with other disorders. *British Journal of Hospital Medicine*, *58*(4), 154–155. PMID:9373405

Robinson, M. A., Jones-Eversley, S., Moore, S. E., Ravenell, J., & Adedoyin, A. C. (2018). Black male mental health and the black church: Advancing a collaborative partnership and research agenda. *Journal of Religion and Health*, *57*(3), 1095–1107. doi:10.100710943-018-0570-x PMID:29417396

Rodríguez-Pichardo, A., Hoffner, M. V., García-Bravo, B., & Camacho, F. M. (2010). (19976-2006) Dermatitis artefacta of the breast: A retrospective analysis of 27 patients. Eur. *J. Acad Dermatol Venereol*, *24*(3), 270–274. doi:10.1111/j.1468-3083.2009.03403.x PMID:19694893

Roffman, J. L., Weiss, A. P., Goff, D. C., Rauch, S. L., & Weinberger, D. R. (2005). Neuroimaging-Genetic Paradigms: A new approach to investigate the pathophysiology and treatment of cognitive deficits in schizophrenia. *Harvard Review of Psychiatry*, *14*(2), 78–91. doi:10.1080/10673220600642945 PMID:16603474

Rogan, R. G., & Hammer, M. R. (1998). An exploratory study of message affect behavior: A comparison between African Americans and Euro-Americans. *Journal of Language and Social Psychology*, *17*, 449–464.

Rogers, B. K., Sperry, H. A., & Levant, R. F. (2015). Masculinities among African American men: An intersectional perspective. *Psychology of Men & Masculinity*, *16*(4), 416–425. doi:10.1037/a0039082

Romano, A., Alqahtani, S., Griffith, J., & Koubeissi, M. Z. (2014). Factitious psychogenic nonepileptic paroxysmal episodes. *Epilepsy & Behavior Case Reports*, *2*, 184–185. doi:10.1016/j.ebcr.2014.08.006 PMID:25667902

Rosenfarb, I. S., Bellack, A. S., & Aziz, N. (2006). Family interactions and the course of schizophrenia in African American and White patients. *Journal of Abnormal Psychology*, *115*(1), 112–120. doi:10.1037/0021-843X.115.1.112 PMID:16492102

Ross, C. C. (2019). African-American women and eating disorders: Depression, and the strong Black woman archetype. *Eating Disorders Review*, *30*(5), 1–1.

Rotton, J., Foos, P. W., Van Meek, L., & Levitt, M. (1995). Publication practices and the file drawer problem: A survey of published authors. *Journal of Social Behavior and Personality*.

Rowan, K., Alphine, D., & Blewett, L. (2013, October 1). Access and cost barriers to mental health care, by ... - health affairs. *Health Affairs*. https://www.healthaffairs.org/doi/10.1377/hlthaff.2013.0133

Roxburgh, S., & MacArthur, K. R. (2020). Racial Differences in the Salience of Social Support for Mental Health: An Intersectional Approach. *Michigan Sociological Review*, *34*, 46–72.

Ruffins, P. (1998). The Tuskegee experiment's long shadow. *Black Issues in Higher Education*, 26. https://link.gale.com/apps/doc/A53257761/ITOF?u=txshrpub100292&sid= bookmark-ITOF&xid=e83e0d32

Rumans, L. W., & Vosti, K. L. (1978). Factitious and fraudulent fever. *The American Journal of Medicine*, *65*(5), 745–755. doi:10.1016/0002-9343(78)90792-1 PMID:707533

Sacks, J. J., Gonzales, K.R., Bouchery, E.E., Tomedi, L,E., & Brewer, R.D. (2010) National and State Costs of Excessive Alcohol Consumption. *American Journal Preventative Medicine*, *49*(5), e73–e79.

Saiyasombat, M. I., & Satyanarayan, M. (2012). Pancytopenia secondary to cyclophosphamide in a case of factitious breast cancer. *The Primary Care Companion for CNS Disorders*, *14*(2). doi:10.4088/PCC.11l01301 PMID:22943027

Sakado, K., Kuwabara, H., Sato, T., Uehara, T., Sakado, T., & Someya, T. (2000). The relationship between personality, dysfunctional parenting in childhood, and lifetime depression in a sample of employed Japanese adults. *Journal of Affective Disorders*, *60*(1), 47–51. doi:10.1016/S0165-0327(99)00150-0 PMID:10940447

Salami, B., Denga, B., Taylor, R., Ajayi, N., Jackson, M., Asefaw, M., & Salma, J. (2021). Original qualitative research-Access to mental health for Black youths in Alberta. *Health Promotion and Chronic Disease Prevention in Canada: Research. Policy & Practice*, *41*(9), 245.

Saloner, B., & Lê Cook, B. (2013). Blacks And Hispanics Are Less Likely Than Whites To Complete Addiction Treatment, Largely Due To Socioeconomic Factors. *Health Affairs*, *32*(1), 135–145. https://doi-org.proxy.tamuc.edu/10.1377/hlthaff.2011.0983. doi:10.1377/hlthaff.2011.0983 PMID:23297281

Samuel, I. A. (2015). Utilization of mental health services among African American male adolescents released from juvenile detention: Examining reasons for within-group disparities in help-seeking behaviors. *Child & Adolescent Social Work Journal*, *32*(1), 33–43. doi:10.100710560-014-0357-1

Sanders, M. (2002). The Response of African American Communities to Alcohol and Other Drug Problems: An Opportunity for Treatment Providers. *Alcoholism Treatment Quarterly*, *20*(3/4), 167–174. https://doi-org.proxy.tamuc.edu/10.1300/J020v20n03_11. doi:10.1300/J020v20n03_11

Sandlund, H., Hetta, J., Nilsson, G., Ekstedt, M., & Westman, J. (2017). Group treatment for insomnia and impact on daytime symptomatology associated with insomnia: Analyses from a randomized controlled trial in primary care. *Sleep Medicine*, *40*, e291–e292. doi:10.1016/j.sleep.2017.11.856

Sandoiu, A. (2019, November 21). Borderline personality disorder: Trauma raises risk by 13-fold. *Medical News Today*. https://www.medicalnewstoday.com/articles/327084

Satcher, D. (2013). Addressing racial and ethnic disparities in health: The need for a national agenda. *Journal of the National Medical Association*, *105*(2, Suppl), 1S–2S.

Savino, A. C., & Fordtran, J. S. (2006). Factitious disease: Clinical lessons from case studies at Baylor University Medical Center. *Proceedings - Baylor University. Medical Center*, *19*(3), 195–208. doi:10.1080/08998280.2006.11928162 PMID:17252033

Sbrocco, T., Osborn, R., Clark, R. D., Hsiao, C. W., & Carter, M. M. (2012). Assessing the stages of change among African American women in a weight management program. *The Journal of Black Psychology*, *38*(1), 81–103. doi:10.1177/0095798411403618 PMID:24683280

Schmidt, F., Strutz, F., Quellhorst, E., & Müller, G. A. (1996). Nephrectomy and solitary kidney biopsy in a patient with Munchausen's syndrome. *Nephrology, Dialysis, Transplantation*, *11*(5), 890–892. doi:10.1093/oxfordjournals.ndt.a027424 PMID:8671920

Schulz, B., & Strauch, R. J. (2008). A case of factitious subfascial emphysema. *Orthopedics*, *31*(5), 495. doi:10.3928/01477447-20080501-26 PMID:19292308

Schwartz, B., & Fuller, K. (2022, June 9). *Impulsive borderline personality disorder (BPD)*. Choosing Therapy. https://www.choosingtherapy.com/impulsive-borderline-personality-disorder/

Schwartz, B., Bernal, D., Smith, L., & Nicolas, G. (2014). Pathways to understand help-seeking behaviors among Haitians. *Journal of Immigrant and Minority Health*, *16*(2), 239–243. doi:10.100710903-012-9751-y PMID:23192378

Schwartz, R. C., & Blankenship, D. M. (2014). Racial disparities in psychotic disorder diagnosis: A review of the empirical literature. *World Journal of Psychiatry*, *4*(4), 133–140. doi:10.5498/wjp.v4.i4.133 PMID:25540728

Scott, T. N., Gil-Rivas, V., & Cachelin, F. M. (2019). The need for cultural adaptations to health interventions for African American women: A qualitative analysis. *Cultural Diversity & Ethnic Minority Psychology*, *25*(3), 331–341. doi:10.1037/cdp0000228 PMID:30272472

Seidler, Z. E., Dawes, A. J., Rice, S. M., Oliffe, J. L., & Dhillon, H. M. (2016). The role of masculinity in men's help-seeking for depression: A systematic review. *Clinical Psychology Review, 49*, 106–118. doi:10.1016/j.cpr.2016.09.002 PMID:27664823

Seidler, Z. E., Rice, S. M., River, J., Oliffe, J. L., & Dhillon, H. M. (2017). Men's mental health: The case for a masculinities model. *Journal of Men's Studies, 26*(1), 92–104. doi:10.1177/1060826517729406

Senol, S. (2023, March 28). *Borderline personality disorder*. Encyclopedia Britannica. https://www.britannica.com/science/borderline-personality-disorder

Shangani, S., van den Berg, J. J., Dyer, T. V., Mayer, K. H., & Operario, D. (2022). Childhood sexual abuse, alcohol and drug use problems among Black sexual minority men in six US Cities: Findings from the HPTN 061 study. *PLoS One, 17*(12), 1–13. https://doi-org.proxy.tamuc.edu/10.1371/journal.pone.0279238. doi:10.1371/journal.pone.0279238 PMID:36548261

Shannon, J., Seward, D. X., Liu, Y., & Stigma, M. L. (2022, October). help-seeking, and counseling with African American male college students. *Journal of Counseling and Development, 100*(4), 421–432. Advance online publication. doi:10.1002/jcad.12435

Sheridan, M. S. (2003). The deceit continues: An updated literature review of Munchausen syndrome by proxy. *Child Abuse & Neglect, 27*(4), 431–451. doi:10.1016/S0145-2134(03)00030-9 PMID:12686328

Sibrava, N. J., Bjornsson, A., Perez Benitez, C. I., Moitra, E., Weisberg, R. B., & Keller, M. B. (2019). Posttraumatic stress disorder in African American and Latinx adults: Clinical course and the role of racial and ethnic discrimination. *The American Psychologist, 74*(1), 101–116. doi:10.1037/amp0000339 PMID:30652903

Sileo, K. M., & Kershaw, T. S. (2020). Dimensions of masculine norms, depression, and mental health service utilization: Results from a prospective cohort study among emerging adult men in the United States. *American Journal of Men's Health, 14*(1), 1557988320906980. doi:10.1177/1557988320906980 PMID:32079448

Sinha, S., & Warfa, N. (2013). Treatment of eating disorders among ethnic minorities in western settings: A systematic review. *Psychiatria Danubina, 25*(Suppl 2), S295–S299. PMID:23995197

Skalamera, J., & Hummer, R. A. (2016). Educational attainment and the clustering of health-related behavior among US young adults. *Preventive Medicine, 84*, 83–89. doi:10.1016/j.ypmed.2015.12.011 PMID:26740348

Sloan, C., Conner, M., & Gough, B. (2015). How does masculinity impact on health? A quantitative study of masculinity and health behavior in a sample of U.K. men and women. *Psychology of Men & Masculinity, 16*(2), 206–217. doi:10.1037/a0037261

Smedley, B. D., Stith, A. Y., & Nelson, A. R. (2003). Racial and ethnic disparities in diagnosis and treatment: a review of the evidence and a consideration of causes. *Unequal treatment: Confronting racial and ethnic disparities in health care.*

Smith, A. R., Zuromski, K. L., & Dodd, D. R. (2018). Eating disorders and suicidality: What we know, what we don't know, and suggestions for future research. *Current Opinion in Psychology*, *22*, 63–67. doi:10.1016/j.copsyc.2017.08.023 PMID:28846874

Snowden, L. R. (2003). Bias in mental health assessment and intervention. *American Journal of Public Health*, *93*(2), 239–243. doi:10.2105/AJPH.93.2.239 PMID:12554576

Snowden, L. R., Catalano, R., & Shumway, M. (2009). Disproportionate use of psychiatric emergency services by African Americans. *Psychiatric Services (Washington, D.C.)*, *60*(12), 1664–1671. doi:10.1176/ps.2009.60.12.1664 PMID:19952158

Soo, S., Zhang, Z., Jia, S., & Khong, E. (2018). Randomized Controlled Trials of Psychoeducation Modalities in the Management of Bipolar Disorder: A Systematic Review. *Journal of Clinical Psychiatry*.

Sowislo, J. F., & Orth, U. (2013). Does low self-esteem predict depression and anxiety? A meta-analysis of longitudinal studies. *Psychological Bulletin*, *139*(1), 213–240. doi:10.1037/a0028931 PMID:22730921

Stansbury, P., Peterson, T. L., & Beecher, B. (2013). An exploration of mental health literacy among older African Americans. *Aging & Mental Health*, *17*(2), 226–232. doi:10.1080/13607863.2012.724652 PMID:23067011

Staples, R. F. (1978). Masculinity and race: The dual dilemma of Black men. *The Journal of Social Issues*, *34*(1), 169–183. doi:10.1111/j.1540-4560.1978.tb02547.x

Stare, B. G., & Fernando, D. M. (2019). Black American men's treatment experiences in mental health court: A phenomenological analysis. *Journal of Addictions & Offender Counseling*, *40*(1), 17–35. doi:10.1002/jaoc.12054

Staton-Tindall, M., Duvall, J., Stevens-Watkins, D., & Oser, C. B. (2013). The Roles of Spirituality in the Relationship Between Traumatic Life Events, Mental Health, and Drug Use Among African American Women from One Southern State. *Substance Use & Misuse*, *48*(12), 1246–1257. https://doi doi:org.proxy.tamuc.edu/10.3109/10826084.2013.799023

Steel, R. M. (2009). Factitious disorder (Munchausen's syndrome). *Journal of the Royal College of Physicians of Edinburgh*, *39*(4), 343–347. doi:10.4997/JRCPE.2009.412 PMID:21152477

Stern, E., & Nellis, M. (2017). The intersection of race and diagnosis among individuals with severe mental illness: A review. *Journal of Clinical Psychology*, *73*(12), 1671–1682.

Stiles, A., Mitrirattanakul, S., & Sanders, B. (2001). Munchausen syndrome presenting in a patient who has undergone temporomandibular joint surgery. Oral surgery, oral medicine, oral pathology, oral radiology, and. *Endodontology*, *91*(1), 20–22.

Stiles-Shields, C., Hoste, R. R., Doyle, P. M., & Le Grange, D. (2012). A review of family based treatment for adolescents with eating disorders. *Reviews on Recent Clinical Trials*, *7*(2), 133–140. doi:10.2174/157488712800100242 PMID:22353196

Stinson, F. S., Dawson, D. A., Goldstein, R. B., Chou, S. P., Huang, B., Smith, S. M., Ruan, W. J., Pulay, A. J., Saha, T. D., Pickering, R. P., & Grant, B. F. (2008). Prevalence, correlates, disability, and comorbidity of DSM-IV narcissistic personality disorder: Results from the wave 2 national epidemiologic survey on alcohol and related conditions. *The Journal of Clinical Psychiatry*, *69*(7), 1033–1045. doi:10.4088/JCP.v69n0701 PMID:18557663

Stokes, P., Bell, K., & Mellman, T. A. (2022). Strategies for Controlling Unwanted Intrusive Thoughts and Insomnia Severity in Urban-Residing Young Adult African Americans. *Behavioral Sleep Medicine, ahead-of-print*(ahead-of-print), 1–8. doi:10.1080/15402002.2022.2057986

Storch, E. A., De Nadai, A. S., Jacob, M. L., Lewin, A. B., Muroff, J., Eisen, J., & Murphy, T. K. (2014). Phenomenology and correlates of insight in pediatric obsessive-compulsive disorder. *Science Direct, 55*, 613-620. http://dx.doi.org/. 2013.09.014 doi:10.1016/j.comppsych

Stroud, C. B., Davila, J., & Moyer, A. (2008). The relationship between stress and depression in first onsets versus recurrences: A meta-analytic review. *Journal of Abnormal Psychology*, *117*(1), 206–213. doi:10.1037/0021-843X.117.1.206 PMID:18266498

Substance Abuse and Mental Health Service Administration. (2023, April 24). *Borderline personality disorder*. SAMHSA. https://www.samhsa.gov/mental-health/borderline-personality-disorder

Substance Abuse and Mental Health Services Administration. (2013). Addressing the Specific Behavioral Health Needs of Men. Treatment Improvement Protocol (TIP) Series 56. HHS Publication No. (SMA) 13-4736. Rockville, MD: Substance Abuse and Mental Health Services Administration.

Substance Abuse and Mental Health Services Administration. (2015). *Racial/ethnic differences in mental health service use among adults.* SAMHSA. https://www.integration.samhsa.gov/MHServicesUseAmongAdults.pdf

Substance Abuse and Mental Health Services Administration. (2019). Results from the 2018 National Survey on Drug Use and Health: Mental Health Detailed Tables. *Table 8.17B*. [Data set]. SAMHSA. https://www.samhsa.gov/data/report/2018-nsduh-detailed-tables

Substance Abuse and Mental Health Services Administration. (2023). *Key Substance Use and Mental Health Indicators in the United States: Results from the 2021 National Survey on Drug Use and Health.* SAMHSA. https://www.samhsa.gov/data/sites/default/files/reports/rpt39443/2021NSDUHFFRRev010323.pdf

Sule, E., Sutton, R. M., Jones, D., Moore, R., Igbo, I., & Jones, L. A. (2017). The past does matter: A nursing perspective on Post Traumatic Slave Syndrome (PTSS). *Journal of Racial and Ethnic Health Disparities*, *4*(5), 779–783. doi:10.100740615-016-0328-7 PMID:28078658

Sulkowski, M. L., Dempsey, J., & Dempsey, A. G. (2011). Effects of stress and coping on binge eating in female college students. *Eating Behaviors*, *12*(3), 188–191. doi:10.1016/j.eatbeh.2011.04.006 PMID:21741016

Sun-Kyung Shin, M. S. W. (2002). Effects of Psychoeducation for Korean Americans with Chronic Mental Illness. *Psychiatric Services*. doi:10.1176/appi.ps.53.9.1125

Sussman, L. K. (2004). The role of culture in definitions, interpretations, and management of illness. In U. P. Gielen, J. M. Fish, & J. G. Draguns (Eds.), *Handbook of culture, therapy, and healing* (pp. 37–65). Lawrence Erlbaum Associates Publishers.

Sutherland, Amanda J., & Rodin, G. (1990). Factitous Disorder in a General Hospital Setting: Clinical Features and a Review of the Literature. *Psychosomatics*, *31*(4), 392–399. doi:10.1016/S0033-3182(90)72133-0 PMID:2247566

Sutherland, M. E. (2013). Overweight and obesity among African American women: An examination of predictive and risk factors and weight-reduction recommendations. *Journal of Black Studies*, *44*(8), 846–869. doi:10.1177/0021934713511639

Svirsky, J. A., & Sawyer, D. R. (1987). Dermatitis artefacta of the paraoral region. *Oral Surgery, Oral Medicine, and Oral Pathology*, *64*(2), 259–263. doi:10.1016/0030-4220(87)90101-0 PMID:3476905

Swami, V. (2016). Masculinities and ethnicities: Ethnic differences in drive for muscularity in British men and the negotiation of masculinity hierarchies. *British Journal of Psychology*, *107*(3), 577–592. doi:10.1111/bjop.12162 PMID:26592864

Talleyrand, R. M. (2011). Eating disorders in African American girls: Implications for counselors. *Journal of Counseling and Development*, *88*(3), 319–324. doi:10.1002/j.1556-6678.2010.tb00028.x

Talleyrand, R. M., Gordon, A. D., Daquin, J. V., & Johnson, A. J. (2017). Expanding our understanding of eating practices, body image, and appearance in African American women: A qualitative study. *The Journal of Black Psychology*, *43*(5), 464–492. doi:10.1177/0095798416649086

Taylor, R., Nguyen, A., Sinkewicz, M., Joe, S., & Chatters, L. (2013). Comorbid mood and anxiety disorders, suicidal behavior, and substance abuse among Black Caribbeans in the U.S.A. *Journal of African American Studies*, *17*(4), 409–425. doi:10.100712111-012-9237-y

Team, O. P. I. (2018, July 16). *What is impulsive borderline personality disorder?* OPI Residential Treatment Center for Young Adults - Private Pay Mental Health Program. https://www.optimumperformanceinstitute.com/bpd-treatment/impulsive-borderline-personality-disorder/

Terrell, F., & Terrell, S. L. (1981). An inventory to measure cultural mistrust among Blacks. *The Western Journal of Black Studies*, *5*, 180–184.

The Office of Minority Health. (2008). *African American Profile.* U.S. Department of Health & Human Services. http:// www.omhrc.gov/templates/browse.aspx?lvl =2&lvlID=51

The Office of Minority Health. (2008). *Stroke and African Americans. Rockville, MD: U.S. Department of Health & Human Services.* Office of Minority Health. http://www.omhrc.gov/templates/content.aspx?lvl=2&lvlID=51&ID=3022

Thompson, V., & Bazile, A. (2004, February 1). *African Americans' perceptions of psychotherapy and psychotherapists*. ResearchGate. https://www.researchgate.net/publication/232423919_African_Americans%27_Perceptions_of_Psychotherapy_and_Psychotherapists

Thompson-Brenner, H., Franko, D. L., Thompson, D. R., Grilo, C. M., Boisseau, C. L., Roehrig, J. P., Richards, L. K., Bryson, S. W., Bulik, C. M., Crow, S. J., Devlin, M. J., Gorin, A. A., Kristeller, J. L., Masheb, R., Mitchell, J. E., Peterson, C. B., Safer, D. L., Striegel, R. H., Wilfley, D. E., & Wilson, G. T. (2013). Race/ethnicity, education, and treatment parameters as moderators and predictors of outcome in binge eating disorder. *Journal of Consulting and Clinical Psychology*, *81*(4), 710–721. doi:10.1037/a0032946 PMID:23647283

Thompson, C., & Park, S. (2016). Barriers to access and utilization of eating disorder treatment among women. *Archives of Women's Mental Health*, *19*(5), 753–760. doi:10.100700737-016-0618-4 PMID:26971265

Thornton, L. M., Watson, H. J., Jangmo, A., Welch, E., Wiklund, C., von Hausswolff-Juhlin, Y., Norring, C., Herman, B. K., Larsson, H., & Bulik, C. M. (2017). Binge-eating disorder in the Swedish national registers: Somatic comorbidity. *International Journal of Eating Disorders*, *50*(1), 58–65. doi:10.1002/eat.22624 PMID:27642179

Thorpe, R. J. Jr, Kennedy-Hendricks, A., Griffith, D. M., Bruce, M. A., Coa, K., Bell, C. N., Young, J., Bowie, J. V., & LaVeist, T. A. (2015). Race, social and environmental conditions, and health behaviors in men. *Family & Community Health*, *38*(4), 297–306. doi:10.1097/FCH.0000000000000078 PMID:26291190

Thriveworks. (2021, August 30). *Borderline personality disorder*. Thriveworks. https://thriveworks.com/borderline-personality-disorder-symptoms-facts/

Thynne, T., White, G. H., & Burt, M. G. (2014). Factitious Cushing's syndrome masquerading as Cushing's disease. *Clinical Endocrinology*, *80*(3), 328–332. doi:10.1111/cen.12343 PMID:24111609

Tolin, D. F., McKay, D., Forman, E. M., Klonsky, E. D., & Thombs, B. D. (2015). Empirically supported treatment: Recommendations for a new model. *Clinical Psychology: Science and Practice*, *22*(4), 317–338. doi:10.1037/h0101729

Tyler, R. E., & Williams, S. (2014). Masculinity in young men's health: Exploring health, help-seeking and health service use in an online environment. *Journal of Health Psychology*, *19*(4), 457–470. doi:10.1177/1359105312473784 PMID:23493865

U.S. Census Bureau. (2005-2013). *American Community Survey 1-Year PUMS file*. US Census Bureau. http://www.census. gov/programs-surveys/acs/data/ pums.html

U.S. Department of Health and Human Services Office of Minority Health. (2021). *Mental and Behavioral Health – African Americans*. US DOHH. https://minorityhealth.hhs.gov/omh/browse.aspx?lvl=4&lvlid=24

U.S. Department of Health and Human Services. (n.d.). *Publications about borderline personality disorder*. National Institute of Mental Health. https://www.nimh.nih.gov/health/publications/borderline-personality-disorder-listing

Udo, T., & Grilo, C. M. (2018). Prevalence and correlates of DSM-5-defined eating disorders in a nationally representative sample of U.S. adults. *Biological Psychiatry*, *84*(5), 345–354. doi:10.1016/j.biopsych.2018.03.014 PMID:29859631

Udo, T., & Grilo, C. M. (2019). Psychiatric and medical correlates of DSM-5 eating disorders in a nationally representative sample of adults in the United States. *International Journal of Eating Disorders*, *52*(1), 42–50. doi:10.1002/eat.23004 PMID:30756422

Udo, T., White, M. A., Lydecker, J. L., Barnes, R. D., Genao, I., Garcia, R., Masheb, R. M., & Grilo, C. M. (2016). Biopsychosocial correlates of binge eating disorder in European American and African American women with obesity in primary care settings. *European Eating Disorders Review*, *24*(3), 181–186. doi:10.1002/erv.2417 PMID:26640009

United States Renal Data System. (2005). *Home*. National Institute of Diabetes and Digestive and Kidney Diseases. Available at: http://www.usrds.org/

Usher, K. (2001). Taking neuroleptic medications as the treatment for schizophrenia: A phenomenological study. *The Australian and New Zealand Journal of Mental Health Nursing*, *10*(1), 145–155. doi:10.1046/j.1440-0979.2001.00205.x PMID:11493286

Vaduganathan, M., McCullough, S. A., Fraser, T. N., & Stern, T. A. (2014). Death due to Munchausen syndrome: A case of idiopathic recurrent right ventricular failure and a review of the literature. *Psychosomatics*, *6*(55), 668–672. doi:10.1016/j.psym.2014.05.013 PMID:25262044

Van Alsten, S. C., & Duncan, A. E. (2020). Lifetime patterns of comorbidity in eating disorders: An approach using sequence analysis. *European Eating Disorders Review*, *28*(6), 709–723. doi:10.1002/erv.2767 PMID:32748537

van Amsterdam, J., & van den Brink, W. (2013). The high harm score of alcohol. Time for drug policy to be revisited? *Journal of Psychopharmacology (Oxford, England)*, *27*(3), 248–255. https://doi-org.proxy.tamuc.edu/10.1177/0269881112472559. doi:10.1177/0269881112472559 PMID:23325370

Van Boekel, B. & Van Weeghel, G. (2013). Stigma among health professionals towards patients with substance use disorders and its consequences for healthcare delivery: systematic review. *Drug Alcohol Depend*, *131*, 23-35. doi:10.1016/j.drugalcdep.2013.02.018

van den Berk-Clark, C., Patterson Silver Wolf, A. U. W. D. A., & Williams, S.-L. (2017). Impact of Race on the Implementation of Empirically Supported Treatments in Substance Abuse Treatment. *Journal of Social Work Practice in the Addictions*, *17*(1/2), 36–56. https://doi-org.proxy.tamuc.edu/10.1080/1533256X.2017.1302883. doi:10.1080/1533256X.2017.1302883 van der Feltz-Cornelis, C. M. (2002). The Impact of Factitous Disorder on the Physician-Patient Relationship. An Epistemological Model, Medicine, Heatlth. *Care and Philosophy*, *5*, 253–261. PMID:12517033

Van Gundy, K. T., Howerton-Orcutt, A., & Mills, M. L. (2015). Race, Coping Style, and Substance Use Disorder Among Non-Hispanic African American and White Young Adults in South Florida. *Substance Use & Misuse*, *50*(11), 1459–1469. https://doi-org.proxy.tamuc.edu/10.3109/10826084.2015.1018544. doi:10.3109/10826084.2015.1018544 PMID:26549159

van Hoeken, D., & Hoek, H. W. (2020). Review of the burden of eating disorders: Mortality, disability, costs, quality of life, and family burden. *Current Opinion in Psychiatry*, *33*(6), 521–527. doi:10.1097/YCO.0000000000000641 PMID:32796186

van Maanen, M., Meijer, A. M., van der Heijden, K. B., & Oort, F. J. (2016). The effects of light therapy on sleep problems: A systematic review and meta-analysis. *Sleep Medicine Reviews*, *29*, 52–62. doi:10.1016/j.smrv.2015.08.009 PMID:26606319

van Manen, M. (1990). *Researching lived experience: Human science for an action sensitive pedagogy*. State University of New York Press.

van Manen, M. (1997). *Researching the lived experience: Human science for an action sensitive pedagogy* (2nd ed., rev.). Althouse.

Vance, T. (2019, February 8). *Addressing mental health in the Black Community*. Columbia University Department of Psychiatry. https://www.columbiapsychiatry.org/news/addressing-mental-health-black-community

Van-Eerven Ludolf, N., do Carmo Silva, M., Simões Gomes, C. F., & Oliveira, V. M. (2017). The Organizational Culture and Values Alignment Management Importance for Successful Business. *Brazilian Journal of Operations & Production Management*, *14*(2), 272–280. https://doi-org.proxy.tamuc.edu/10.14488/BJOPM.2017.v14.n2.a15. doi:10.14488/BJOPM.2017.v14.n2.a15

Varcarolis, E. M., & Halter, M. J. (2010). *Foundations of psychiatric mental health nursing: A clinical approach* (6th ed.). Saunders.

Verywell Mind. (2023). Doctor discussion guides. *Verywell Mind*. https://www.verywellmind.com/doctor-discussion-guides-4797486

Vidourek, R. A., King, K. A., Burbage, M., & Okuley, B. (2018). Impact of Parenting Behaviors on Recent Alcohol Use Among African American Students. *Child & Adolescent Social Work Journal*, *35*(3), 271–282. https://doi-org.proxy.tamuc.edu/10.1007/s10560-017-0524-2. doi:10.100710560-017-0524-2

Vogel, D. L., Heimerdinger-Edwards, S. R., Hammer, J. H., & Hubbard, A. (2011). "Boys don't cry": Examination of the links between endorsement of masculine norms, self-stigma, and help-seeking attitudes for men from diverse backgrounds. *Journal of Counseling Psychology*, *58*(3), 368–382. doi:10.1037/a0023688 PMID:21639615

Volpe, U., Tortorella, A., Manchia, M., Monteleone, A. M., Albert, U., & Monteleone, P. (2016). Eating disorders: What age at onset? *Psychiatry Research*, *238*, 225–227. doi:10.1016/j.psychres.2016.02.048 PMID:27086237

Wade, J. C., & Rochlen, A. B. (2013). Introduction: Masculinity, identity, and the health and well-being of African American men. *Psychology of Men & Masculinity*, *14*(1), 1–6. doi:10.1037/a0029612

Walker, R. (2020). *The unapologetic guide to Black mental health : Navigate an unequal system, learn tools for emotional wellness, and get the help you deserve*. EBSCO Host. https://search.ebscohost.com/login.aspx?direct=true&db=nlebk&AN=2267576&site=ehost-live

Walton, M. F. (2014). *Betrayal trauma, experiences of racism, resilience, and borderline personality characteristics in African-Americans* (Order No. 3623046). Available from ProQuest Dissertations & Theses Global. (1548306775). https://go.openathens.net/redirector/ace.edu/login?url=https://www.proquest.com/dissertations-theses/betrayal-trauma-experiences-racism-resilience/docview/1548306775/se-2

Wang, J., Patten, S. B., Lam, R. W., Attridge, M., Ho, K., Schmitz, N., Marchand, A., & Lashewicz, B. M. (2016). The effects of an e-mental health program and job coaching on the risk of major depression and productivity in Canadian male workers: Protocol for a randomized controlled trial. *JMIR Research Protocols*, *5*(4), e6350. doi:10.2196/resprot.6350 PMID:27847352

Ward, E. (2013, June 1). African American men and women's attitude toward mental. *Nursing research*. https://journals.lww.com/nursingresearchonline/Abstract/2013/05000/African_American_Men_and_Women_s_Attitude_Toward.6.aspx

Ward, E. C., & Heidrich, S. M. (2009, July 31). African American women's beliefs about mental illness, stigma, and preferred coping behaviors. *Research in Nursing & Health*, *32*(5), 480–492. doi:10.1002/nur.20344 PMID:19650070

Ward, E. C., Wiltshire, J. C., Detry, M. A., & Brown, R. L. (2013). African American men and women's attitude toward mental illness, perceptions of stigma, and preferred coping behaviors. *Nursing Research*, *62*(3), 185–194. doi:10.1097/NNR.0b013e31827bf533 PMID:23328705

Ward, E. G. (2005). Homophobia, hypermasculinity and the US black church. *Culture, Health & Sexuality*, *7*(5), 493–504. doi:10.1080/13691050500151248 PMID:16864218

Ward, E., Clark, L. O., & Heidrich, S. (2009). African American women's beliefs, coping behaviors, and barriers to seeking mental health services. *Qualitative Health Research*, *19*(11), 1589–1601. doi:10.1177/1049732309350686 PMID:19843967

Washington, H. (2006). *Medical apartheid: The dark history of medical experimentation on black Americans from colonial times to the present*. Random House.

Watkins, D. C., Green, B. L., Rivers, B. M., & Rowell, K. L. (2006). Depression and black men: Implications for future research. *Journal of Men's Health & Gender*, *3*(3), 227–235. doi:10.1016/j.jmhg.2006.02.005

Watkins-Hayes, C. (2009). Raceing the bootstrap climb: Black and Latino bureaucrats in post-reform welfare offices. *Social Problems*, *56*(2), 285–310. doi:10.1525p.2009.56.2.285

Watkins-Hayes, C. (2011). Race, respect, and red tape: Inside the black box of racially representative bureaucracies. *Journal of Public Administration: Research and Theory*, *21*(Suppl. 2), i233–i251. doi:10.1093/jopart/muq096

Watson, J. (2014). Young African American males: Barriers to access to health care. *Journal of Human Behavior in the Social Environment*, *24*(8), 1004–1009. doi:10.1080/10911359.2014.953416

Watson, L. B., Ancis, J. R., White, D. N., & Nazari, N. (2013). Racial identity buffers African American women from body image problems and disordered eating. *Psychology of Women Quarterly*, *37*(3), 337–350. doi:10.1177/0361684312474799

Waxenbaum, J., Reddy, V., & Varacallo, M. (2020). *Anatomy, Autonomic Nervous System*. NCBI. https://www.ncbi.nlm.nih.gov/books/NBK539845/#:~:text=The%20autonomic%20nervous%20system%20is,sympathetic%2C%20parasympathetic%2C%20and%20enteric

Webb Hooper, M., Nápoles, A. M., & Pérez-Stable, E. J. (2020). COVID-19 and racial/ethnic disparities. *Journal of the American Medical Association*, *323*(24), 2466. doi:10.1001/jama.2020.8598 PMID:32391864

Weigel, A., Lowe, B., & Kohlmann, S. (2019). Severity of somatic symptoms in outpatients with anorexia and bulimia nervosa. *European Eating Disorders Review*, *27*(2), 195–204. doi:10.1002/erv.2643 PMID:30318829

Weiss-Gal, I. (2008). The Person-in-Environment Approach: Professional Ideology and Practice of Social Workers in Israel. *Social Work*, *53*(1), 65–75. https://doi-org.proxy.tamuc.edu/10.1093/sw/53.1.65. doi:10.1093w/53.1.65 PMID:18610822

Welch, E., Jangmo, A., Thornton, L. M., Norring, C., von Hausswolff-Juhlin, Y., Herman, B. K., Pawaskar, M., Larsson, H., & Bulik, C. M. (2016). Treatment-seeking patients with binge-eating disorder in the Swedish national registers: Clinical course and psychiatric comorbidity. *BMC Psychiatry*, *16*(1), 1–8. doi:10.118612888-016-0840-7 PMID:27230675

Wexler, R., Elton, T., Pleister, A., & Feldman, D. (2009). Barriers to blood pressure control as reported by African American patients. *Journal of the National Medical Association*, *101*(6), 597–603. doi:10.1016/S0027-9684(15)30947-0 PMID:19585931

Whaley, A. (2001). Cultural mistrust and mental health services for African Americans: A review and meta-analysis. *The Counseling Psychologist*, *29*(4), 513–531. doi:10.1177/0011000001294003

Whaley, A. L. (2001a). Cultural mistrust and the clinical diagnosis of paranoid schizophrenia in African American patients. *Journal of Psychopathology and Behavioral Assessment*, *23*(2), 93–100. doi:10.1023/A:1010911608102

Whaley, A. L. (2001b). Cultural mistrust: An important psychological construct for diagnosis and treatment of African Americans. *Professional Psychology, Research and Practice*, *32*(6), 555–562. doi:10.1037/0735-7028.32.6.555

Wheaton, M., Berman, N., Fabricant, L., & Abramowitz, J. (2013). Differences in obsessive–compulsive symptoms and obsessive beliefs: A comparison between African Americans, Asian Americans, Latino Americans, and European Americans. *Cognitive Behaviour Therapy*, *42*(1), 9–20. doi:10.1080/16506073.2012.701663 PMID:23134374

Wheeler, J. R., & Nahra, T. A. (2000). Private and public ownership in outpatient substance abuse treatment: Do we have a two-tiered system? *Administration and Policy in Mental Health*, *27*(4), 197–209. doi:10.1023/A:1021357318246 PMID:10911669

Whisman, M. A., Sheldon, C., & Goering, P. (2000). Psychiatric disorders and dissatisfaction with social relationships: Does type of relationship matter? *Journal of Abnormal Psychology*, *109*(4), 803–808. doi:10.1037/0021-843X.109.4.803 PMID:11196008

White, A. (2008). *Ain't I a feminist? African American men speak out on fatherhood, friendship, forgiveness, and freedom*. State University of New York Press.

White, T. (2017). *Semi-structured interviews: African American clergy perceptions regarding mental health*. Sage Publications. doi:10.4135/9781526424136

Williams, E. C., Gupta, S., Rubinsky, A. D., Jones-Webb, R., Bensley, K. M., Young, J. P., & Harris, A. H. S. (2016) Racial/ethnic differences in the prevalence of clinically recognized alcohol use disorders among patients from the U S Veterans Health Administration Alcoholism. *Clinical and Experimental Research*, *40*(2), 359–366 https://doi 12950 PMID:26842254 doi:org/101111/acer

Williams, M. (2022, November 2). Why African Americans avoid psychotherapy. *Psychology Today*. https://www.psychologytoday.com/us/blog/culturally-speaking/201111/why-african-americans-avoid-psychotherapy

Williams, M. T. (2007). *Racial differences in the assessment of obsessive-compulsive disorder* (Publication No. 3294804). [Doctoral dissertation, University of Virginia] Proquest Dissertations and Thesis.

Williams, Perlis, M., Castor, C., Barnes, A., Chung, A., Kalinowski, J., Roseus, J., Rogers, A., & Jean-Louis, G. (2018). 0193 An Exploratory, Descriptive Study Of African American's Experiences Of Insomnia Symptoms And Treatment. *Sleep (New York, N.Y.)*, *41*(suppl_1), A75–A76. doi:10.1093/sleep/zsy061.192

Williams, D. R. (2018). Stress and the Mental Health of Populations of Color: Advancing Our Understanding of Race-related Stressors. *Journal of Health and Social Behavior*, *59*(4), 466–485. doi:10.1177/0022146518814251 PMID:30484715

Williams, J. E., Newby, R. G., & Kanitz, H. E. (1993). Assessing the Need for Alcohol Abuse Programs for African-American College Students. *Journal of Multicultural Counseling and Development*, *21*(3), 155–167. https://doi-org.proxy.tamuc.edu/10.1002/j.2161-1912.1993.tb00595.x. doi:10.1002/j.2161-1912.1993.tb00595.x

Williams, M. T., La Torre, J. T., & Sharif, N. (2020). Cultural competency in the treatment of obsessive-compulsive disorder: Practitioner guidelines. *Cognitive Behaviour Therapist*, *13*(e48), 1–25. doi:10.1017/S1754470X20000501

Williams, M. T., & Mohammed, S. A. (2009). Discrimination and racial health disparities: Evidence and needed research. *Journal of Behavioral Medicine*, *32*(1), 20–47. doi:10.100710865-008-9185-0 PMID:19030981

Williams, M. T., Printz, D. M. B., & DeLapp, R. C. T. (2018). Assessing racial trauma with the trauma symptoms of discrimination scale. *Psychology of Violence*, *8*(6), 735–747. doi:10.1037/vio0000212

Williams, M. T., Taylor, R. J., George, J. R., Schlaudt, V. A., Ifatunji, M. A., & Chatters, L. M. (2021). Correlates of obsessive-compulsive symptoms among Black Caribbean Americans. *International Journal of Mental Health*, *40*(1), 53–77. doi:10.1080/00207411.2020.1826261 PMID:33840831

Williams, S.-L. L., & Cabrera-Nguyen, E. P. (2016). Impact of lifetime evaluated need on mental health service use among African American emerging adults. *Cultural Diversity & Ethnic Minority Psychology*, *22*(2), 205–214. https://doi-org.proxy.tamuc.edu/10.1037/cdp0000040. doi:10.1037/cdp0000040 PMID:25844566

Wilson, M., Gwyther, K., Swann, R., Casey, K., Featherston, R., Oliffe, J. L., Englar-Carlson, M., & Rice, S. M. (2022). Operationalizing positive masculinity: A theoretical synthesis and school-based framework to engage boys and young men. *Health Promotion International*, *37*(1), daab031. doi:10.1093/heapro/daab031 PMID:33842967

Wilson, P. L., O'Connor, D. P., Kaplan, C. D., Bode, S., Mama, S. K., & Lee, R. E. (2012). Relationship of fruit, vegetable, and fat consumption to binge eating symptoms in African American and Hispanic or Latina women. *Eating Behaviors*, *13*(2), 179–182. doi:10.1016/j.eatbeh.2012.01.007 PMID:22365808

Windsor, L. C., Jemal, A., & Alessi, E. J. (2015). Cognitive Behavioral Therapy: A Meta-Analysis of Race and Substance Use Outcomes. *Cultural Diversity & Ethnic Minority Psychology*, *21*(2), 300–313. https://doi-org.proxy.tamuc.edu/10.1037/a0037929. doi:10.1037/a0037929 PMID:25285527

Wojewoda, K., Brenner, J., Kąkol, M., Naesström, M., Cubała, W. J., Kozicka, D., Nowicki, R., Sokołowska-Wojdyło, M., & Barańska-Rybak, W. (2012). A cry for help, do not omit the signs. Dermatitis artefacta — Psychiatric problems in dermatological diseases (a review of 5 cases). *Medical Science Monitor*, *18*(10), CS85–CS89. doi:10.12659/MSM.883474 PMID:23018360

Wolny, J., Moussa-Tooks, A. B., Bailey, A. J., O'Donnell, B. F., & Hetrick, W. P. (2023). Race and self-reported paranoia: Increased item endorsement on subscales of the SPQ. *Schizophrenia Research, 253*, 30–39. doi:10.1016/j.schres.2021.11.034 PMID:34895794

Wong, C. A., Eccles, J. S., & Sameroff, A. (2003). The influence of ethnic discrimination and ethnic identification on African American adolescents' school and socioemotional adjustment. *Journal of Personality, 71*(6), 1197–1232. doi:10.1111/1467-6494.7106012 PMID:14633063

Wong, E. C., Derose, K. P., Miles, J. N. V., & Litt, P. (2018). Sources of Care for Alcohol and Other Drug Problems: The Role of the African American Church. *Journal of Religion and Health, 57*(4), 1200–1210. https://doi-org.proxy.tamuc.edu/10.1007/s10943-017-0412-2. doi:10.100710943-017-0412-2 PMID:28502023

Wong, M. D., Chung, A. K., Boscardin, J. W., Li, M., Hsieh, H.-J., Ettner, S. L., & Shapiro, M. F. (2006). The contribution of specific causes of death to sex differences in mortality. *Public Health Reports (Washington, D.C.), 121*(6), 746–754. doi:10.1177/003335490612100615 PMID:17278410

Wong, Y. J., & Rochlen, A. B. (2005). Demystifying Men's Emotional Behavior: New Directions and Implications for Counseling and Research. *Psychology of Men & Masculinity, 6*(1), 62–72. doi:10.1037/1524-9220.6.1.62

Wong, Y. J., & Wester, S. R. (2016). *APA Handbook of Men and Masculinities*. American Psychological Association. doi:10.1037/14594-000

Woods-Giscombe, C., Robinson, M., Carthon, D., Devane-Johnson, S., & Corbie-Smith, G. (2016). Superwoman schema, stigma, spirituality, and culturally sensitive providers: Factors influencing African American women's use of mental health services. *Journal of Best Practices in Health Professions Diversity : Research, Education and Policy, 9*(1), 1124–1144. PMID:33043323

World Health Organization. (1948). The sixth revision of the International Statistical Classification of diseases, injuries and causes of death (ICD-6),

World Health Organization. (1992). *The ICD-10 classification of mental and behavioural disorders: clinical descriptions and diagnostic guidelines*. World Health Organization.

World Health Organization. (2022). *Drugs Impact*. WHO. https://www.who.int/health-topics/drugs-psychoactive#tab=tab_2

World Health Organization. (2022, March 2). *Mental health and COVID-19: early evidence of the pandemic's impact: scientific brief.* WHO. https://apps.who.int/iris/handle/10665/352189

World Health Organization. (2023). *Alcohol Overview*. WHO. https://www.who.int/health-topics/alcohol#tab=tab_1

World Health Organization. (2023). *Schizophrenia*. WHO. https://www.who.int/news-room/fact-sheets/detail/schizophrenia

Xanthos, C., Treadwell, H. M., & Holden, K. B. (2010). Social determinants of health among African–American men. *The Journal of Men's Health*, *7*(1), 11–19. doi:10.1016/j.jomh.2009.12.002

Yeh, C. J., Hunter, C. D., Madan-Bahel, A., Chiang, L., & Arora, A. K. (2004). Indigenous and interdependent perspectives of healing: Implications for counseling and research. *Journal of Counseling and Development*, *82*(4), 410–419. doi:10.1002/j.1556-6678.2004.tb00328.x

Yelton, B., Friedman, D. B., Noblet, S., Lohman, M. C., Arent, M. A., Macauda, M. M., Sakhuja, M., & Leith, K. H. (2022). Social determinants of health and depression among African American adults: A scoping review of current research. *International Journal of Environmental Research and Public Health*, *19*(3), 1498. doi:10.3390/ijerph19031498 PMID:35162519

Yılmaz, E., & Kavak, F. (2018). Effects of Mindfulness-Based Psychoeducation on the Internalized Stigmatization Level of Patients with Schizophrenia. *Clinical Nursing Research*, 105477381879787–. https://www.bap.org.uk/articles/mental-health-stigma/ https://www.nami.org/Blogs/NAMI-Blog/October-2018/Overcoming-Stigma doi:10.1177/1054773818797871

Yourstone, J. Y., Lindholm, T., Grann, M., & Fazel, S. (2009). Gender differences in diagnoses of mentally disordered offenders. *International Journal of Forensic Mental Health*, *8*(3), 172–177. doi:10.1080/14999010903199316

Yu, Y., Matlin, S. L., Crusto, C. A., Hunter, B., & Tebes, J. K. (2022). Double Stigma and Help-Seeking Barriers Among Blacks With a Behavioral Health Disorder. *Psychiatric Rehabilitation Journal*, *45*(2), 183–191. https://doi doi:org.proxy.tamuc.edu/10.1037/prj0000507

Zai, G. C. M. (2016). *Genetics of obsessive-compulsive disorder: From phenotypes to pharmacogenetics* (Order No. 10140946). Sci Tech Premium Collection.

Zamir, E., Read, R. W., & Rao, N. A. (2001). Self-inflicted anterior scleritis. *Ophthalmology*, *108*(1), 192–195. doi:10.1016/S0161-6420(00)00480-2 PMID:11150288

Zapolski, T. C. B., Pedersen, S. L., McCarthy, D. M., & Smith, G. T. (2014). Less Drinking, Yet More Problems: Understanding African American Drinking and Related Problems. *Psychological Bulletin*, *140*(1), 188–223. https://doi-org.proxy.tamuc.edu/10.1037/a0032113. doi:10.1037/a0032113 PMID:23477449

Zeigler-Hill, V., & Wallace, M. (2011). Racial differences in narcissistic tendencies. *Journal of Research in Personality*, *45*(5), 456–467. doi:10.1016/j.jrp.2011.06.001

Zeinscott, T. (2022, June 30). How to motivate someone with borderline personality disorder? *Heart Eyes Magazine*. https://www.hearteyesmag.com/how-to-motivate-someone-with-borderline-personality-disorder/

Zemore, S. E., Mulia, N., Williams, E., & Gilbert, P. A. (2017). Job loss and alcohol dependence among Blacks and Whites in a National Longitudinal Survey. *Journal of Ethnicity in Substance Abuse*, *16*(3), 314–327. https://doi-org.proxy.tamuc.edu/10.1080/15332640.2016.1209144. doi:10.1080/15332640.2016.1209144 PMID:27594166

Zerhouni, E. (2002). Prostate Cancer Research Plan FY 2003-FY 2008. NIH., Available at http:// planning.cancer.gov/ pdfprgreports/prostateplan.pdf, Retrieved January 4, 2010, from.

Zheng, Q., Qin, Y., Lyu, Y., Li, L., Chen, Y., & Yao, Z. (2021). Community promotion and application of Wuqinxi combined with brief behavioral therapy for insomnia: A study protocol. *Medicine, 100*(49), e28046–e28046. doi:10.1097/MD.0000000000028046 PMID:34889248

Zoubaa, S., Dial, B., Ryan-Jones, L., Shah, V., & Yanos, P. T. (2022). On the relationship between experienced microaggressions and mental health stigma among members of marginalized groups. *Counselling Psychology Quarterly, 35*(4), 867–879. doi:10.1080/09515070.2021.1968795

Zwick, J., Appleseth, H., & Arndt, S. (2020). Stigma: How it affects the substance use disorder patient. *Substance Abuse Treatment, Prevention, and Policy, 15*(1), 1–4. https://doi-org.proxy.tamuc.edu/10.1186/s13011-020-00288-0. doi:10.118613011-020-00288-0 PMID:32718328

About the Contributors

***

Jovaria Baig is a licensed professional counselor and licensed chemical dependency counselor who is Gottman Level-1 certified. Dr. Baig has been in private practice for more than six years. She enjoys working with young adults, students and couples, and clients experiencing addiction-related issues or diagnoses, including but not limited to depression, anxiety, adjustment disorders, post-traumatic stress disorder, veteran issues and trauma. She is passionate about teaching and providing the tools necessary for students to succeed in counseling. She encourages students to find their passion and fulfill their educational dreams.

Daniel Bates earned his Ph.D. in Counselor Education from the University of Cincinnati and holds professional licenses in several states. Daniel is also a nationally board-certified counselor. His research, advocacy, and published work explores the intersection between men's mental health, access to services and masculine norms.

Marvin Bellows is a Doctoral Student, Counselor Education and Supervision.

Marcus K. Bills M.Ed., LCDC, has a career in Addiction & Chemical Dependency. His Bachelor's degree is in Kinesiology and his Master's degree is in Student Affairs of Counseling. He currently works as a LCDC in the outpatient department of Homeward Bound Inc.

Gracie Brownell is an Associate Professor, Director, and Advisor of the Master of Social Work (MSW) program at Texas at A&M University-Commerce. Dr. Brownell is passionate about helping marginalized populations, especially minorities, abused and neglected children, children affected by war and families experiencing immigration issues and other social problems. She is committed to preparing globally minded social workers to practice locally and internationally. Her experience includes working directly with abused and neglected children and their families, and indirectly in administration, planning and research. Dr. Brownell earned her BSW from Shorter University, her MSW from Baylor University and her Ph.D. from University of Texas at Arlington.

James Devlin is an Assistant Professor, Department of Counseling, Texas A&M University-Commerce.

Samone Donald is a Doctoral Student, Counselor Education and Supervision.

Marian Ellis is an educator, writer, and researcher. She has 26 years of combined experience in public school and higher education. She has been a high school teacher working in DAEP and correctional education settings. Her experience in leadership includes school principal and Director of Curriculum, Instruction, State and Federal Programs. She spent several years molding future educators in higher education classrooms. Dr. Ellis is currently the Superintendent of Clarksville ISD in Clarksville, TX.

Anissa Guerin has over a decade of experience serving in various academic and leadership roles; assisting higher education institutions develop creative initiatives to raise completion rates, address diversity inequalities, improve skills training programs, and expand educational experiences for aspiring leaders. Although she has worn many hats, teaching, and research is her passion. She is devoted to helping students overcome the most challenging obstacles and she embraces academia's mission with lucidity and compassion.

Elizabeth Malveaux-Hudson, Ph.D. has spent most of her career in school counseling. She has been a public secondary school counselor where she worked with students as they explored which career path to take. Elizabeth Malveaux-Hudson, Ph.D. now uses her vast experience to work with students at Texas A&M University-Commerce where she teaches students strategies to be successful as school counselors.

Rahmatu Kassimu is an educator, researcher, public health consultant, and change agent. She has spent the last nine years educating students and training teachers to advocate for themselves in their educational trajectories. Her degrees in Sociology, Public Health, Health Studies, and Educational Leadership have allowed her to combine her passion for education, increasing the quality of life, and increasing health equity into her labor of love, Dr. K.'s Health Minute, which provides easily accessible and digestible health and wellness information on a variety of topics with concentrations on mental health, Black maternal health, and health inequities.

Avril W. Knox, DSW, ACSW, CSW Assistant Professor/ MSW Field Education Director_ Avril W. Knox, a mother and wife possesses a Doctor of Social Work degree from Walden University. She specialized in social work administration and engaged in research studies implementing social and global change. In addition, she holds a Master of Social Work degree and a Bachelor of Arts in Psychology, with a minor in Biology, from Southern University in New Orleans, Louisiana. Dr. Knox has been working in higher education since 2006. She has held Adjunct Professor positions at Dallas College, Virginia Commonwealth University, and Texas A&M University-Commerce (TAMUC) in the School of Social Work. At TAMUC, Dr. Knox holds the position of Assistant Professor and Master Social Work Field Education Director. Before her tenured track appointment, Dr. Knox was the Director of Programs for one of Dallas's most influential and reputable non-profit organizations. She was the overseer of seven departments; Refugee Resettlement Services, Disaster Relief and Preparedness Services, Financial Stability and Career Services, Hunger Services, Housing, and Border Crisis Intervention Services; seventeen programs within these departments. She successfully led these departments while serving as a Co-Facilitator of the Dallas Area Refugee Forum. Dr. Knox also once held the Director of Case Management position for the most prominent family violence shelter in Dallas. She has over 20 years of exemplary senior leadership in social work and exemplifies a history of proficiency in administration, planning, and organizing social service agencies. In 2014, she was awarded the Distinguished Human Service Professional Award through the Community Council of Greater Dallas, one of the most exclusive honors held in social work in its service area. Dr. Knox's repertoire includes a collective interest and clinical expertise in family reunification, domestic violence, sexual assault, crisis intervention, health/mental health, gerontology, and refugee services. Dr. Knox's most recent scholarly publication illustrates the ability to study and unveil the integration of social work practices in working with refugee families.

John Kuykendall graduated from the University of Arkansas at Pine Bluff with a secondary education (biology) degree. He earned his master's at Christian Brothers University in Educational Leadership and Doctorate in Higher Education Administration from Indiana University. He has a research background in college student success, preparing culturally relevant teachers, and preparing high school students for college. Dr. Kuykendall has held faculty appointments at Marquette University, where he coordinated the college student affairs program, and the University of Arkansas at Little Rock, where he earned tenure and served as the inaugural Director of the School of Education. Dr. Kuykendall's research focuses on the following areas: College Preparation for High School Students, Culturally Relevant Teacher

Preparation (Novice Teachers), High School to College Transitions for Black Males, African-African Male Student Success, and Engagement.

LaShondra P. Manning is an Assistant Professor of Counseling in the College of Health Sciences at Tarleton State University. Her research interests include crisis and trauma in forgotten populations. She is also a licensed professional counselor supervisor in the state of Texas.

Karl Mitchell is an Assistant Professor at Texas A&M University – Commerce with over 15 years of experience serving and working within the Mental Health field, and with clients and communities from various populations. Professional and research interests include service-learning in counselor education, multiculturalism, multicultural competence/counseling, social justice advocacy, globalization of counseling, interventions for quality care of clients and communities we work with, and treatments to help eliminate misdiagnosis.

Sindu Padmanabhan is a highly skilled researcher in Education & Health Psychology with experience in educational institutions and organizations and possessing a strong interest in health and cognitive psychology. I have a proven track of various research work, education delivery, as well as outstanding analytical and observational skills. Reviewer for International Journals. Highly proficient in using industry research software packages. Now seeking to advance my research career and take on further responsibilities.

Marcella Smith is an Associate Professor and Department Head for the School of Social Work at Texas A&M University-Commerce. Prior to her current leadership position, she served as the MSW Program Director for 2 years. She earned her Ph.D. in Social Work from The University of Texas at Arlington (UTA), holds a MSW in Social work from UTA, and a Bachelor of Science in Business Administration from Louisiana State University in Shreveport (LSUS). Her research interests include minority and adolescent health, health disparities, and immigration issues.

Kayla Solomon received her Bachelor's degree in both Psychology and Criminal Justice from the University of Texas at San Antonio in 2017. Her passion to assist others led her to the Texas A&M Commerce Counseling program, where she is a graduate student seeking her Master's degree in Clinical Mental Health counseling. She has always had a desire to be a "helper" and with her degree, she will help individuals by providing therapeutic services.

David Tolliver, PhD most recently served as the Assistant Director of Graduate Recruitment and Outreach at the University of Arkansas' Graduate School and International Education, where he managed domestic graduate student recruitment and outreach initiatives, including those related to increasing the diversity of students in graduate programs. Dr. Tolliver completed his PhD in Public Policy as an SREB Doctoral Scholar from the University of Arkansas' interdisciplinary Public Policy PhD Program, with a specialization in higher education policy. Prior to his position at the University of Arkansas, Dr. Tolliver, worked in administrative and instructional roles in post-secondary student success in the Minnesota State University System and has previous experience in secondary education, brand strategy, and the United States Air Force.

Elizabeth Wachira is an Associate Professor at Texas A&M University-Commerce and Public Health program director. Her research aims to understand the often-covert pathways of oppression and injustices that marginalized populations face. She aims to inform and expand authentic, lived-experienced knowledge on health vulnerabilities as determinants of health among marginalized individuals. As an educator, through service-learning, her students do a community needs assessment to implement initiatives that have community impact, such as a peer-led mental health promotion program for campus students.

Priscilla Wachira is a Nationally Certified Counselor, a Licensed Professional Counselor. She holds a Bachelor's Degree in Psychology with a minor in Spanish/Behavior Analysis from the University of North Texas and a Master's degree in Clinical Mental Health from Texas Woman's University. Her research interests include health equity as it pertains to women's health, and exploring the stigma of mental health within the African, immigrant community. She believes that people begin to heal the moment they feel seen for whom they are & heard! This healing results from a safe environment (space) that is created to provide emotional healing and connection instead of judgment or shame.

Index

(CBT) 45, 54-55, 60, 79, 92, 124

A

Abnormal Motor Behavior 217-218
African American 9, 22-27, 33, 36-43, 48-53, 58-60, 63-64, 67-83, 85-90, 93-96, 112, 115-123, 125-126, 128, 130, 132-138, 140-146, 149, 151-159, 161-162, 166-170, 172-174, 176, 178-181, 183-184, 194, 196, 204-214, 221-222, 225, 229-237, 239-240, 243-244, 248-249, 251, 253, 256-259, 261-266, 269-272, 274-275, 277-281, 288, 292, 294
African American Culture 38, 68, 112, 123, 146, 234, 259
African American Mental Health 36, 50, 144, 172-174
African Americans 1, 8-12, 17-18, 22-28, 30-42, 48-51, 53-55, 59-60, 62, 64, 67-68, 72-82, 84, 88, 93-96, 104, 112, 115-119, 121-125, 129-131, 133-146, 149, 151-157, 159, 161, 163-178, 180, 202, 205, 209, 212-213, 216, 222, 224, 233, 235-236, 239-241, 247-250, 254-256, 258-263, 265-267, 272-274, 278, 288, 294
anorexia nervosa 64-66, 68, 150
Anxiety 3, 13-14, 20, 26-28, 44, 46-47, 50, 52-53, 61-62, 69, 74, 78, 93, 108, 110, 112-113, 115, 121, 123, 125, 130, 133-134, 139, 151, 177, 186, 192, 203, 218, 224-225, 229, 257-258, 266, 272, 289
Avolition 216, 218

B

binge-eating 64-79, 84, 89-90
Black 8-11, 19-22, 24, 29, 33, 36, 40-42, 48-51, 67, 70-71, 74-77, 79, 82-84, 86-89, 116-119, 121-124, 128-139, 142-145, 149, 153, 156, 158-161, 166-167, 175-178, 183-184, 190, 194-196, 201, 203-205, 207-212, 214, 216, 221-229, 233, 235-237, 239-240, 242-244, 249-258, 260-263, 265-277, 279-280, 287-288, 293
bulimia nervosa 65-68, 86, 90

C

Care 1, 8, 10-12, 14, 16, 18, 20-21, 25, 29, 32-34, 50, 62, 74, 76-79, 81, 83-85, 89, 92-96, 104, 109-110, 124, 136-138, 140, 142, 144, 152, 155-156, 159, 165, 168-175, 177-178, 187, 191, 194, 204, 211-212, 214, 222, 226, 228-229, 231-235, 243-244, 249-250, 262-266, 270-271, 274-275, 281, 283, 285-286, 288-289
Church 9, 23, 39-40, 42, 74-75, 77, 79-82, 87, 122, 135, 137-138, 142, 144, 154-158, 160-161, 168, 177, 214, 225, 236, 246, 249, 253, 261-262, 266, 269, 281
Cognitive Behavioral Therapy 45, 47-48, 54-60, 79, 124, 261, 281
Consequences 47, 64, 76-77, 107, 118, 136, 140, 189, 201, 238, 252-255, 258-260, 264, 269, 279, 283, 286, 289
contamination 117-118, 123

COVID-19 19, 24, 112, 114-115, 131, 147, 160, 165-166, 169, 172, 176-179, 243
curriculum development 112, 123, 131-132

D

Delusions 216-218, 220
Discrimination 23, 25-26, 28, 30, 38-42, 64, 73, 75, 77, 80-82, 85-86, 94, 116-117, 119, 131, 135, 137, 140, 144-145, 147, 152-153, 158, 168-169, 173-174, 177, 183-184, 187-189, 193, 202, 205-206, 209, 211, 214, 224-225, 235, 250, 258, 265-266, 272, 274-275, 283-287, 289-293
disorder 1-6, 8, 11-16, 18-24, 36-37, 40-42, 44-45, 48-49, 58-59, 61, 64-67, 69-73, 76-87, 89-97, 99-108, 110, 112-114, 116, 119, 123-124, 126-128, 130-135, 139, 142, 144, 146-147, 150-151, 153, 155, 158-161, 163-164, 170, 176-178, 217-218, 224-225, 229, 235, 238, 240, 244-245, 248, 250, 255-256, 258, 262, 267, 273, 280-283, 290-291, 293-294
Drug and alcohol 252-255, 258-261, 269, 274, 277

E

eating disorders 64-69, 71-73, 76-90
Education 2, 10-11, 28, 30, 41, 46, 56, 58, 60, 89, 93, 97, 115, 124-125, 133, 140, 142, 144, 157, 160-162, 165, 167, 169, 172-174, 196, 203, 228, 235, 242, 247, 251, 255, 257-258, 265, 267-268, 276, 284-286, 288-290, 294
Expressed Emotion 232, 237-238

F

factitious 91-106, 108-110
First-episode Psychosis 227-228, 236

H

Hallucinations 217-218, 220
Health Disparities 10, 42, 133, 145, 163, 168, 170, 172, 176, 178, 184, 188-190, 192, 206, 236, 257, 288, 293
hemodynamic 126, 133

I

impairment of daily functioning 45
Impulsivity 1, 5, 12-14
inequities 10, 135, 147, 167, 216, 222, 224, 235, 239, 244
Insomnia 43-48, 50-63
International OCD Foundation 114
Intersectionality 24-25, 41, 82

M

Major Depressive Disorder 24, 87, 163-164, 176-178, 238
Masculinity 153, 171, 183-185, 188-209, 211-215
mental health 2-4, 8-11, 15-16, 18, 20-23, 27, 30-45, 48, 50, 52-54, 58-60, 62, 66-67, 69, 74-85, 87-89, 91-93, 95-97, 112, 116, 119-124, 130-132, 134, 136-145, 147, 149-162, 164-180, 183-192, 196-202, 205-206, 209-217, 221-222, 226-228, 230, 232, 234-236, 239-241, 243-244, 248-249, 251-255, 257, 259-260, 263, 265-268, 270-273, 275, 277-281, 284-294
Mental Health Illness 249
mental health perceptions 252-253
Mental Health Promotion 183, 291, 294
misdiagnosis 115, 155, 171, 174-176, 225, 250

N

Narcissistic Personality Disorder 146-147, 158-159, 161
NAVIGATE 25, 60, 134, 196, 228
neuroablation 132
Neurodevelopment 242
Neurodevelopmental disorder 8, 244

O

OCPD 114, 128, 132, 150
OCRD 113, 124, 126-127
Oppression 24-26, 28, 38, 40, 71, 73, 141, 167, 183-184, 190, 193, 195-196, 200, 243

P

Paranoia 135-136, 138-141, 143-145, 224, 241
Pathway 242-243, 256
PCP 234
person in environment 269
Post Traumatic Slave Syndrome 25, 42
Post-Traumatic Stress Disorder 23, 36-37, 261
Psychiatric diagnoses 14, 142
Psychoeducation 266, 269, 283, 289-294
PTSD 23-26, 28-31, 33, 36-37, 40-42, 71, 192
PTSS 26, 37, 40-42

R

Race-Based Trauma 25, 28
Racial disparities 10-11, 19-20, 80, 137, 144, 207, 229, 237-238, 240, 273
Racial Trauma 42
racism 10-11, 19, 22, 24-26, 28, 30, 37-39, 49, 64, 70, 72-73, 75-78, 80-81, 94, 112, 116, 118-119, 136, 140-141, 143-144, 153, 163-167, 169-172, 177, 180, 188, 206, 224-225, 228, 235, 239, 243, 249, 258, 260, 262, 265, 277, 287, 289, 293
RAISE-ETP 228, 239
religion 38, 42, 74-75, 129, 131-132, 138, 154, 158, 161, 199, 256, 266, 269, 272, 281

S

Schizotypal Personality Questionnaire 224
sleep disturbance 14, 43-45, 54, 60
Stigma 8-9, 20, 22-23, 33-36, 40-42, 58, 74-77, 80-82, 87, 90, 96, 112, 117, 130, 137, 142-143, 151, 153, 156, 162, 166-168, 171-176, 179-180, 187-189, 191, 196, 214, 225, 228, 235, 249, 264, 266, 279-294
Substance Abuse 14-15, 21, 66, 94, 122-123, 134, 140, 165, 171, 189, 197, 200, 212-213, 240, 253-257, 260-265, 267-270, 273-282, 291

T

treatment 6, 8-9, 11-12, 14-15, 17-21, 23, 28, 31-38, 40, 43-45, 47-50, 53-60, 62-63, 66, 76-79, 82-83, 85-86, 88-89, 92-97, 115, 117, 119-128, 131-134, 136-142, 144-145, 148-151, 153-155, 157-161, 164, 166-167, 170-178, 184-186, 188-190, 200-201, 204-205, 208-210, 212, 216, 221-229, 231-236, 238-241, 244, 250-253, 255, 258, 261-265, 267-270, 272-280, 282-286, 289-291
trichotillomania 113, 124-125, 127, 132-133

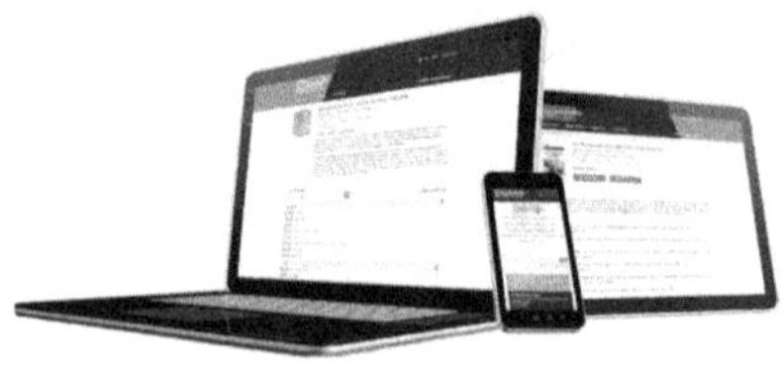

www.ingramcontent.com/pod-product-compliance
Lightning Source LLC
LaVergne TN
LVHW080602300926
849162LV00005B/1029
* 9 7 8 1 6 6 8 4 8 9 1 8 5 *